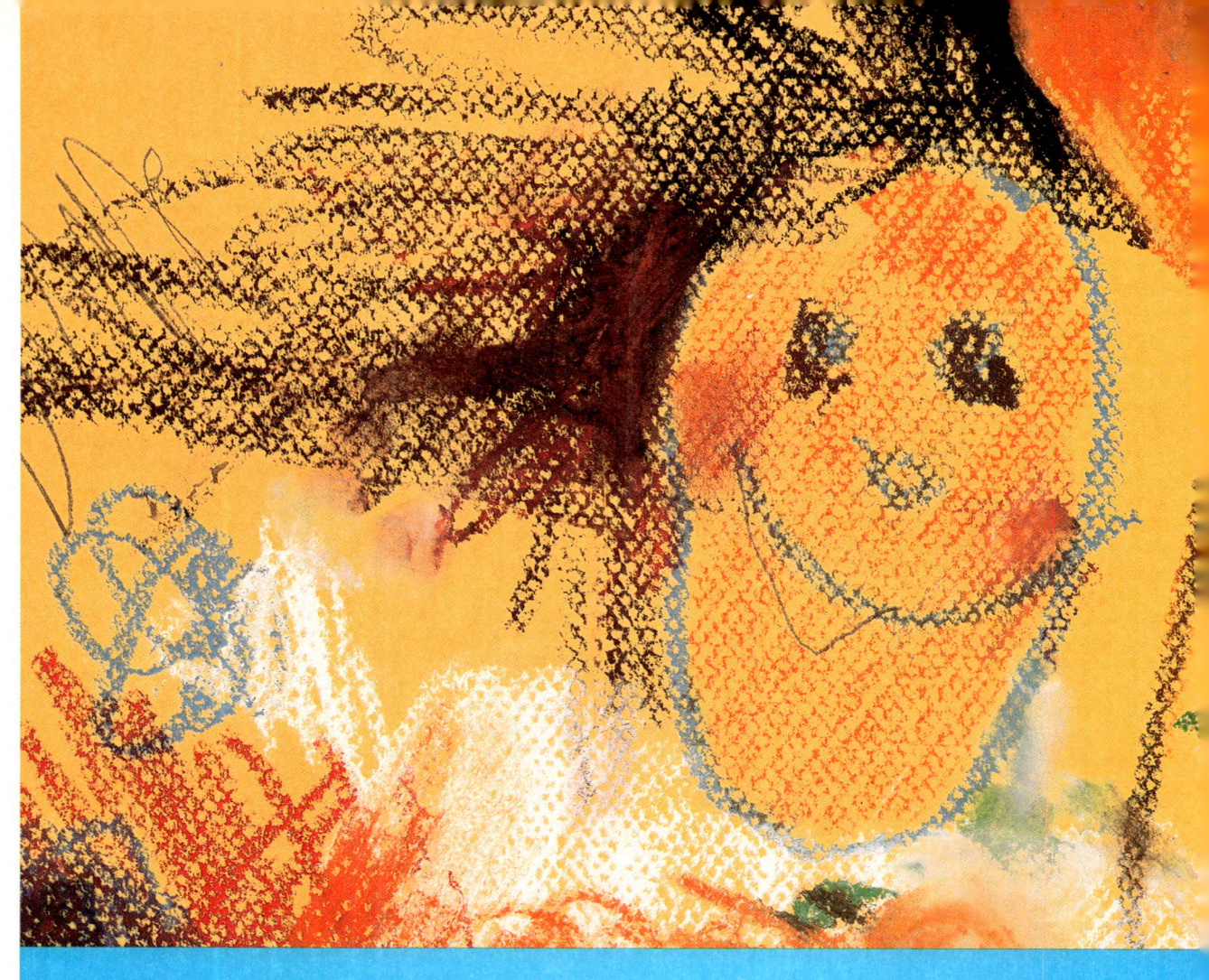

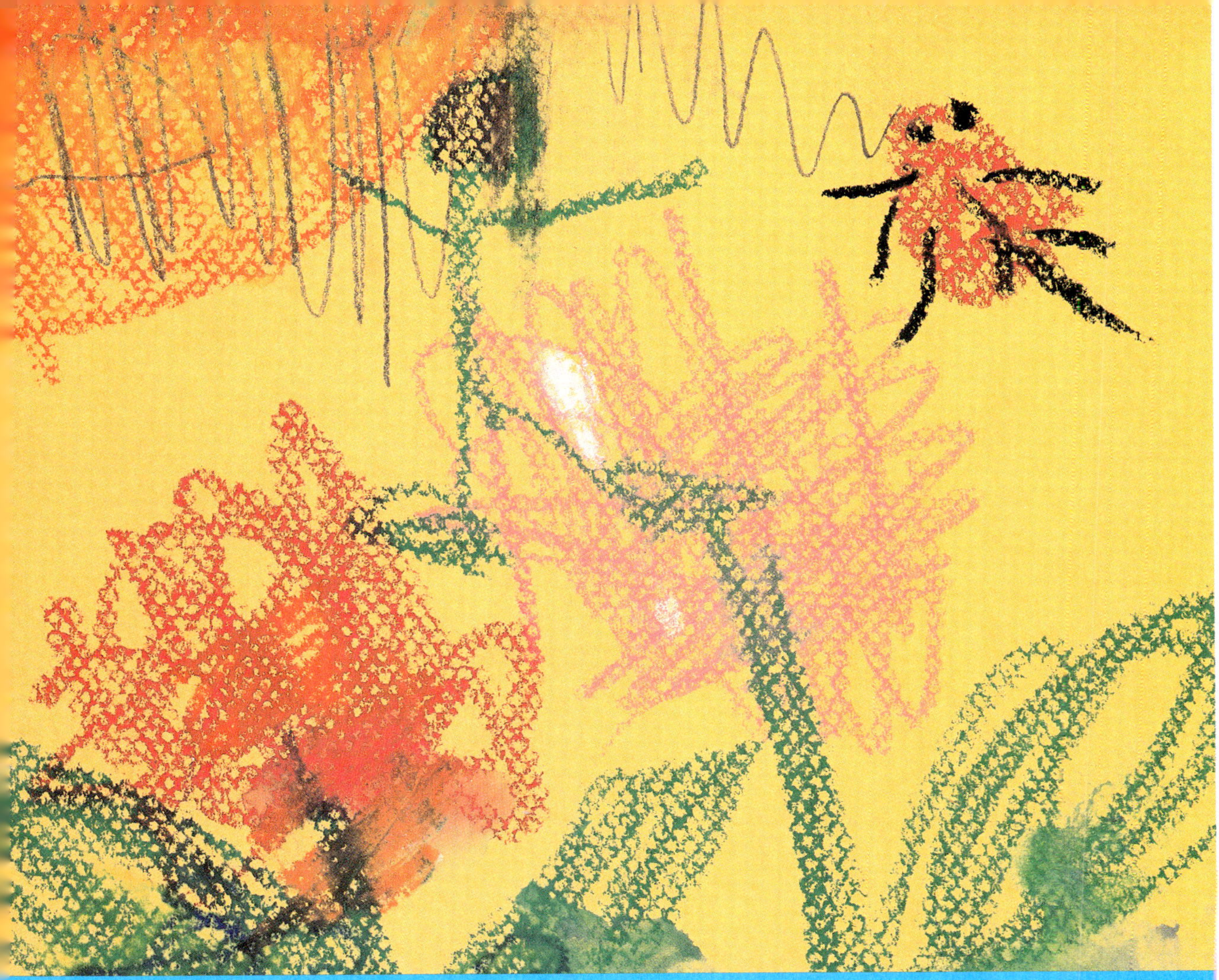

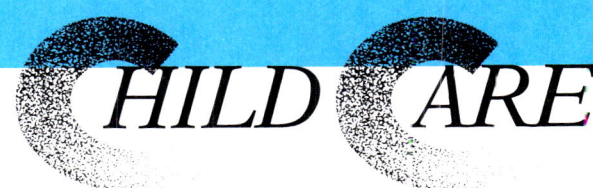

CHILD CARE

Genelle Felio, CFLE, CHE

Chairperson and Child Care Teacher
Department of Home Economics
Odessa High School
Odessa, Texas

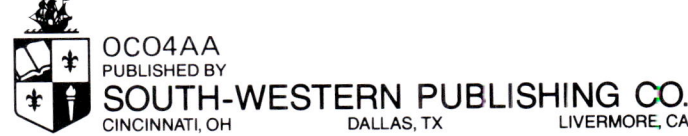

OCO4AA
PUBLISHED BY
SOUTH-WESTERN PUBLISHING CO.
CINCINNATI, OH   DALLAS, TX   LIVERMORE, CA

Acquisitions Editor: Carolyn Love
Production Editor: Rhonda Eversole
Cover and Internal Designer: Elaine Lagenaur
Photo Researcher: Kathryn Russell
Cover Photographer: Diana Fleming
Marketing Manager: Don Fox

Consulting Editor

Kay Clayton, Ph.D., CHE
Professor and Chair
Department of Home Economics
Texas A&I University

Content Reviewers

Katherine H. Brophy   Gloria McGrath
State Supervisor   Supervisor
Hartford, Connecticut   Consumer and Home Economics
                             Omaha Public Schools
                             Omaha, Nebraska

ISBN: 0-538-60255-4

Library of Congress Catalog Card Number: 89-60846

1 2 3 4 5 6 7 8 RN 7 6 5 4 3 2 1 0
Printed in the United States of America

TO THE STUDENT

You enrolled in child care because you love young children and are concerned for their future. I share that love and concern. *Child Care* provides as much information as possible about how you can successfully make young children a part of your future.

The chapters in this book have been set up to make learning about young children easier and more enjoyable. At the beginning of each chapter is a list of objectives. Throughout each chapter some words appear in **bold type** like these. You will want to learn these to help you speak the language of caring for children. The chapter summaries will help you remember the important things the text has presented. The questions and problems at the end of each chapter will give you an opportunity to go back over important ideas. They will also help you develop some ideas of your own.

This book also has some special features you will enjoy. In each chapter a story about a family or caregivers represents the ideas being presented. The Hands On features present skills that will help you do a good job with young children. You will enjoy discussing some of the issues in the Something to Think About features with your teacher and classmates. You will also get acquainted with some individuals and organizations considered leaders in the child development profession.

Every person is important. Parents, children, teachers, and students each have a unique and irreplaceable position in life. You count. Children count. Parents, caregivers, and teachers count. As you read *Child Care*, keep this idea in mind. If you understand this, you will gain more from your reading.

Welcome to this field of study. I hope you find the work challenging and the children delightful. Most of all, if you decide to become a child care professional, I wish you much success!

Cordially,

Genelle Felio

PREFACE

When a textbook is written, it is intended to provide students with the best knowledge that is available at the time. Writers are like other people; they have main points of view. *Child Care* is written with the idea that every person is important. Everyone counts—parents, caregivers, children, teachers, and students—and each person is unique and irreplaceable.

The content of *Child Care* and its accompanying supplementary materials have been developed to make learning about young children easier and more enjoyable. The text is also developed to pique interest in those who are thinking of making child care their profession. Through their study of *Child Care*, students will gain a greater appreciation and understanding of the children in their lives.

AN OVERVIEW OF THE CONTENT

Some families in which children live work well for them; others do not. The first five chapters (Part 1) of *Child Care* deal with children's needs, how families meet needs and challenges, and how growth and development occur in children under six.

Because of demands of careers or jobs, many parents place children in child care centers. The second part of *Child Care* deals with caring for children in group settings. The ways child care centers are organized and how careers and leadership are developed are covered in Chapter 6. Providing adequate health care and handling illnesses are dealt with in Chapter 7, and Chapter 8 covers safety and emergencies.

The best child care programs are those that also provide for children's learning needs. The third part of *Child Care* deals with teaching small children in groups. The topics of guidance, discipline, and abuse are addressed in Chapter 9. The text concludes with individual chapters on caring for and teaching each age group—infants, toddlers, and preschoolers.

ORGANIZATION AND FEATURES OF CHAPTERS

Chapters are organized to make learning as enjoyable as possible. Objectives are listed at the beginning of each chapter, and key terms are in bold type. Each chapter begins and ends with a short story line that involves people who use some of the skills or face issues the chapter addresses. As reinforcements, chapter summaries restate the main ideas presented in the text.

Leadership at a Glance. A person or an organization considered a leader in the profession of child development is featured in each Leadership at a Glance. If their study of the profession continues beyond *Child Care,* students will see or hear these names many times and may perhaps become members of one or more of the organizations.

Hands On with Children. The Hands On with Children feature at the end of each chapter introduces a skill for working with children. Although there are many more skills for preschool teachers to learn, mastering those presented will give students a start in working skillfully with young children.

Something to Think About. Many issues about children, families, and child care in general are currently discussed in homes or schools and covered in the media. Some of these issues are presented in the Something to Think About features. Some of the issues will be new to students; about others, students may already hold very strong opinions. If discussion of the issues is allowed in the classroom, you will want to remember they are *issues,* and therefore there is more than one side to consider. As pre-professionals in child care, students will want to exercise self-control and demonstrate maturity as they discuss these issues with classmates. They may also want to ask their parents and other significant people in their lives to express opinions. Ultimately, though, they will have to decide for themselves what they think.

Terms and Concepts. Each profession has its own terms. Important terms and concepts are set in bold type throughout each chapter and are also listed in a separate section following the summary. When students finish reading the chapter, they should review these terms. If they cannot recall any of them, they should go back and reread the relevant section(s) of the text. If necessary, they can refer to the glossary located at the end of the book, which lists all the terms and their definitions in alphabetical order.

Checking Your Understanding. Checking Your Understanding follows the list of terms and concepts in each chapter and allows students to do what its title says. Understanding involves more than rote memorizing and recall of terms, concepts, and principles. Completing the items in Checking Your Understanding will help students recognize and appreciate the applications of the concepts presented and the impact on them as future child care professionals.

ACTIVITY GUIDE

The *Activity Guide* available for use with *Child Care* is filled with exercises and activities to perform in or outside of the classroom environment. The *Activity Guide* broadens their understanding of concepts in the text.

INSTRUCTOR'S RESOURCE GUIDE

Also available for use with *Child Care* is the *Instructor's Resource Guide*. In addition to an overview of the text and materials and answer keys to the text and *Activity Guide*, the *Instructor's Resource Guide* includes sections on entrepreneurship (the business of child care), on planning skills, on skills for teaching infants, toddlers, and preschoolers, on caregiving skills, on lab experiences and management, and on student evaluation, including printed chapter tests.

ACKNOWLEDGMENTS

When a book is published, the author receives credit as well as responsibility for its contents. In reality, the contents of any book, particularly a textbook, are based on the work of many people. *Child Care* has many contributors, and I would like to thank them.

Dr. Kay Clayton, chair of the home economics department at the University of Southern Mississippi and later at Texas A&I University and 1990 president of the American Vocational Association, is the consulting editor of *Child Care*. Her recommendations for the content strengthened the text and helped balance its treatment of men and women. Her contribution to the issues section of each chapter and to the structure itself has significantly added to the depth of the text. I appreciate her efforts very much.

The people and organizations whose research and efforts are described in the Leadership at a Glance features are also valued contributors, because their work contributed to the content of *Child Care*. They are Dr. T. Berry Brazelton, Dr. James C. Dobson, Dr. Maria Montessori, Dr. Jean Piaget, Dr. Gerald Powell, Dr. Nick Stinnett, Dr. David Weikart, and Dr. Burton White; The American Academy of Pediatrics, The Future Homemakers of America, Inc., The National Association for the Education of Young Children, The National Committee for the Prevention of Child Abuse, and The National Council on Family Relations. Others whose work contributed are credited in the text.

On the Personal Side. Dr. Marion P. Hardman, professor emeritus of New Mexico State University, has believed in me and encouraged this authorship. She taught me to teach the tough issues with perseverance and strength and approach them boldly in the classroom. She, more than any other, pointed the direction and set the standard. Then she—perhaps very wisely—left me to complete the text on my own. I have missed her tremendously.

No one has given more to this effort than my husband, Larry. His example as a committed husband and father has provided a living example for establishing and maintaining a strong family. He has sacrificed hundreds of hours of personal time and his own interests to encourage my writing. Only those who have writing spouses know how much time, effort, and money are poured into an authorship. Larry has paid the price and has provided all the support possible. I wish to thank him publicly for his private contributions.

Our children, Shariene and David, gave me the joy of raising children. Each day they challenged and delighted me. They were the ones who lived through the tests of my evolving theories of child growth and development and prodded me to keep working.

My parents, Ed and Robbie Nelle Hamilton, gave me the kind of childhood in which strong family values were lovingly but firmly followed. They did not waiver, and I thank them. Along with Roxanna Douglas Felio, they have also read and responded to parts of the manuscript for *Child Care*.

Friends and colleagues who have contributed by providing information or reading copy include the following: James and Jody Adams, Willie Adams, Linda Allen, Kathryn Gibson, Maryln Hair, Mary Joyce Harding, Jon Harrington, Joellen Hill, Eunice Kaiser, Lori Nelson, Don Palmer, and Steve and Margaret Stratton.

Administrators in my school district who allowed me to pilot the text in my classroom and have supported my writing efforts include Raymond Starnes, Principal of Odessa High School; Marc Ramage, Instructional Services Director; and Bob Durrett, then Director of Secondary Education.

Finally, I wish to thank my students in the pre-employment child care laboratory at Odessa High School for piloting *Child Care* and giving perhaps the most honest feedback a teacher or writer could have. They told it like it is, and I thank them.

Genelle Felio

Meet the Author

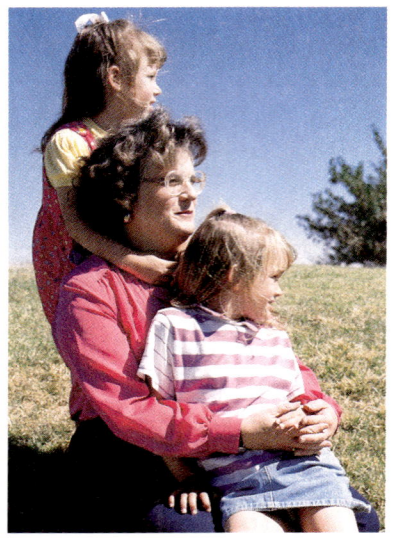

Genelle Felio is a Certified Family Life Educator and a Certified Home Economist. She blends her training and experience in early childhood education and in vocational home economics as author of *Child Care*. Mrs. Felio has taught for more than twenty years, half of those as a teacher of child development at the high school level. Four years were invested in the child development program at Odessa College, where she directed the child development lab and helped develop and teach the child care program. During that time she served as a trainer for candidates seeking CDA (Child Development Associate) credentials and as validator for Texas CDA materials. Currently Mrs. Felio teaches the pre-employment child care laboratory at Odessa High School.

Mrs. Felio has written nationally for teachers' periodicals and has written a column on parenting for local newspapers. Her graduate study was in the area of parental commitment, and her thesis was published by the ERIC Clearinghouse on Early Childhood Education.

Mrs. Felio has been on community boards serving both private and public agencies concerned with the care of young children. She has served on school district committees concerned with parental involvement and programs for teenage parents. She has been actively involved in developing child care facilities for four different community programs.

Mrs. Felio holds a bachelor of science degree in Vocational Home Economics Education from New Mexico State University and a master of arts degree in Early Childhood Education from the University of Texas of the Permian Basin. She is a member of the National Association for the Education of Young Children and the National Council on Family Relations.

CONTENTS

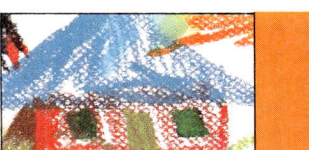

PART 1 Understanding Children

PART 2 Caring for Children

PART 3   Teaching Children

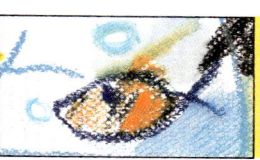

FEATURES

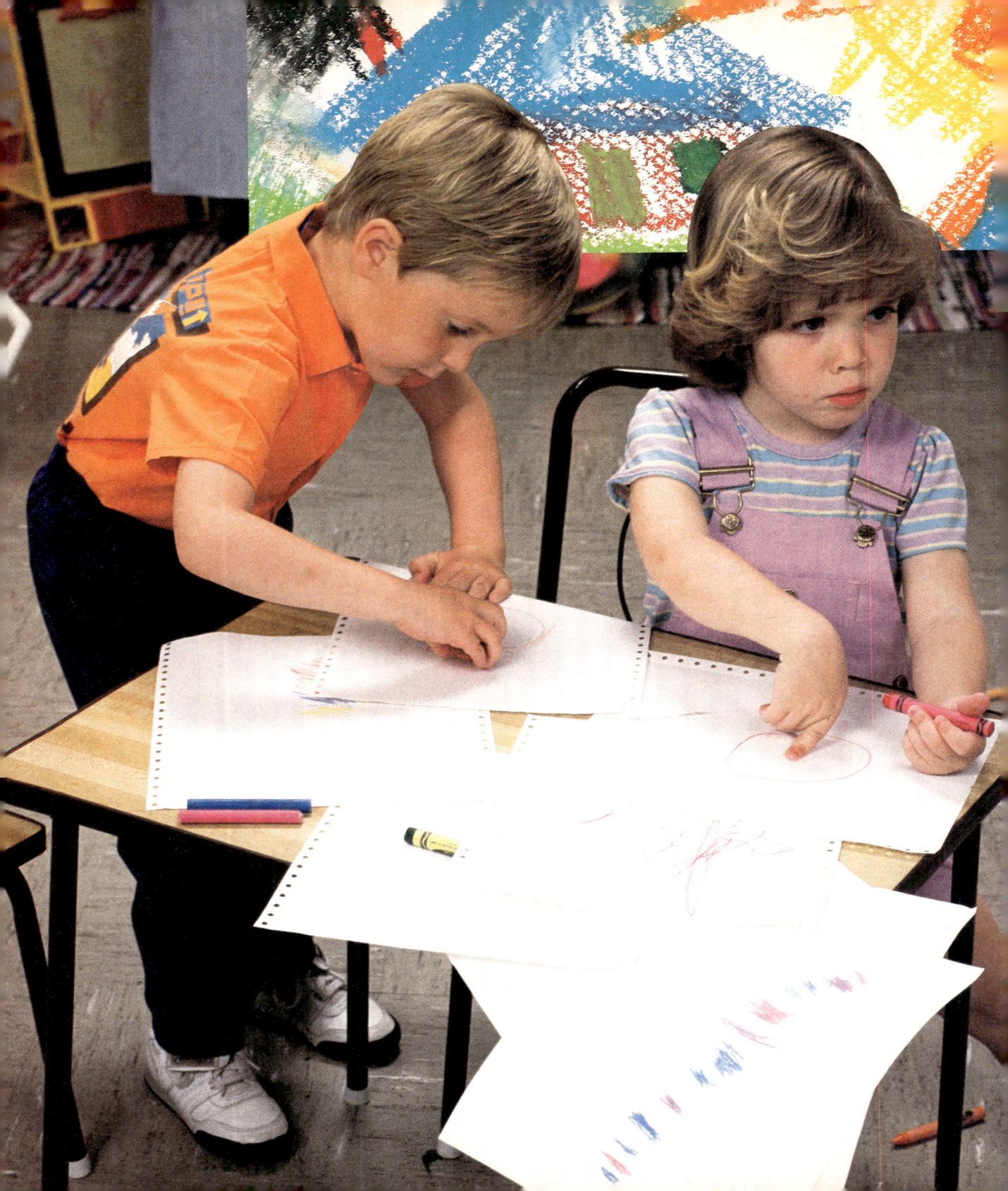

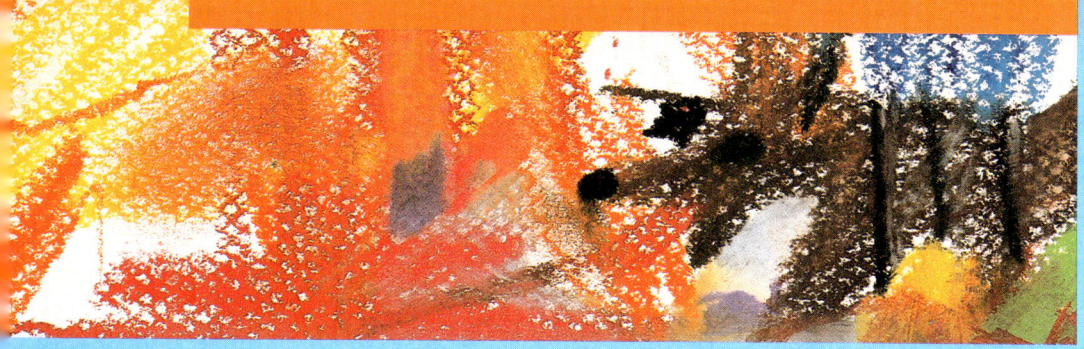

PART 1
Understanding Children

CHAPTER 1
Fathers, Mothers, and the Needs of Children

OBJECTIVES

After you have finished this chapter, you will be able to

- List and briefly discuss the needs of young children
- Explain the difference between parenting goals and goals for children
- Describe some ways in which parents can meet children's needs
- Identify the functions of parents and relate them to the needs of children
- Compare the kinds of parental leadership
- Analyze the roles of parents
- Discuss the role of commitment in effective parenting

Brad stretched out his arms awkwardly toward his five-minute-old daughter. "Come meet your dad," he said nervously. He placed her head in the bend of his arm and spoke her name, "Sarah." Sarah stopped crying and gazed into his eyes.

"Can she see me?" he asked the nurse, without taking his eyes off his daughter.

The nurse moved confidently closer to Brad and Sarah. "Of course! Especially right after birth," she responded.

"Do you think she knows who I am?" Brad asked, addressing no one in particular. Without waiting for a reply, he continued, "You're beautiful—just beautiful—just like your mom."

Brad bent down so that his wife, Monica, could see Sarah. He wondered how he would ever be able to take care of her and teach her what he wanted her to know. How would he protect her from the things that could hurt her? Becoming a parent was a more wonderful and yet more frightening experience than he had imagined it would be.

Monica was relieved that the birth was over and was as excited as Brad about Sarah's finally being there. She placed her finger in Sarah's tiny hand, and immediately the baby responded by squeezing her mother's finger. Intense new feelings of awe and amazement filled Monica. A few hours earlier she had been huge with the long-awaited baby—now there was a new person in her life. Both Monica and Brad were aware that Sarah would have many needs, which they must learn to meet. Some of those needs would be much like their own; others would be unique to young children.

CHILDREN HAVE SPECIAL NEEDS

Children's greatest need is to live with parents who love them, who are available to lend support as they grow, and who are committed to helping them become healthy adults. Parents are expected to take responsibility for meeting their children's needs. Some of these needs are discussed in this section.

Children Need to Belong to a Secure Family

Families come in all shapes and sizes. Children need families who will provide for their basic needs, who truly want them, and who are willing to invest themselves in children's lives. Although most children would prefer to live with both their mother and their father, other forms of families can provide a happy and secure place for them to grow. Grandparents, foster families, adoptive families, blended families, and single-parent families may also provide them with a secure environment and help meet their needs.

Whatever form a family takes, children need to feel that they are members of their family and to sense its loyalty to them. They need to learn about their roots and to get to know their relatives, to be a part of family celebrations, and thus to become aware of what others in the family think and believe. They need to respect and enjoy their family name.

It is necessary that children feel sure of their parents' love in all circumstances, that they know it will always be there, no matter what happens or what they do. This kind of love is called **unconditional love.** Children also need parents who are committed to them as persons and committed to meeting their needs.

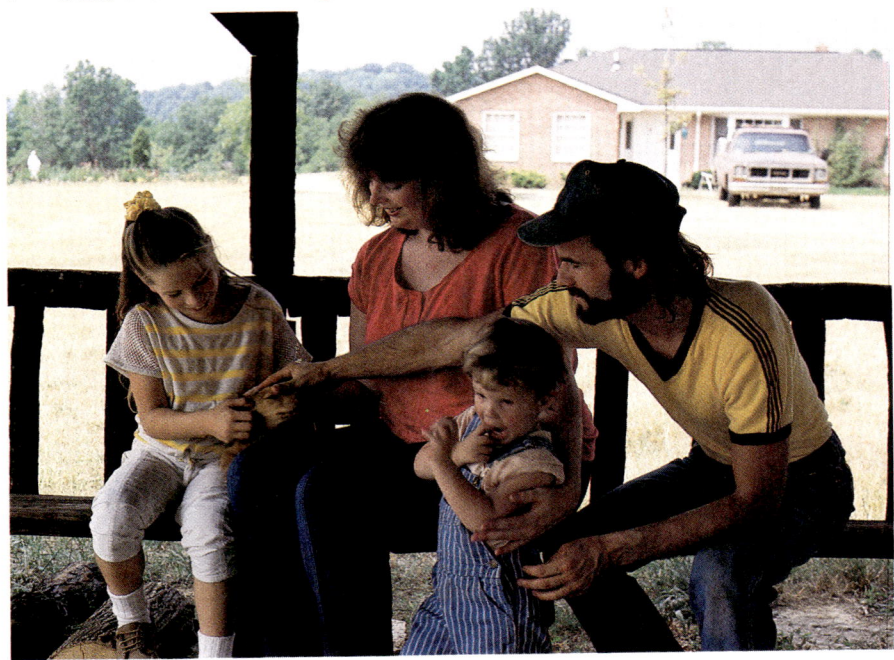

FIGURE 1-1   Enjoying happy times with both parents helps children feel secure.

Children Need a Sense of Worth

Parents who see each child as a unique person and value that child because he or she has life communicate to the child a sense of personal worth. A child who is valued and loved just for being has a sense of satisfaction other children do not experience.

CHILDREN NEED TO KNOW THAT THEY ARE VALUABLE

There are two ways of valuing people—**extrinsic valuing** and **intrinsic valuing.** When children are valued for extrinsic reasons, emphasis is placed on their talents, their appearance, or their accomplishments—what they can *do*. Being important in this sense alone does not satisfy a child's heart or emotional needs.

Children also need to be valued for intrinsic reasons. Parents who value children as unique persons, persons who have an important place in their lives, give children a deeper joy about themselves and a sense of security with regard to their relationship with their parents.

CHILDREN NEED TO LEARN TO RESPECT THEMSELVES AND OTHERS

Self-respect confirms self-worth. Learning to respect others helps children learn to value life, to get along with people and to make friends, and to express feelings and communicate in a pleasing and nonmanipulating way.

CHILDREN NEED TO LEARN TO BE RESPONSIBLE

Children need to be given responsibilities they can handle and be expected to carry them out to the best of their ability. They need to be praised when they accomplish a task. Being responsible and accomplishing tasks gives them a feeling of **competence.** Competence means feeling or being capable. This feeling supports a child's sense of worth.

Children Need to Learn

Young children have an enthusiastic interest in the world around them, particularly the natural world. It is important for parents to arrange safe opportunities for children to explore and to experiment, to try out new skills. Parents also serve as resources to help children understand the world they are discovering.

CHILDREN NEED TO LEARN IN A PEACEFUL ENVIRONMENT

Children learn best in surroundings that are free of violence and unnecessary tension. Parents need to provide a home where children are free enough from anxiety that they can learn. Children who come from a peaceful home environment do better in day care or in school.

CHILDREN NEED TIME WITH THEIR PARENTS

Availability is one characteristic of parents. Children need parents who are available to them. Parents who are available spend enough time with their children, are attentive, and listen carefully, even when the children are too young to speak well.

The amount of time parents spend with children is called **quantity time.** It is measured in hours.

More important than the number of hours parents spend with their children is how that time is spent. **Quality time** is measured in the benefits derived from time spent together. When there is a sense of closeness between children and parents, when communication is effective, when parents and children learn from one another, and when time spent together is enjoyable, quality time is being shared.

When the time parents are able to spend with children is limited, it is especially important that it be quality time. When it is not, little benefit results. Quality time requires that quantity time be invested in ways that will satisfy children's eagerness to learn and their desire to be with their parents.

You might put these ideas about the time parents and children spend together into an equation:

Quality time + Quantity time = Learning + Relationship

FIGURE 1-2 Helping to cook something provides a chance to learn new skills and share time with a parent.

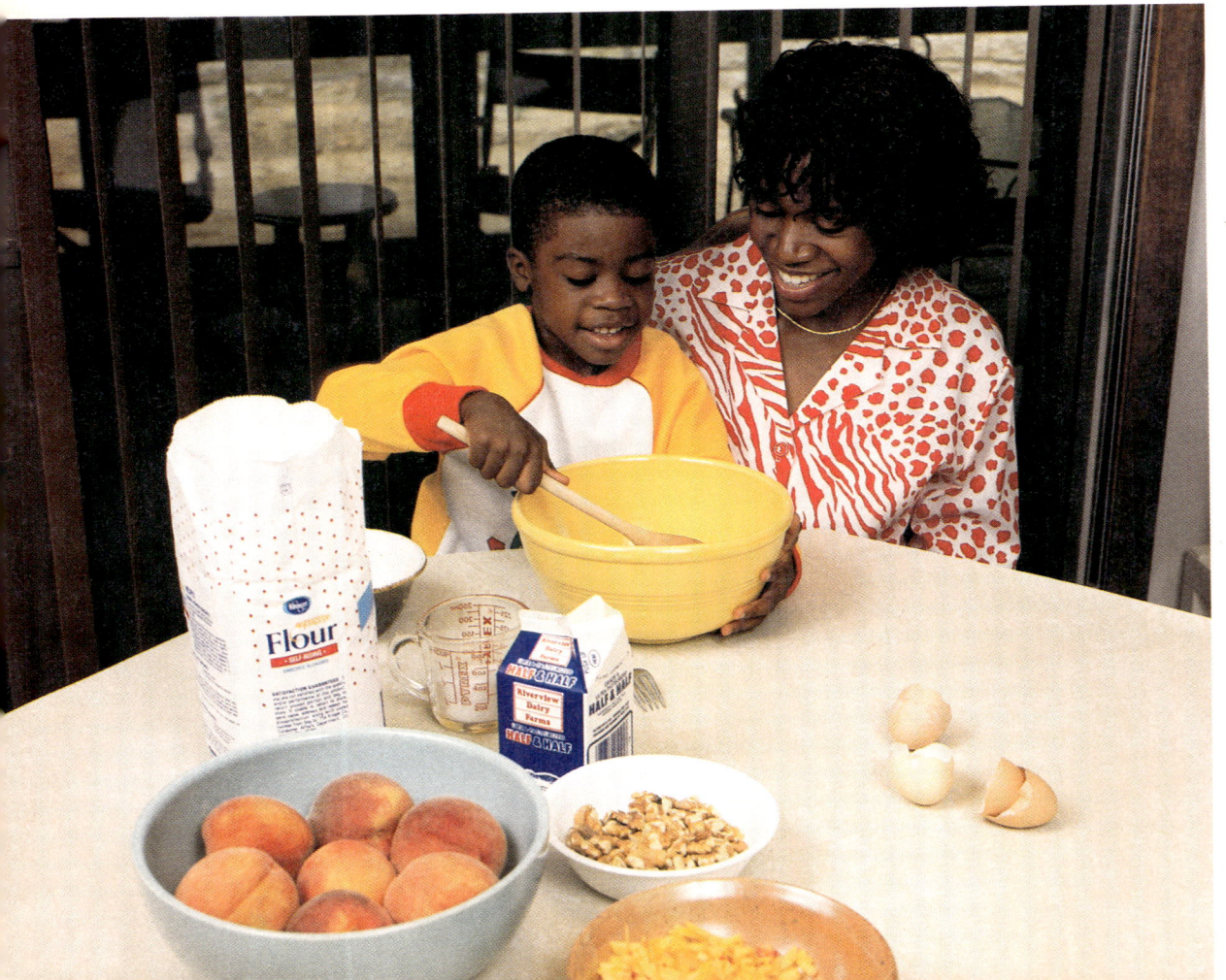

CHILDREN NEED ENCOURAGEMENT

Children need parents who encourage their efforts to learn. Praise is especially helpful when parents notice that a child's attempts to learn have been successful. When children are having a difficult time, clear support for their efforts, along with redirection when called for, is far more helpful than criticism. **Redirection** is giving a child another option for his or her effort or behavior when it is not successful or desirable.

Children Need to Be Protected

One characteristic of children is **vulnerability.** Children are vulnerable to the world around them, which means they can be easily hurt. Small children need to be protected from hurting themselves physically and from being hurt by other people or objects in their surroundings.

CHILDREN NEED TO BE PROTECTED FROM DANGER

Keeping children safe is sometimes difficult. When they are small, they are unaware of danger. Even when they are older and are aware of danger, they may not know how to keep themselves safe. Traffic, electricity, water, medications, and household products are just a few of the potential dangers children do not handle well alone. (The leading cause of death for children under six is accidents.)

CHILDREN NEED TO BE PROTECTED FROM ILLNESS

Children need proper preventive health care and appropriate care when they do become ill. Parents can sometimes provide the needed care themselves, but medical attention is necessary at other times.

CHILDREN NEED TO BE PROTECTED FROM VIOLENCE

Children need to be protected from violence both within and outside the family. Children suffer greatly in times of war and community violence. Also, many suffer from child abuse.

CHILDREN NEED TO BE PROTECTED FROM MENTAL AND EMOTIONAL ABUSE

They need to be shielded from inappropriate information and from their own ignorance. Children also need to be protected from people who might manipulate them or play mind games. Physical violence, neglect, sexual abuse, and being used for child pornography all result in emotional abuse.

Children should not be allowed to witness adult sexual acts first-hand or in the media. Because they are not equipped for handling these situations, they can become upset and confused.

Children need to be protected from abusive speech, particularly verbal abuse that leaves them feeling guilty or worthless. But they do need to be noticed in an appropriate way by parents. Being ignored can be emotionally painful to children. Parents need to protect children from this hurt and recognize them in appropriate ways.

Children Need to Have Their Physical Needs Met

Basic physical needs of children include the following:

- Food
- Shelter
- Clean water
- Appropriate touching
- Clothing
- Rest
- Clean air

Young children can neither feed nor clothe themselves. They are not able to provide themselves with clean air or water or a proper place to rest. Adults must provide these necessities for them. Children who are homeless often do not have even their basic physical needs met. Those who are neglected do not receive the physical or emotional support they need.

Physical touch stimulates children's appetites. That means touching stimulates growth. Babies who do not receive enough appropriate touching may stop eating, which may lead to malnutrition or even death.

What is appropriate touching? **Appropriate touching** means physical contact that feels safe to children. The Hands On with Children feature of the end of this chapter discusses appropriate touching in more depth.

Children Need Guidance

Children need parents to point a direction for their lives. They need positive **guidance** based on parents' wisdom and experience. Guidance also means providing children with the time and space to do their own thinking and asking them questions that will direct their thoughts in productive ways. Children need opportunities to learn meanings and beliefs and to ponder the important questions of life. Parents help their children develop desirable character traits when they provide these opportunities.

CHILDREN NEED DISCIPLINE

Discipline is training and correcting children in a way that encourages them to mature—to become responsible and self-sufficient. It is important that parents set and enforce reasonable limits consistently. Children need parents who help them understand the nature of authority—who model reasonable and proper authority and who teach them how to deal with those who misuse authority.

CHILDREN NEED GUIDANCE IN THEIR MENTAL AND PHYSICAL DEVELOPMENT

Children need parents who will help them develop and build on their strengths. When their interests stray from being healthy, children need parents who will redirect them.

CHILDREN NEED GUIDANCE IN THEIR SOCIAL AND MORAL DEVELOPMENT

Children need parents who will teach them how to get along with other people and to be responsible members of society. This training includes instilling respect for the law and fostering character development. Table 1-1 lists character traits parents may be concerned with developing. Which of these do you feel are important? Which are unimportant?

TABLE 1-1   Desirable Character Traits for Children to Develop

▪ Generosity	▪ Patience
▪ Honesty	▪ Gentleness (not weakness)
▪ Truthfulness	▪ Self-control
▪ Dignity	▪ Faithfulness
▪ Honor	▪ Forgiveness
▪ Loyalty	▪ Moderation
▪ Kindness	▪ Sense of humor

Parents' job is to meet the needs of their children. Some parents do a better job than others. How do parents accomplish this task? One way is to set goals.

THE PARENTING TASK

A person has to learn to be a good parent. Being able to give birth has very little to do with being able to raise a child. What makes an effective parent? Let's examine some of the possibilities.

New parents typically think about what the future will hold for their child. As they care for the baby and become acquainted with the child's special ways, you might hear them say, "She's strong-willed like her mother," or "Look how long he is! I'll bet he'll play basketball for the Broncos."

In quiet moments alone with the baby, parents often imagine what the child may become. Parents who imagine good life stories for their children tend to communicate those ideas to them. A parent who dreams of higher education for a child might say, "You learn easily. I think you could do well in college." Children often pick up on these dreams and make them their own.

Unfortunately, some parents to not see the good possibilities for their children. Instead they think about the bad things that can happen or the unacceptable things the child might do. Parents who say things like "You're no good—you'll probably end up in prison" also plant dreams in their children's minds; unhappily, some of these ill-fated imaginings do happen.

Parents can help, then, by looking for the potential good in their children rather than the opposite. Parents who can imagine good possibilities for their children's lives can set better goals for parenthood.

Goals for Parenthood

A **goal** is something a person wants to accomplish. Parents have goals for themselves as parents as well as goals for their children. They also help their children to develop their own goals for their lives. What kinds of goals are helpful for parents?

PARENTING GOALS

The goals parents have for themselves concern the ways they want to behave as parents. These include how they will provide for, protect, discipline, nurture, guide, and teach their children and how they will provide for the children's security and en-

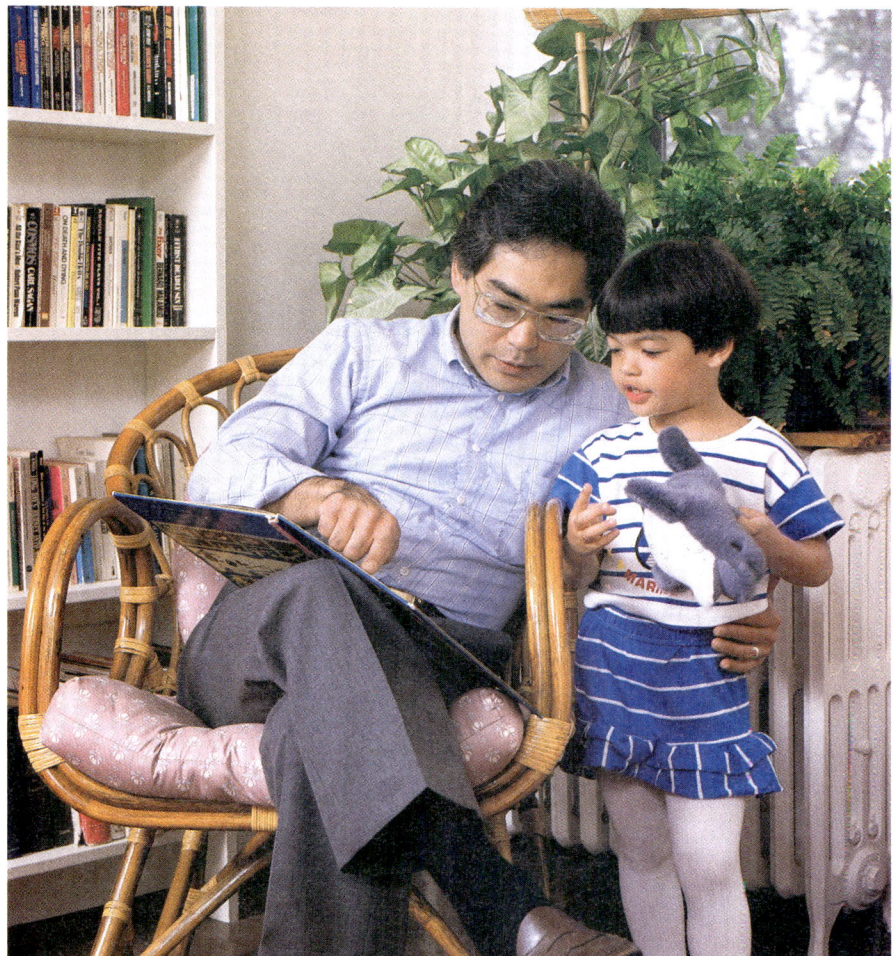

FIGURE 1-3 Reading books with children is one way parents may work toward their goals of guiding and teaching.

courage their sense of self-worth. Parents have a great deal of choice in planning and carrying out activities that will accomplish these goals.

PARENTS' GOALS FOR CHILDREN

The kinds of goals parents have for their children are based on what they hope the children will do and become. These goals concern how children's talents will be developed, what level of education they will attain, whom they will choose for friends, and what they will believe about life. Parents may have many hopes for their children, yet they often have little control over the achievement of these goals.

Even so, parents who do the job well tend to be goal-directed. They work hard at the goals they have set for themselves as parents, and as a result they tend to be more effective. Parents whose hopes for their children help those children set the pace for their own lives tend to accomplish more as parents. As children grow, however, their input becomes increasingly powerful. When older children and teenagers disagree with their parents about goals, wise parents give them room to make some choices, while providing enough guidance to keep them moving in a positive direction.

Meeting Children's Needs

The first task of a parent is to meet the child's needs. Parents are ultimately responsible for children's well-being. When parents are involved in meeting children's needs in a committed and caring way, children benefit. A father and a mother working together can form a powerful team.

FUNCTIONS OF PARENTS

The duties of parenthood, or the **functions of parents,** are related to children's needs. Parents' functions include the following:

- Establishing and maintaining a secure family
- Helping children develop a sense of self-worth
- Teaching children and providing for learning
- Protecting children
- Providing for children's physical needs
- Guiding and disciplining children

Parents Establish and Maintain a Secure Family

It is important that parents create a secure family—one in which children learn to value the family name and history, in which parents demonstrate loyalty, and in which children are introduced to the family tradition. Children also benefit if the family has financial security.

FAMILY NAME AND HISTORY

Children develop a sense of family membership by knowing, using, and finding pleasure in their family name. A child's first name may also have a family origin, which can be explained to the child.

Parents can tell stories about people in the family, places they live or have lived, and things they have done. This helps children

FIGURE 1-4   At an early age a child can begin establishing a sense of family membership by spending time with grandparents and other relatives.

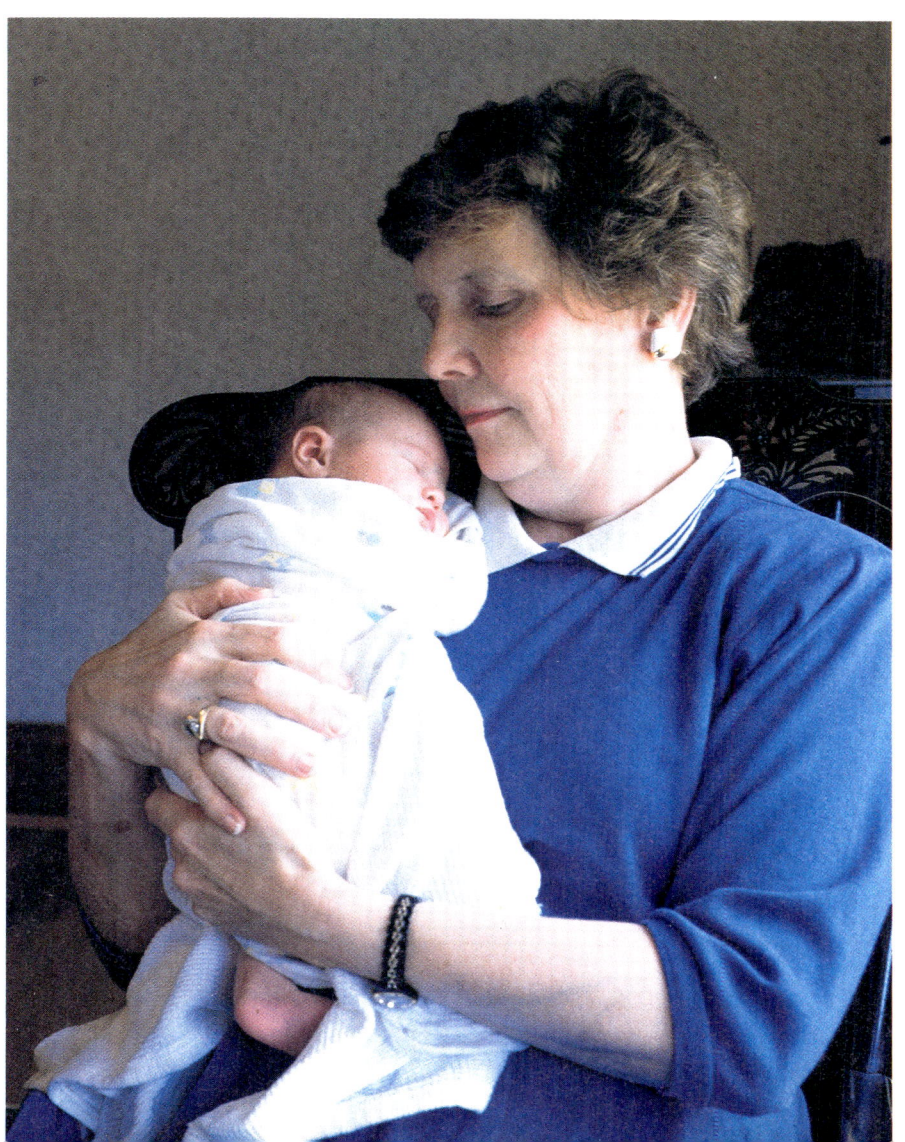

build a sense of who they are. Parents can help children put together and look at simple books that tell stories about themselves and their family.

Parents can make it possible for children to know members of their extended families. The **extended family** includes relatives other than parents and children. For example, grandparents and cousins are members of the extended family. Knowing and being around these relatives strengthens the child's idea of family.

LOYALTY AND TRADITION

Parents who are loyal to one another and to their families lead their children to develop loyalty, which strengthens relationships. A secure relationship between parents fosters security for their children. Parents who show themselves to be persons of good character have the qualities that strengthen families.

Parents can plan family celebrations that pass on traditions to children. By participating in and blending traditions that originate in both the father's and the mother's family, children build a sense of family identity. This adds to their feeling of security.

Parents can further their children's sense of being part of a secure family by introducing them to the culture of which they are a part. Participating in community festivals, helping to prepare and sharing traditional food, and learning music, dances, poetry, and literature from the family's cultural heritage can strengthen a child's sense of family identity, and thus his or her security.

FINANCIAL SECURITY

Parents who can establish and maintain financial security contribute to a child's sense of security. Children do not have to know the details of parents' financial records to sense that their family is secure.

Parents Help Children Develop a Sense of Self-Worth

Every child needs to develop a sense of self-worth early in life. A sense of self-worth is developed when a child has acceptance from parents and others and the opportunity to gain some sense of competence.

THE IMPORTANCE OF ACCEPTANCE

The kind of acceptance children crave from parents is unconditional love. Unconditional love is constant, no matter what the

Leadership at a Glance

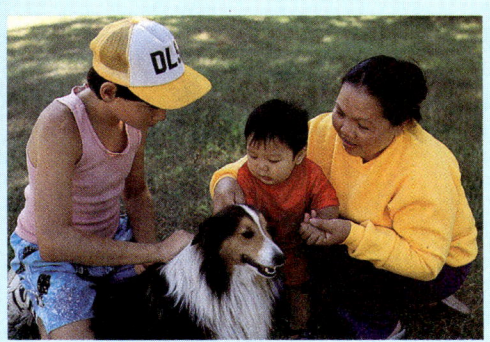

National Council on Family Relations

The National Council on Family Relations (NCFR) is an organization of people who care about and work with families. The members are from many different professions. The organization studies issues related to the family. It also identifies current legislation that is of concern to families and expresses views to members of Congress.

NCFR publishes journals and newsletters and holds conferences to discuss family-related issues. The organization has developed guidelines for family life education. Some of the ideas in this chapter were based on those guidelines.

NCFR has developed the only certification program for family life educators. This program certifies professionals who are qualified to teach family life education.

To learn more about NCFR, write to the following address:

National Council on Family Relations
1910 West Count Road B, Suite 147
St. Paul, MN 55113

Source: Family Matters 36, no. 1 (January 1987). Copyright 1987 by the National Council on Family Relations, 3989 Central Ave. NE, Suite 550, Minneapolis, MN 55421.

circumstances. Parents who accept a child unconditionally discipline him or her in a way that maintains personal dignity. This means that the parents correct the child's behavior with firmness, but continue loving the child and expressing that love freely. They care enough for the child to risk the child's temporary anger with them when discipline is needed. Chapter 9 deals more completely with the issue of discipline.

Developing a sense of self-worth also involves learning how to respect and be accepted by other people. Children need to learn how to make, keep, and end friendships. Parents need to help children learn how to handle conflicts with other children and how to restore relationships that have been damaged by conflict. Children need to learn skills that enable them to express respect for other people and express their feelings in acceptable ways.

A FEELING OF COMPETENCE

Feeling competent means feeling good about one's own abilities. Children need to feel that their competence is growing in order to have a sense of self-worth. Developing feelings of competence depends on having manageable challenges available and having the freedom to practice new skills. Parents who encourage children, who accept their attempts to succeed and urge them to continue to try, contribute to their developing sense of self-worth.

Parents help children develop feelings of competence by assigning them responsibilities and then following through to see that these tasks are completed. Feelings of competence also develop when parents help children learn to make choices and to live with the consequences of their choices.

Parents Teach Children and Provide for Learning

Parents are children's first and most powerful teachers. The first love bonds that are formed between children and their parents are very important. A parent's example is more powerful to a child than anyone else's, and his or her teaching is more fully utilized than anyone else's will be.

Parents can create an atmosphere that is helpful for learning or one that works against it. The child's ability to learn at school or at a child care center is affected by the atmosphere in the home. When that atmosphere promotes learning, children learn more readily. What do parents do to aid the learning process?

THE LEARNING ENVIRONMENT

Parents create an environment that promotes learning when they establish a peaceful atmosphere in the home. In addition, they provide a safe place to play, appropriate toys and materials, and a variety of experiences to expand children's understanding of the world. Children are allowed to work at their own pace and are given time to finish a task to their own satisfaction.

ENCOURAGEMENT

The way in which parents interact with their children makes an important difference in how well the children learn. Parents promote learning by fostering curiosity and encouraging children to try new things and take risks they can handle. Parents need to provide help, but just enough to encourage children to succeed on their own. Parents need to supervise children's activities, supporting and redirecting them rather than criticizing them when they are unable to complete a task. It is important for parents to praise children's accomplishments.

THE TIME FACTOR

Parents who spend as much quality time as possible with their children promote learning. One highly effective technique for encouraging children's learning is for parents to include them in as many of their own activities as possible, being sure that children participate as fully as they are able to. Time spent with children gives parents an opportunity to set a good example for children's behavior. Parents who are gracious to their children and who act with loving-kindness toward them make their children want to be with them and to learn from them.

HOME SCHOOLING

Some parents today have chosen to teach their children completely at home rather than sending them out to school. This is called **home schooling.** Some parents choose their own materials and make their own schedules for home schooling. Others teach from a purchased home-school curriculum designed to match the material being taught at the various grade levels in public schools. Table 1-2 gives some advantages and disadvantages of home schooling.

Suzanna Wesley, a mother in eighteenth-century England, spent one hour each week with each of her nineteen children. She taught them to read, write, spell, and do arithmetic, and she taught them about her religious faith. Two of her sons, John and Charles, went on to lead a movement called the Great Awakening, which resulted in the founding of a large Protestant denomination. Abraham Lincoln was also taught at home by his mother.

TABLE 1-2   Advantages and Disadvantages of Home Schooling

Advantages	Disadvantages
Children receive individual attention.	Children have fewer peers to play with and to learn to get along with.
Children can study subjects not taught in schools.	Children may fall behind peers or get ahead of them, making entering schools difficult.
Parents are always aware of what children are learning.	Parents may not be skilled teachers or enjoy teaching. Parents not suited to teaching may harm children's learning.
Families may have closer relationships, giving society stronger families.	Families who choose home schooling will bear extra costs (school taxes must still be paid).
Significant numbers of children being schooled at home might reduce the tax burden.	Home schooling is not legal in some states.

Parents Protect Children and Keep Them Safe

Protection of children has historically been considered one of parents' primary tasks. Parents have accomplished this task by defending children from harm and being advocates for children. They also teach children to protect themselves.

DEFENDING CHILDREN FROM HARM

Parents defend children from diseases by providing for health check-ups and inoculations. Parents defend children from harm when they defend their country against invasion and make the home secure from weather and safe from intruders. Parents also protect children from abuse by outsiders or other family members and from manipulation by people who come in contact with them.

Children need to be shielded during their early years because they are more vulnerable to harm than adults are. Children do not have sufficient strength or experience to handle some types of situations. Therefore, parents arrange for children's safety. The first step in providing for safety is to child-proof the home and play space.

BEING ADVOCATES FOR CHILDREN

An **advocate** is a person who speaks for, supports, and intercedes for another person or group of people. Parents become advocates for their own children and other children by initiating and supporting community programs that benefit children. They also become advocates for children by supporting legislation and government policies that protect all children. Advocates for children support laws that prevent children from becoming victims of molesters, child pornographers, and other criminals and that forbid exploitation of children through unfair labor practices, improper advertising, and media programming injurious to them.

Parents Provide for Children's Physical Needs

Providing for children's physical needs is the most basic and obvious of parenting tasks. The specific elements of this necessary task are meeting physical needs, teaching children to care for possessions, and giving appropriate affection.

MEETING PHYSICAL NEEDS

Parents provide the basic raw materials with which the family can meet its physical needs and purchase necessary goods and services. Parents provide physical care, including medical care, for children until they can care for themselves. They also teach children self-help skills.

TEACHING CHILDREN TO CARE FOR POSSESSIONS

Parents teach children to care for their possessions and use them appropriately. They help children learn to use community resources such as the public library and medical facilities.

GIVING APPROPRIATE AFFECTION

Parents provide children with generous amounts of affectionate, appropriate touching. Appropriate affection strengthens feelings of security by increasing children's trust in parents. Parents' trustworthiness permits a child to develop a sense of self-worth. Parents who provide affection and security provide an environment that is safe both physically and emotionally.

Parents Guide and Discipline Children

Children expect parents to guide them—to point them in a particular direction and help them manage a world they do not

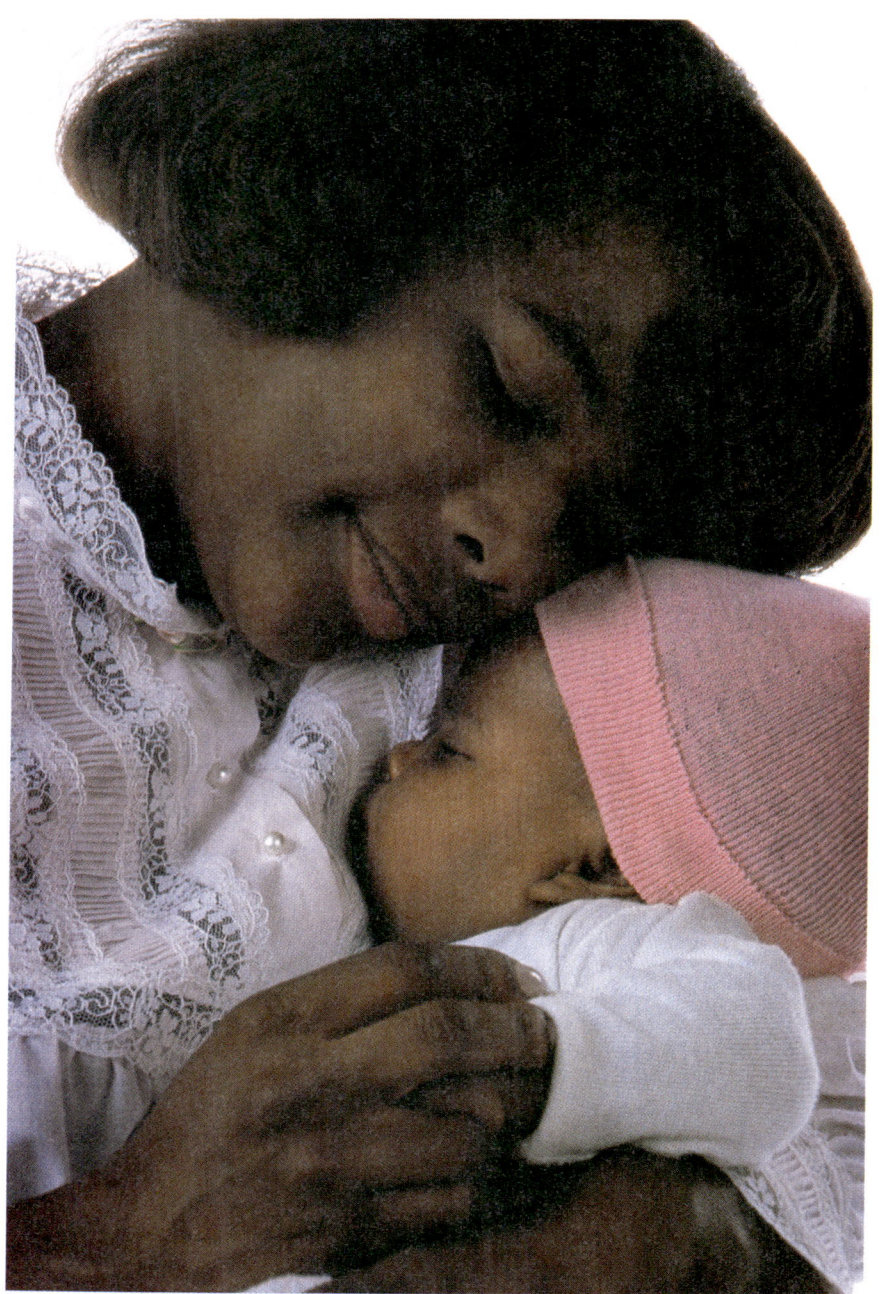

FIGURE 1-5 All children—and especially infants—need affectionate touching.
Source: Good Samaritan Hospital

fully understand. Effective parents spend more time guiding children than disciplining them.

Guiding children includes setting a standard for their behavior in one's own behavior. Parents who are secure in their own beliefs and set an example for their children teach them values, fairness, and justice. They teach them how to get along with other people. Good guidance includes building on children's personal strengths.

Discipline includes setting and enforcing reasonable limits. Parents must decide what is safe and unsafe. They must also decide what they believe to be right and wrong and what they—and other people—find to be acceptable and unacceptable behavior. They then communicate the set limits clearly and consistently to the child.

Skillful parents are able to provide leadership and guidance without being overbearing. They are able to discipline children when the situation calls for it without being abusive. Parents approach guidance in one of three ways: as strong leaders, as oppressive leaders, or as irresponsible leaders.

STRONG LEADERSHIP

Parents who give strong leadership have a healthy understanding of authority and how it is best used with children. Children need parents who set and enforce reasonable limits on a consistent basis. They need to know from the beginning that mom and dad are in charge and that the rules are to be respected. The best leadership comes when both parents are in agreement about the rules and stand together as a team.

Strong leadership can afford to be democratic. Parents who are strong leaders are not afraid to allow children to express their wishes and thoughts. They listen to children's opinions and, whenever possible, incorporate them into their decisions. But they are definitely the leaders of the home. They discipline children as needed and may even spank them occasionally in an appropriate manner.

Parents who are strong leaders perform some of the following tasks:

- They establish reasonable rules.
- They enforce those rules consistently.
- They demonstrate the consequences of children's actions.

- They establish and maintain order in the household and in family relationships.
- They teach children to respect all persons and that all persons have rights.
- They identify children's strengths and build on those strengths.
- They take responsibility for their own actions and teach children to take responsibility for theirs.
- They teach children to understand and to respect the law.
- They teach children how to handle oppressive leadership in other people.
- They give additional rights and responsibilities as children grow.
- They teach children to act with consideration for themselves and others.
- They teach children when and how to share their ideas and feelings with others.
- They establish routines.
- They teach children self-care.
- They provide a model for a personal philosophy and system of beliefs.

OPPRESSIVE LEADERSHIP

Parents who are oppressive leaders are actually abusive. They punish children rather than disciplining them. Oppressive leaders may perform any of a number of undesirable actions. These are some of the most common ones:

- Labeling
- Accusations and put-downs
- Denying children choices
- Withholding love
- Denying children their basic needs
- Making fun of children
- Trying to force their own philosophy or beliefs on children
- Criticizing children's ideas and wishes
- Playing favorites
- Playing power games
- Locking children in closets
- Inappropriate spanking

- Slapping a child's face
- Beating, as well as other forms of physical abuse
- Emotional abuse
- Sexual abuse

IRRESPONSIBLE LEADERSHIP

When parents are irresponsible leaders, they really abdicate their leadership position in the family. (Abdicate means to step down from or resign from a position of responsibility.) Not only do such parents not lead children, they fail even to supervise them. Although they may give them many toys and beautiful clothes, they often neglect them in more meaningful ways.

Children whose parents are irresponsible as leaders grow up without guidance. A rosebush that is neglected becomes a weed. Children who do not have guidance grow up like weeds, with no direction for their lives.

Parents who are strong leaders discipline children rather than punishing them. Discipline aims at developing self-controlled and self-responsible children. **Punishment** is correcting children in ways that are harmful and do not contribute to growth. Punishment occurs when parents take out their anger and frustration on their children. It is irresponsible and abusive.

Parents make mistakes; and because they are human, they do not always act in a consistent manner. When parents who are strong leaders are tired or stressed, they may become oppressive or even irresponsible for a time. On the other hand, parents who start out as oppressive or irresponsible leaders sometimes develop into strong and capable leaders. Strong leadership is a goal for parents to strive toward, even though it may be difficult to maintain at all times. And parents, like everyone else, need to be forgiven for their mistakes.

ROLES OF PARENTS

The ways parents have functioned have been somewhat consistent throughout history. The **roles of parents** are society's conceptions of what mothers or fathers do. These expectations may change with each new generation of parents.

Earlier in the twentieth century, most men would not even have considered attending classes to prepare them to be present at the birth of their own child. Today, many fathers desire that privilege. In the recent past, many fathers felt that they would be doing "women's work" if they changed a diaper or helped with laundry or dishwashing. Today many mothers work outside the home and cannot do all the household chores as well; they need help from fathers and, when possible, children. More than half of the mothers of preschool children now work outside the home, and that percentage is expected to increase in the years ahead.

FIGURE 1-6 Many fathers are finding that they enjoy helping with child-rearing tasks and that it makes them feel closer to their children.

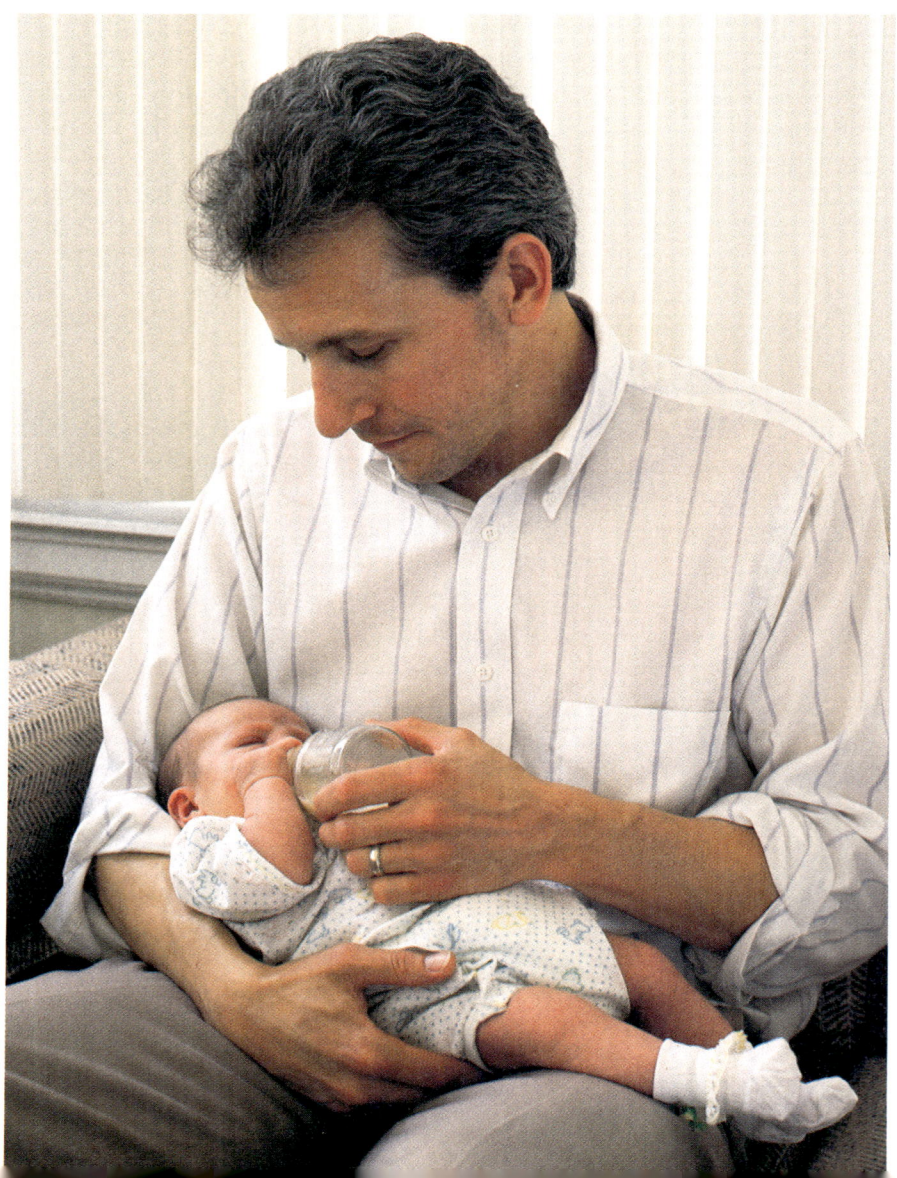

Changing roles have freed family members to do many things they have always been capable of doing. Mothers have been able to extend their talents to the workplace and to increase the family income; at the same time fathers have become more involved with their children. In many families, however, the transition has been difficult and has caused a great deal of conflict and stress.

Regardless of society's expectations of the roles of mothers and fathers, each parenting team must negotiate its own roles and style. Parents make these decisions based on what they think is best for themselves and their children. The section of this chapter called "Something to Think About" presents some aspects of the issue of parents' roles. What do you think is best for children and families?

COMMITMENT TO CHILDREN AND PARENTHOOD

Parental commitment is a choice parents make to act in a child's best interests in spite of the cost to themselves. When parents commit themselves to a child, they choose to be the best parents possible. Not only do they want to learn how to be good parents, they also focus on discovering the special talents and abilities of their child. For committed parents love is unconditional.

Being committed as a parent means being actively involved with one's child and acting in the child's best interests. Being committed costs parents. They often give up interests of their own in behalf of the child. If it is to be functional, parental commitment must be a father's and mother's top priority. If other commitments become a higher priority, particularly commitments that are inconsistent with their functions as parents, the child becomes an interest rather than a commitment. Parents who are committed to the family and the needs of their children as their first priority tend to be more successful parents over the years than those who put other things first.

THE ROLE OF CAREGIVERS AND TEACHERS

People who care for children away from home will be called **caregivers** in this book. Such people provide for basic physical and emotional needs when a child is away from his or her parents. Caregivers who also teach and guide children will be called **teachers** in this book. Teachers address more of children's needs than do caregivers.

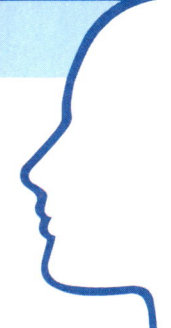

Something to Think About

Parents versus Fathers and Mothers

Much discussion has taken place in recent years about the roles of men and women, fathers and mothers. Women have demanded equal opportunities in the workplace, and men have demanded custody rights of children. During the search for equality, many have said that men and women, and therefore fathers and mothers, are the same. Some women say that they can do anything a man can do, plus give birth. Men have retaliated that anything women can do they can do better, plus sire children. Other people say that only women can change diapers, wipe noses, prepare meals, and keep an orderly home, and only men should earn a living, defend the home, and tell the wife and children what to do. Many have rebelled against this stereotypical image of their roles.

What talents might be wasted if men and women are limited to the stereotypical roles described above? If parents are limited to developing themselves according to these definitions, what will their children miss?

Are there any unique and special contributions to be made individually by fathers or mothers? What do children need? Can either parent fulfill all the needs of children? What particular strengths do children receive from mothers or from fathers? When a mother and a father work together as a team on behalf of children, what are the special benefits?

If you believe that children draw some strengths from mothers and others from fathers, what kind of burden is placed on single parents to meet the needs of children? How might caregivers and teachers of young children assist parents, particularly single parents, in meeting the needs of young children?

Or perhaps you think that mothers and fathers are essentially the same—their only difference being their biological contribution to the forming of life. The issue, then, for equality of mothers and fathers is really one of sameness versus specialness. What do you think?

Children generally have more of their needs met when they are with parents who care a great deal about them and can give them an abundance of quality time. This arrangement is not always possible. An increasing number of children under six are cared for outside the home for some part of the time. What is the role of caregivers and teachers in the lives of children?

Caregivers and teachers assist parents with their parenting functions. The more time children spend with caregivers, the more of these tasks will have to be done by them. It is important for those who care for children outside the home to work harmoniously with parents. In some cases parents are very busy, or even absent. Caregivers may be the only parenting person in children's lives. When this occurs, the role of caregiver or teacher becomes even more important.

Brad and Monica made a commitment to be good parents to Sarah. They knew they had a great deal to learn and would need assistance. They promised themselves that as Sarah grew, they would watch other parents—the ones they felt were successful—in order to shape their own parenting to meet Sarah's changing needs.

Summary

Children need a sense of worth and opportunities to learn. They need to be protected, to have their physical needs met, and to feel secure. Parents are usually the people best qualified to meet those needs. Parents who envision good things for their children and who set goals to help their children achieve are usually more effective.

Parents have functions that meet children's needs. They provide a secure family, establish a sense of self-worth, teach children basic skills and values, arrange for further learning, protect children, provide for their physical needs, and give guidance and discipline. Parents' roles are changing, and these changes affect children.

Parental commitment involves choosing to be committed, focusing on the child as a person, providing unconditional love, acting in the child's best interest, placing children ahead of conflicting interests, and making family and child-rearing their first priority in life.

Caregivers and teachers can assist with parenting at times when parents do not or cannot fulfill their functions.

Terms and Concepts

Unconditional love	Discipline
Extrinsic valuing	Goal
Intrinsic valuing	Functions of parents
Competence	Extended family
Availability	Home schooling
Quantity time	Advocate
Quality time	Punishment
Redirection	Roles of parents
Vulnerability	Parental commitment
Appropriate touching	Caregivers
Guidance	Teachers

Checking Your Understanding

1. Name and briefly describe each of the needs of young children.

2. Explain the difference between parenting goals and goals for children.

3. Select one of the needs of children discussed in the chapter and explain how parents meet that need.

4. List the functions of parents and how each relates to the needs of children.

5. List the three kinds of parental leadership. Discuss how each kind of leadership affects children.

6. Write a paper describing how fathers and mothers should work out their roles so both children and parents can have their needs met within the family.

7. Contrast the strengths of families in which parents are committed to children with those of families in which parents are not committed. Why is commitment a necessary ingredient in effective parenting?

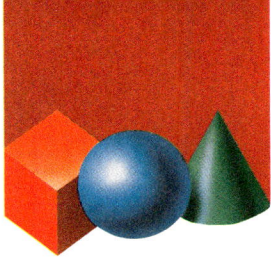

1 HANDS ON WITH CHILDREN

TOUCHING CHILDREN APPROPRIATELY

Children need to be touched, but the touching should be appropriate. Appropriate touching includes these forms of contact:

- Cuddling
- Holding
- Hugging
- Kissing on the cheek
- Bathing
- Cleaning diaper area

Inappropriate touching includes the following, which are forms of child abuse:

- Using force
- Hitting or beating
- Pinching
- Shaking
- Stimulating nipples or genitals

Can you think of other examples of appropriate and inappropriate touching?

Caregivers touch children as they care for them. When caregivers change diapers and assist with toileting, they need to be especially careful to touch children only in appropriate ways.

The following is an acceptable procedure for changing diapers:

Step 1   Wash your hands thoroughly before you begin.

Step 2   If the baby has had a bowel movement, clean as much from the skin as possible with the unsoiled area of the diaper. Wipe any remaining feces from the skin with a disposable towelette, a moistened paper towel, or toilet tissue.

Step 3   Use a clean, dampened cloth to thoroughly clean the whole genital area. Dispose of the soiled cloth properly.

Step 4   Rub diaper cream onto the skin surrounding the genitals and the baby's bottom.

Step 5   Place a clean diaper on the infant and put the soiled diaper in an appropriate place.

Step 6   Disinfect the diaper change area.

Step 7   Wash your hands thoroughly before changing another baby or moving on to another task.

Once toddlers are toilet-trained, they need a different kind of assistance. Teach them to wipe themselves with toilet paper. Follow through by checking to see if they have cleaned adequately. If they have not, do it for them, and then wash your hands.

Preschoolers should be fairly experienced at going to the toilet themselves. They may need to be supervised and sometimes reminded to clean themselves. For most of them, this will be adequate.

CHAPTER 2
Parents and Families

OBJECTIVES

When you have finished this chapter, you will be able to

- Point out factors of the choice to become parents
- Describe the adjustments necessary when a baby joins the family
- Discuss problems and choices concerning childlessness
- Identify the leadership responsibilities of parents
- Describe the characteristics of a strong family
- Summarize the important influences on the children's development
- Identify the unique problems faced by teenage parents and their children

James is Brad's younger brother. James and Vicki had their first baby just after she turned sixteen. He was seventeen and a senior in high school. Vicki was surprised and afraid when she found out she was pregnant. James was nervous, too. He had no idea how he would support a family.

Little Jimmy was born three weeks early and weighed just under five pounds. He had some problems breathing at first, so he had to stay in the hospital for a few extra days. The hospital bill was increased by several thousand dollars because of this extra time and care. James and Vicki did not have hospitalization insurance. They received some help from the state and some from their parents. It took them two years to pay all the hospital costs.

Although the going was tough, they made it because they had encouragement from their parents, and they both worked really hard.

BECOMING A FAMILY

The first step in becoming a family is choosing parenthood. This has to be a mature decision. Giving birth is only the beginning, however. From then on there are many decisions to be made regarding parenthood.

Choosing Parenthood

Vicki and James did not plan her first pregnancy. When they found out she was pregnant, they arranged for medical care and began to adjust their lives to include a baby. They began to think in terms of the needs of three persons rather than just two.

FIGURE 2-1   Choosing to become parents is a mature decision that brings joy and hope.
Source: © Erika Stone 1981

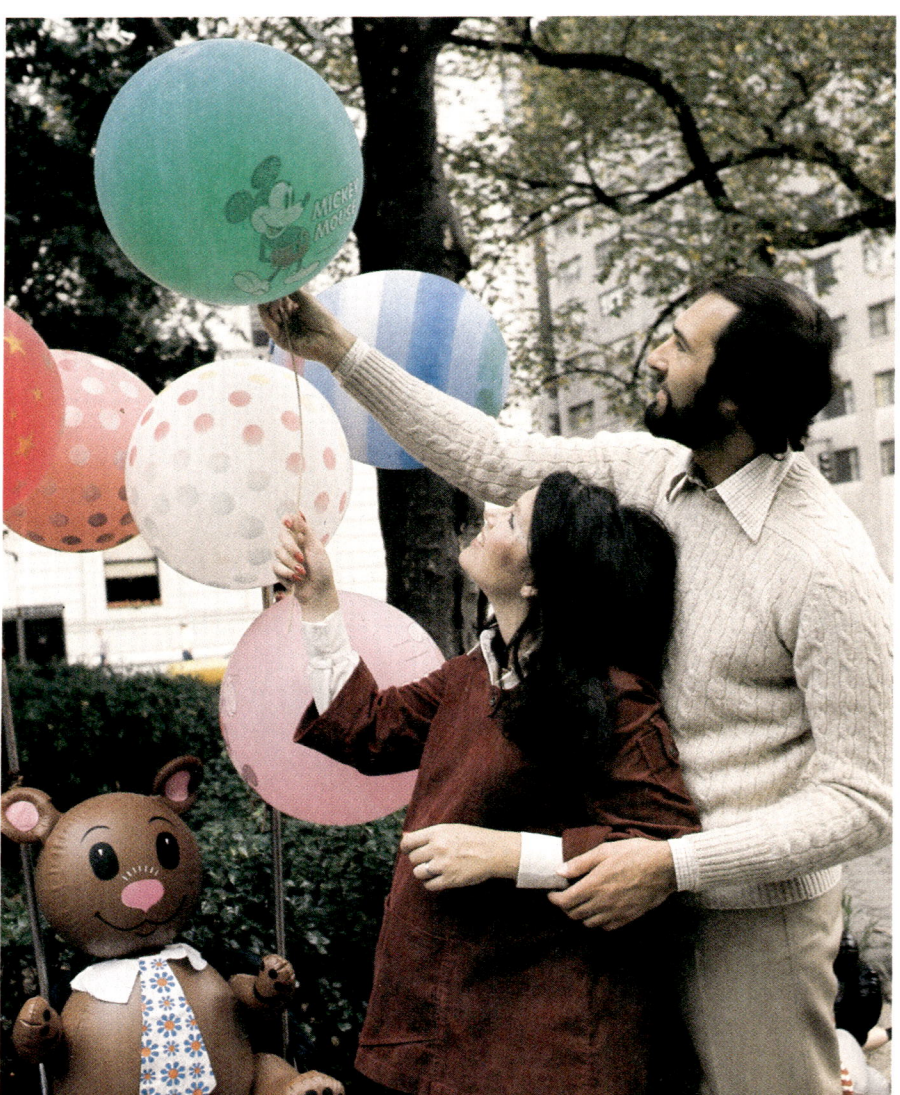

REASONS FOR HAVING A BABY

Whether or not a pregnancy is planned, dealing with the pregnancy must be approached in a mature way. Healthy and unselfish reasons for having a baby include wanting to give life and to care for and teach and love a new person.

Sometimes people have babies for unhealthy or selfish reasons. These include the following:

- To trap someone into marriage
- To prove themselves physically as a man or a woman
- To provide a playmate for other children
- To provide a grandchild
- To improve a problem marriage
- To have someone who will love them
- To be in a weakened position for a while in order to be cared for
- To gain financially (by increasing welfare eligibility or producing a future worker to add to family income)
- To take revenge on parents or others

READINESS FOR PARENTHOOD

Being ready for parenthood not only means wanting a baby for unselfish, mature reasons, but also being prepared to provide for the child. Parents should be able to provide at least the following basic physical necessities: a clean, safe place to live, food, clothing, and medical care. These necessities must be provided continuously for at least eighteen years.

Parents should also be able to provide emotional security. In order to do that, parents must have at least the following:

- Confidence in their ability to be parents
- A home that is emotionally secure
- A few good friends
- Stable jobs they can at least tolerate
- Plans, hopes, and dreams for their own future

Children whose parents have acquired some ideas about how

to be parents and how to rear a child have a clear advantage over other children.

FINANCIAL CONSIDERATIONS

Having children is expensive. During pregnancy, money is necessary for paying the doctor and buying any medications or vitamins prescribed. Most hospitals require a deposit. Even parents who have health insurance often pay a portion of the doctor and hospital bills. These costs vary in different communities. What are the costs for delivering a baby in your part of the country?

If there are problems and the baby must remain in the hospital after the birth, the cost increases. It can be as high as $1,000 per day for time spent in a neonatal intensive care unit (NICU) because of the special skills and equipment offered there. Babies who are very sick and must remain in the hospital for a time can become million-dollar babies. When parents' money runs out, hospitals sometimes must absorb some of these costs.

There are expenses in addition to medical costs. Before the birth, there is the cost of the mother's maternity clothing. Parents spend money for clothing, a bed, a car seat, and other equipment and furniture for the new baby. Supplies for feeding and bathing are also needed.

One expense parents sometimes forget to plan for is the increased cost of housing. Although babies may take up little extra space at first, most families are more comfortable when children do not share a bedroom with parents. One way to estimate this added expense is to figure the difference in the yearly cost of a one-bedroom and a two-bedroom apartment.

The cost of food and diapers for the baby's first year can also be calculated. Babies on formula average one can per day if the formula is premixed or one can per week if it is dry. Feeding costs also include those for baby food for about eight months (the fifth through the twelfth month), a sterilizer, bottles, feeding dishes, and a high chair. The cost of diapers is significant.

Babies quickly outgrow their clothing, so a larger size will be needed at least once and probably twice during the first year. Money spent on supplies such as shampoo, lotions, and powder adds up, too.

During the first year, babies usually have check-ups at the doctor's office at two weeks, six weeks, three months, six months, and one year. In addition, when a baby is sick, a visit to the doctor will be necessary, and medication may be required. Hospital stays may occur during the first year. Immunizations against disease also begin during the first year. These are usually given during the regular check-ups, but they do cost extra.

Nearly all parents want to buy toys for their children. Although this expense does not have to be excessive, most parents will spend more than they expect on toys during the first year.

Although the cost of having and rearing a baby is very high, there are many ways to save money. Having a sound insurance policy that covers a portion of the medical expenses helps to keep those bills manageable. Many parents carry health insurance through their employers. Health insurance policies usually must be in effect for ten months before the birth of a baby. A policy that allows parents to add coverage for a new baby at birth is very helpful.

Money can also be saved by borrowing equipment from other parents and by using secondhand clothes. If it is clean and fits comfortably, used clothing can do as well as new. Parents can save money by taking advantage of sales and by buying some things at thrift stores or garage sales. Can you think of other ways for parents to save money without neglecting a baby's needs?

Adjusting to a New Baby

When Jimmy was born, Vicki and James changed from being a family unit to being a parenting family unit, from being a husband and wife to being parents. This change required many adjustments for them. When parents expect their second child, even more adjustments are necessary. Not only do they need to make room for another child, they have to help the first child adjust to the new baby, too.

ADJUSTMENTS FOR PARENTS

By the time the baby arrives, most couples are really excited about becoming parents. Expectant parents look forward to holding the baby in their arms, seeing what the baby looks like, and talking to the baby. They think about bringing the baby home, pick out names, and talk about who the baby will resemble.

After the birth, excitement settles down, and parents begin to face the reality of caring for the baby's needs. Being responsible for a life can seem overwhelming. Most parents want to do their very best to help their baby grow and thrive.

Care of a small baby is exhausting. He or she demands almost constant care. Attention that a husband and wife once gave only to each other must now be shared with the baby. Immature parents sometimes become jealous of the baby.

If one parent spends too much time with the baby and neglects the marriage partner, problems may arise. Both parents need an opportunity to help with child care, but they also need time alone together. One of the best gifts a parent can give a child is to maintain a strong relationship with the other parent.

New parents are often frustrated by all the demands placed on them. Because of exhaustion from labor and delivery, the new responsibilities of caregiving, and the stress on the couple's relationship, some new mothers experience **postpartum blues.** This period of depression can last a few hours or a few weeks, during which the mother may cry a great deal. If the depression lasts for more than a few days or if it is severe, a doctor should be consulted for help.

ADJUSTMENTS FOR SIBLINGS

Siblings are brothers and sisters. New babies require so much time and attention that older siblings sometimes feel neglected. Jealousy is very common. Older children may need special time and attention from parents at this time to feel that they, too, are special. At the end of this chapter, the special feature called "Hands On with Children" provides some suggestions for helping older children adjust to a new baby. Each time a family member is added, the task of helping the other members adjust to and accept the new baby becomes more complex.

THE ROLE OF GRANDPARENTS

Grandparents can be a special blessing to young children. Most grandparents enjoy being around grandchildren and are more relaxed than they were when they were raising their own children. Children benefit from having someone who loves them a great deal just for who they are. Grandparents often enjoy telling stories about the children's parents and thus are a good source of family history.

Sometimes grandparents have a difficult time accepting their new role because it marks them as being a generation older. New parents who help their own parents enjoy being grandparents will find them a tremendous asset in their children's lives.

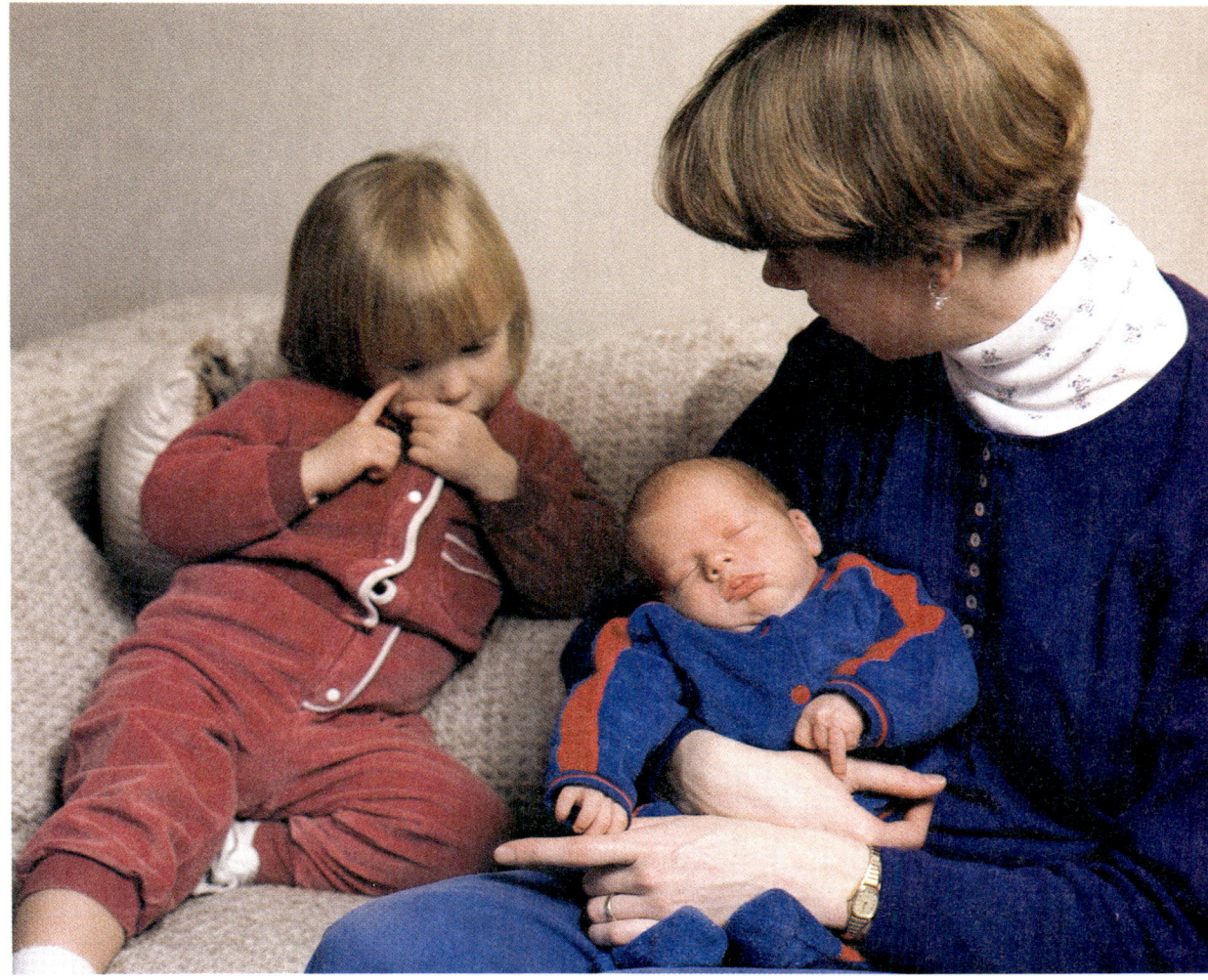

FIGURE 2-2   Jealousy of a new baby in the family is not an unusual
feeling in young children.
Source: © Erika Stone 1987

Childlessness

Many couples who want children are not able to have them.
One couple in ten has difficulty having children. For some of these
couples, longing for a child is deep, and they are very sad because
they cannot have children. When couples adopt babies, their sadness very often turns to joy. Illustration 2-1 is a letter from an
adoptive mother to the baby's birth mother.

Dear birth mother,

Thank you for being able to share your precious baby daughter with us. Only your willingness to do this has allowed us the opportunity to be fulfilled as parents. More than seven years without the sound of a child in our home left us both feeling very empty. Words are extremely inadequate to express our praise and gratitude to you.

We can assure you that our baby will be nurtured and loved. Also, she will know at an early age that we are not her natural parents. Credit will be given where credit is due.

May God bless you in an extra way in the days, months, and years to come.

Lovingly,

Very happy adoptive parents

ILLUSTRATION 2-1   This letter from adoptive parents to their child's birth mother expresses their happiness and gratitude.

In some cases, **childlessness** is not a couple's choice, but some couples choose not to be parents. (Methods of birth control are discussed in Chapter 4.) Couples elect not to be parents for many reasons. Some prefer to focus on careers; others choose to devote their lives to a cause or task that requires the time and energy that would otherwise be given to children. Some people feel they are not suited to being parents; others simply do not want to be.

Adoption

Although they were happy with their decision to become parents, Vicki and James had thought about putting their baby up for adoption before he was born. At that time they learned many things they did not know about the process of adoption. For example, they learned that babies can be adopted through an adoption agency or through private individuals.

ADOPTION AGENCIES

Generally the people best equipped to help with adoption are those working for an agency that has a good reputation and can give a number of references. Many such agencies are operated by churches or private, nonprofit organizations. Reputable adoption agencies have policies that protect all the persons involved—the adoptive parents, the birth parents, and the child. The **adoptive parents** are the people who adopt the baby. The **birth parents** are the people who give the baby up for adoption.

People who handle most agency adoptions are trained to be respectful of both the adoptive family and the birth parents. They employ a screening process that helps them place each baby with the kind of family the birth parents want. Some agencies even allow the birth mother to make the final choice from a selected group of families. Agencies also try to screen for characteristics that the adoptive parents request.

For the benefit of everyone—the birth parents, the adoptive parents, and the baby—usually only the adoption agency keeps a record of the names and addresses of the other people involved.

OPEN ADOPTION

In **open adoption** the agency encourages the birth parents to write a letter to the baby telling him or her why they decided to allow the adoption. Illustration 2-2 is a letter from a birth mother to her baby. As you can see, the letter expresses a great deal of love and caring for the baby. A letter like this can help a child

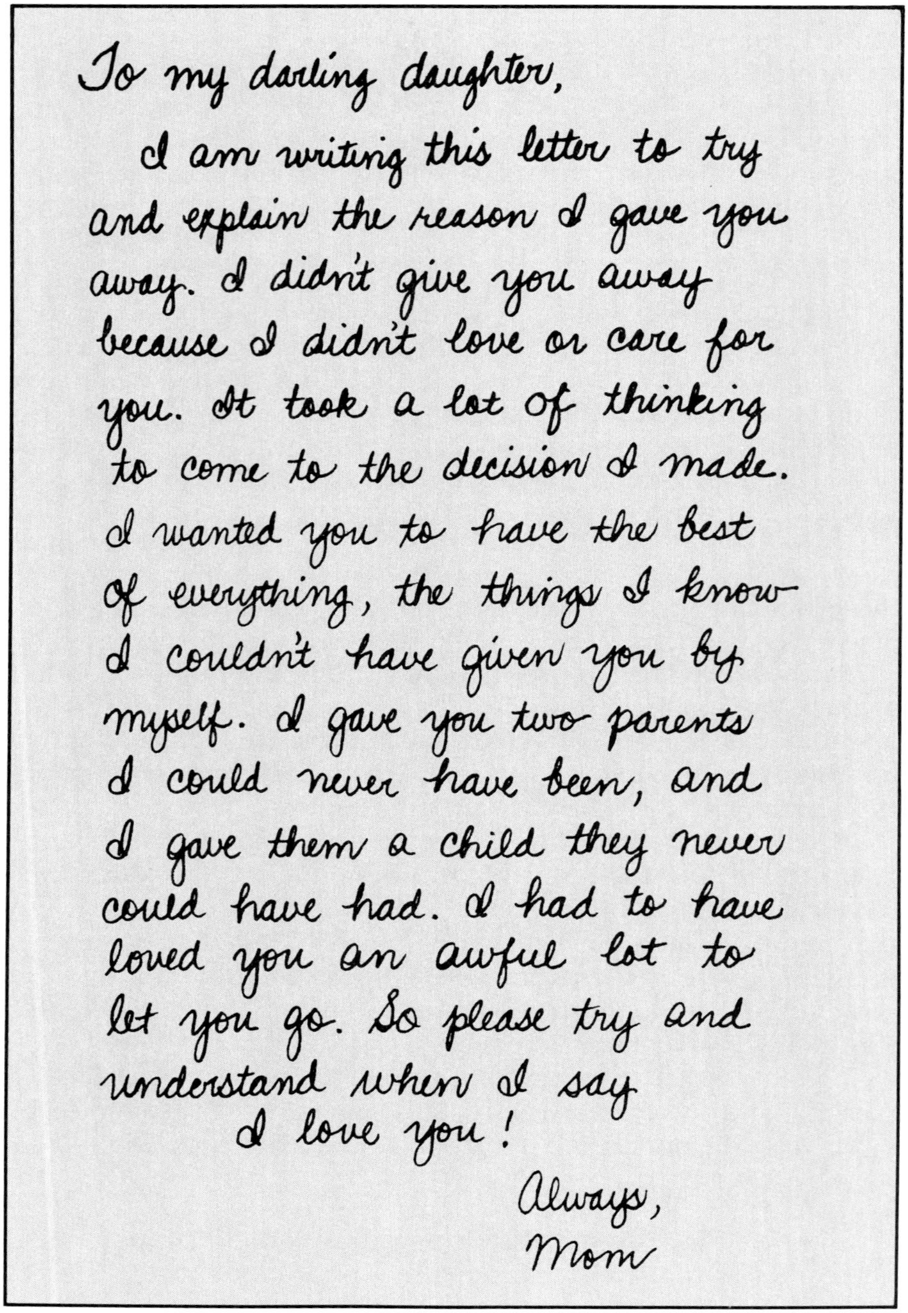

To my darling daughter,

I am writing this letter to try and explain the reason I gave you away. I didn't give you away because I didn't love or care for you. It took a lot of thinking to come to the decision I made. I wanted you to have the best of everything, the things I know I couldn't have given you by myself. I gave you two parents I could never have been, and I gave them a child they never could have had. I had to have loved you an awful lot to let you go. So please try and understand when I say I love you!

Always,
Mom

ILLUSTRATION 2-2   This letter is from a birth mother to the baby she gave up for adoption.

feel that the adoption took place because of love and not because of rejection.

Open adoption allows birth parents and children an opportunity to get to know one another once the child is grown, if they wish to do so. Under these conditions, adoptive parents must accept the fact that their child may also come to love his or her birth parents later in life.

Pregnancy and Child Loss

Not all pregnancies are happy times. Some unborn babies do not grow and develop normally. The expectant mother's life may be endangered. Some pregnancies require specialized medical care or emotional adjustments.

Sometimes unborn babies die or are not carried long enough to survive outside the uterus. When a pregnancy is lost, parents grieve. Sometimes the grief centers on the pregnancy. More often it centers on the lost child.

MISCARRIAGES

Some women tend to have miscarriages. The medical term for a miscarriage is **spontaneous abortion.** Spontaneous abortion occurs when the baby is expelled from the mother's body before the twentieth week of pregnancy. Parents who lose a baby by miscarriage often grieve deeply for the lost baby. Some feel guilty because they wonder if they might have done something to cause the loss. There are, however, many reasons for miscarriage, over which parents have little or no control.

Doctors who care for women's reproductive problems are **gynecologists.** Those who specialize in delivery of babies are called **obstetricians.** Most gynecologists are also obstetricians. This kind of specialist is the most qualified to assist a woman during a pregnancy, when a miscarriage occurs, or when there are decisions to be made about a pregnancy.

STILLBORN BABIES

A baby who is born dead is referred to as stillborn. Sometimes parents know before the birth that the baby is not likely to live. At other times they expect a healthy baby and are shocked when the baby is dead. In some cases a doctor can tell in advance that the baby is not alive and must inform the parents of this very sad circumstance.

EARLY DEATHS

Some babies die within a few hours or days following birth. Usually the cause is a birth defect or problems during the birth process.

ABORTION

Abortion is the term most people use for what doctors call **induced abortion.** Induced abortion means intentionally separating the fetus (or unborn baby) from the mother before it is able to live on its own. Parents who decide on having an abortion, for whatever reason, often grieve for the baby even though they have made this choice.

Choosing not to parent *before* a pregnancy occurs is preferable to making that choice *during* a pregnancy. Choosing abortion is a decision that can have far-reaching consequences. Some of these are presented in the Something to Think About feature.

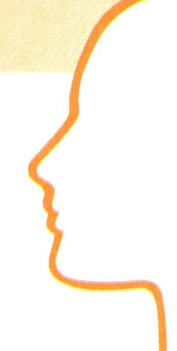

Something to Think About

Deciding About an Unintended or Problem Pregnancy

One of the themes of this text is that each person is unique and irreplaceable. Do you agree? Are unborn children important? Does the life of a pregnant teenager matter? These questions are all involved in deciding what you believe about abortion. It is not the purpose of this feature to discuss whether or not abortion should be legal. The purpose is to help you think through decisions concerning whether abortion is a wise personal choice.

What are the outcomes for the baby? Some people think of an unborn baby as a mass of the mother's body tissue, a potential life. Others think the baby is a person who, from the moment of conception, is intentionally and wonderfully formed in the mother's womb. With either view, any opportunity for life ends with an abortion.

When do you think a baby's life begins? Is it at the moment of conception when the mother's ovum and the father's sperm join and create the first cell? Or does life begin later in prenatal development? A detailed discussion of prenatal development is found in Chapter 4. You will want to study it before deciding what you believe.

The baby responds to objects that touch it in the uterus as early as the eighth week of pregnancy. Does that mean the baby can feel pain? Some people think it does. Others disagree. If an unborn baby can feel pain at eight weeks, abortion procedures after that time are likely to be painful to the baby.

What are the possible outcomes for the parents? There are possible medical complications for the mother. Either during pregnancy or at the time of delivery, there can be complications. Sometimes there are complications from abortion. These can include bleeding, damage to the uterus or cervix, infections, blood clots, and breathing problems. There is usually some pain, depending on the method used. Occasionally a woman dies of complications from abortion procedures.

There is greater risk when the abortion is not performed in a medically safe environment. The woman is less likely to experience complications in the following situations:

- When the abortion is performed before the twelfth week of pregnancy (This means early detection of the pregnancy.)

- When the abortion is performed by an obstetrician or gynecologist who is familiar with the procedure

- When a follow-up visit to the doctor that performed the abortion occurs

- When someone close to the woman having the abortion knows about it, in case complications occur later

- When the doctor performing the abortion has access to the woman's medical history (Usually he or she will be the patient's own doctor or one to whom that doctor has referred the patient.)

Abortions performed later in a pregnancy (after the eighth to twelfth week) are more risky. Most doctors will recommend that an abortion performed after that time take place in a hospital rather than a clinic because hospitals are better regulated and provide more safety for the patient.

There are outcomes concerning the parents' emotions. Most couples faced with an unintended pregnancy expect to experience relief after an abortion. The strongest and most frequent emotion, however, is grief. Other emotional outcomes of abortion can include guilt, an inability to forgive self or others, a desire to end the relationship with one's partner, loss of interest in sex, and depression or thoughts of suicide. Family members may experience grief, concern for the mother's life and health, guilt, an inability to forgive, or depression.

What are the parents' responsibilities? The responsibility for causing a pregnancy is both the father's and the mother's. The responsibility for the outcome of the pregnancy also belongs to both. This means that neither has the right to coerce the other into making a decision that is against his or her will. Each needs to think deeply about what he or she believes to be right and to follow those beliefs. Responsible decision making involves the following:

- Getting good, caring, objective counseling before making any decision (Counseling is more likely to be helpful if it is obtained from a qualified counselor who is not involved with a possible abortion procedure.)
- Being well informed about what the decision involves and what the outcomes can mean
- Accepting responsibility for the decision and its outcomes

Couples facing decisions about unintended pregnancies need the love and support of friends and family even if friends or family members disagree with their choice.

How can teenagers show this kind of care to friends and family members? When do you think a baby's life begins? How can the lives of both the unborn baby and the teenage parents be valued? Is abortion an answer to unintended pregnancy? What do you think?

MOURNING THE LOSS OF A PREGNANCY OR BABY

Parents who have lost a pregnancy or baby will tell you that it is one of the most painful grief experiences possible. When parents have an opportunity to hold and talk to the infant, even if it is stillborn, the grief process is facilitated. Where a miscarriage or abortion has occurred, the parents sometimes have more difficulty dealing with the grief. Sometimes they become very depressed before life feels good again.

There are three steps in mourning the loss of a pregnancy or baby:

▪ *The parents protest the loss of the pregnancy or baby.* They may be angry because of the loss. They are shocked and cannot believe the baby or pregnancy is gone.

▪ *Parents' lives become disorganized.* They are very sad and depressed. Their lives are confused. They struggle to understand why the baby or pregnancy is gone. Many parts of their lives seem not to work. They feel as though they have failed and may feel unworthy.

▪ *Parents begin to reorganize their lives and find new purpose and new directions.* Their lives begin to come together and to work again. Although they still feel sad when they think about their loss, they think about other things most of the time and find good reasons to go on with life. Another pregnancy or birth often helps parents get their lives back together.

Experienced medical personnel and a supportive group of people who have similar problems can be helpful in recovering from the loss of a pregnancy or baby.

BUILDING A FAMILY

Building a family begins with leadership by parents. Families who are strong show commitment, good communication, and other positive qualities.

Parental Leadership

A family needs leadership, and it is up to parents to provide it. The way a couple negotiates the various leadership responsibilities is usually established during the early months of marriage. Partners may share household tasks or divide responsibilities, deciding who is to do each one.

Parents need to decide how they will take care of each of the following:

▪ Providing an income   ▪ Protecting the family

- Caring for and maintaining the household
- Bringing order into family relationships
- Developing a sense of family membership
- Providing a sense of security

- Nurturing the children
- Teaching children
- Guiding and disciplining children
- Caring for the family's health needs
- Providing shelter

In most cases, as the marriage matures, these roles and responsibilities will shift somewhat.

Characteristics of Strong Families

What makes a family strong? Researchers Nick Stinnett and John DeFrain studied 3,000 families from all over the world and found that strong families show the following characteristics: commitment, appreciation, communication, time together, spiritual wellness, and coping skills.[1]

COMMITMENT

In strong families, the family comes first. **Commitment** in strong families tends to last over time and holds them together during difficult times. It includes sexual fidelity. If there is infidelity, there is a time of forgiveness and beginning again. Ongoing traditions are used to strengthen a strong family's commitment.

Commitment is a way of describing the special kind of love that holds families together, a love that does not change as moods shift, as times pass, or as hard times come and go. Commitment involves the unconditional kind of love discussed in Chapter 1. Giving this kind of love tells a person, "I love you even when things go wrong—nothing can take my love away."

APPRECIATION

In strong families, members regularly and genuinely express their **appreciation** of one another. These families often plan in-

---

[1]Nick Stinnett and John DeFrain, *The Secrets of Strong Families* (New York, NY: Little, Brown and Co., 1985).

Leadership at a Glance

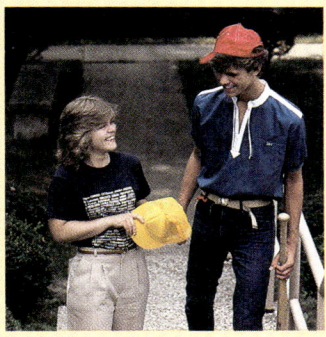

Nick Stinnett, Ph.D.

Dr. Nick Stinnett wants to know what makes good families work. He has spent fifteen years trying to answer that question and teaching about family strength. The results of his study have been published as a book called *The Secrets of Strong Families.* Articles about this work have appeared in popular magazines such as *Reader's Digest* and *Redbook.*

Dr. Stinnett also writes about family strength and other family research topics for professional publications. He teaches at the University of Alabama and is the author of a college textbook called *Relationships in Marriage and the Family.*

Dr. Stinnett is currently studying teenagers. He has noticed that although some teenagers have a very difficult time growing up, others do not. He wants to know what is different about those who do well.

Dr. Stinnett is married. He and his wife have two sons. In all ways, he is someone to look to when thinking about family strength.

tentional activities to show this appreciation. The parents tend to teach appreciation to their children and to create the positive kind of home environment that involves giving and receiving compliments graciously.

COMMUNICATION

Communication is good in strong families. Family members spend time talking together, listening in a way that conveys caring and respect. As they listen, they try to understand how things seem to other family members, and they check messages that are not clear. Communication in strong families is carried on in a caring atmosphere in which members avoid criticizing, evaluating, and acting superior. Communication is honest and kind and deals with only one issue at a time. Family members air grievances while they are current, and they are specific in their communication. They support one another and avoid using what is known about another person as a weapon.

TIME TOGETHER

Strong families share **time together.** Essentially, members share their whole lives—household chores, recreation, meals, family history, relatives, and stories. They talk with one another and tell one another about their day-to-day experiences.

The way families spend their time together makes a difference. Strong families allow for plenty of individual freedom, which results in the development of a family identity. The kinds of things strong families do together include playing together as well as many ordinary things such as eating meals and doing chores. Many strong families attend church or synagogue and school or community activities. Special events such as holidays and birthdays are nearly always observed in strong families.

SPIRITUAL WELLNESS

Strong families share spiritual convictions, which provide purpose or meaning for members' lives. Their convictions are a guide for daily living; they practice what they believe in. Families having **spiritual wellness** tend to experience freedom and peace in their lives and maintain a positive, confident outlook. They engage in prayer and meditation and often enjoy support from other people who share the same religious heritage. Rituals and traditions tend to be an outward expression of a deeper spiritual feeling.

COPING SKILLS

Strong families have developed **coping skills** for dealing with crises and stress. An important characteristic of strong families is the ability to see something positive in a difficult situation and to focus on that aspect. Members provide help for one another during a crisis and do not hesitate to seek support within the family when they need it. During a crisis, strong families draw on their spiritual resources and continue to communicate skillfully. Members are also adaptable and flexible, with each one adjusting to the needs of the others.

Strong families under stress find it helpful to make certain efforts. Members keep things in perspective and find humor in

FIGURE 2-3 Strong families spend time together doing things that are fun for all.
Source: (bottom) © *Ancona 1959/International Stock Photography*

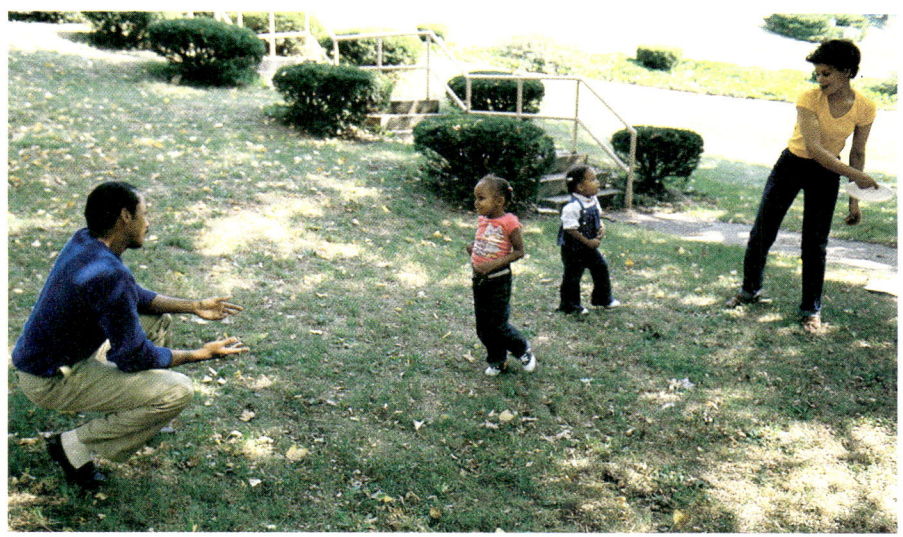

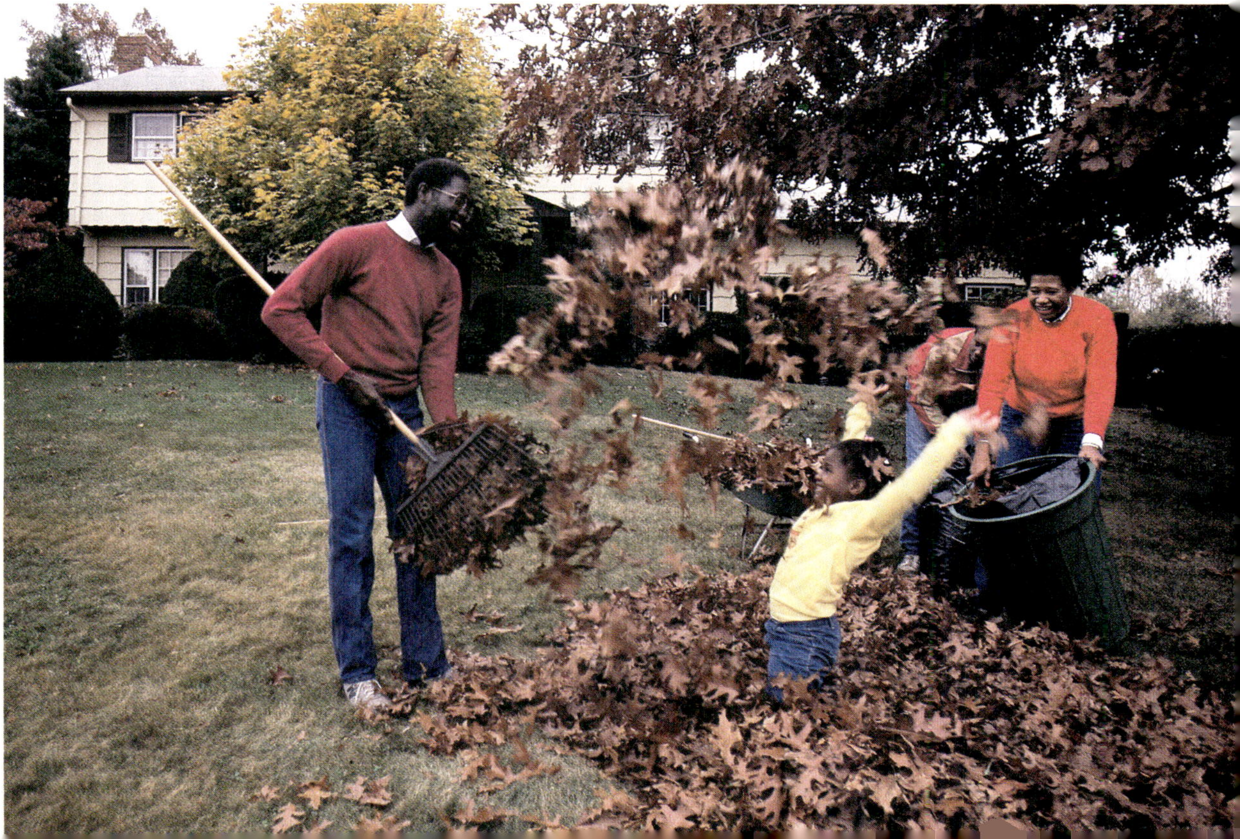

the situation. They avoid worrying and approach big tasks one step at a time. They restore themselves, exercise, enjoy family pets, and engage in outdoor activities together. They involve themselves in worthy projects to which they can give of themselves, without becoming too caught up in things outside the family.

A strong family is not a perfect family, but one in which the members have developed techniques for getting through life together. Most find that the effort required is well worth the price.

INFLUENCES ON CHILDREN'S DEVELOPMENT

What influences a child's development the most? Some people say it is the physical make-up a child inherits from parents. Others say it is the kind of environment a child is reared in. Still others say it is the child's response to inherited traits and environment.

Genetic Inheritance

Heredity, or the characteristics a person inherits from parents through the genes and chromosomes, plays an important role in development. All genetic inheritance is determined at the moment of conception.

Environment

A child's **environment** consists of everything that surrounds and involves the child. The child's environment provides a setting for growing and developing, in which people, places, activities, and learning are all involved to some degree.

PHYSICAL ENVIRONMENT

The first physical environment for a baby is the mother's uterus. Later the child's home, food, water, air, clothing, and community make up the physical environment.

PEOPLE

People are the most powerful influence in a child's environment. Parents influence the baby most. Other family members and caregivers also affect development to a great degree. For a small baby, life literally depends on other people, who do the things that need to be done. Language, values, and the meanings of life are established through early relationships with other people.

PERSONAL HISTORY

Everyone has a personal history. Your personal history not only consists of an account of your own life but also includes the life stories of your parents, grandparents, and ancestors. Can you trace your family tree? How many generations back can you identify? Stories of families can be both fascinating and embarrassing. Sometimes children who have been adopted feel a deep longing to know the history of their birth family.

Whether or not you know your family history, you are affected to some degree by the decisions your ancestors made and the kind of lives they led. Your children will be affected by the choices you make. Personal history, then, is a part of each person's living environment.

CULTURE

Culture has to do with the way families live and their ties to a particular nationality, language, or racial group. It has to do with the customs and traditions families follow. These often involve food, clothing, housing and household practices, religious observances, holidays and other celebrations, and child-rearing practices.

COMMUNITY

The place where a child lives also influences his or her development. Families in rural areas generally hold to their cultural traditions longer than families in urban areas. Children who grow up in rural areas may have more opportunities than city children do to enjoy the out-of-doors. Urban children may have more recreational opportunities and public services.

The Child's Response

Some parts of the environment affect people more than others. How people choose to respond to the environment makes a big difference in how much it affects them. Parents and children choose how they will respond to each other and to the rest of the environment.

Children with the same genetic make-up (identical twins) who live in the same environment do not develop in exactly the same way. What does the individual child contribute?

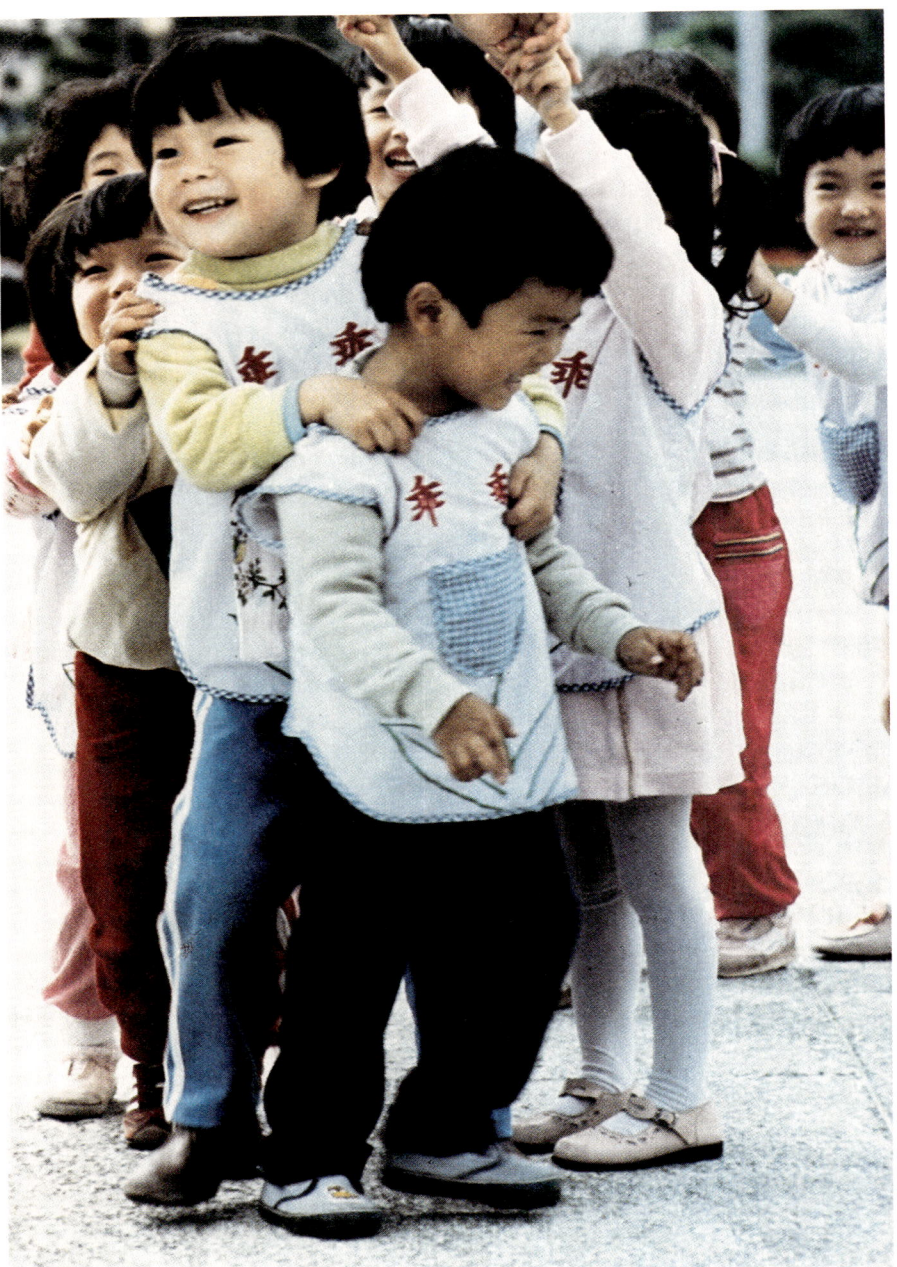

FIGURE 2-4 Some children's environment includes a special cultural influence that may affect some aspects of their development.
Source: Coordination Council for North American Affairs

TEMPERAMENT

Children vary greatly in the way they respond to other people and their environment. **Temperament** has to do with the tendency of a person to act, feel, and think in similar ways throughout a lifetime. When someone makes a statement like "Don't let Sammy bother you—that's just the way he is," the particular behavior being commented on may well reveal something about Sammy's temperament. Understanding their own and their children's temperaments can help parents make discipline more effective and identify strengths and weaknesses.

Florence Littauer has written about four basic temperaments named after those first described by the Greek physician Hippocrates: sanguine (or the popular personality), choleric (the powerful personality), melancholy (the perfect personality), and phlegmatic (the peaceful personality).[2] The strengths and weaknesses of Littauer's personality types are given in Table 2-1. Most people are a blend of these temperaments, with one or two dominating. The many possible combinations of strengths and weaknesses account for the wide variety of personalities.

Both children and adults have temperaments. Some combinations of personalities work together more easily than others. Which personality types do you think you would find easier to work with and which ones would be more difficult?

Although it can be helpful to understand temperaments and to be able to identify them in children, it is important not to stereotype anyone. **Stereotyping** means putting people in categories, labeling them, and then treating them according to the labels rather than as individuals. Understanding children's temperaments should, instead, help adults see their uniqueness. How do you think understanding a child's temperament might affect the method of discipline you would use as a parent or caregiver?

ABILITY TO MAKE CHOICES

Children decide how they will react in a situation or what they will do. Their choices affect their growth, their development, and sometimes their future options. Food choices affect growth. Play choices affect muscular and mental development. Choices

---

[2]Florence Littauer, *Raising the Curtain on Raising Children* (Waco, TX: Word, Inc., 1988).

TABLE 2-1 Strengths and Weaknesses of Four Temperaments, or Personality Types

Temperament	Strengths	Weaknesses	Emotional Needs	Things Avoided
SANGUINE—The Popular Personality (Bright yellow like the sun) The extrovert The talker The optimist	**Baby** Bright and wide-eyed Curious Gurgles and coos Wants company Responsive **Child** Daring and eager Innocent Inventive and imaginative Cheerful Enthusiastic Fun-loving Chatters constantly Bounces back Energized by people	**Baby** Screams for attention Knows is cute Shows off **Child** No follow-through Disorganized Easily distracted Short interest span Emotional ups and downs Wants credit Tells fibs Forgetful	Attention, approval, affection, acceptance, presence of people and activity	Dull tasks, routines, criticism, details, lofty goals

Personality		Needs	Dislikes
CHOLERIC—The Powerful Personality (Hot red like a fire) The extrovert The leader The optimist	Adventuresome Energetic Outgoing Precocious Born leader Daring and eager Productive worker Sees the goal Moves quickly Self-sufficient Competitive Assertive Trustworthy	Appreciation for all achievements, opportunity for leadership, participation in family decisions, something to control (own room, garage, backyard, dog)	Rest, boredom, playing games that can't be won
	Baby Strong-willed Demanding Loud Throws things Not sleepy **Child** Manipulative Temper tantrums Constantly going Insistent Testing Arguing Stubborn		
MELANCHOLY—The Perfect Personality (Deep blue like the ocean) The introvert The leader The pessimist	Serious Quiet Likes a schedule **Baby** Looks sad Cries easily Clings	Sensitivity to deep desires, satisfaction from quality achievement,	Noise, confusion, trivial pursuits,

(continues on next page)

TABLE 2-1 *(Continued)*

Temperament	Strengths	Weaknesses	Emotional Needs	Things Avoided
		Child	own space, security and stability, separation from noisy, messy siblings, support from parents ("I believe in you")	being "jollied"
	Thinks deeply Talented Musical Fantasizes True friend Perfectionist Intense Dutiful and responsible	Moody Whines Self-conscious Too sensitive Fears negatives Avoids criticism Sees problems Won't communicate		
PHLEGMATIC—The Peaceful Personality (Cool green like the grass) The introvert The follower The pessimist	Easy-going Undemanding Happy Adjustable	Baby Slow Shy Indifferent	Peace and relaxation, attention, praise, self-worth, loving motivation	Conflict, confrontation, initiative, decisions, extra work, responsibility, tension, quarrels
	Watches others Easily amused Little trouble Dependable Lovable Agreeable	Child Selfish Teasing Avoids work Fearful Quietly stubborn Lazy Retreats to watch TV		

Source: Florence Littauer, Raising the Curtain on Raising Children *(Waco, TX: Word, Inc., 1988). Used by permission of the author.*

based on temperament can have long-term effects on future decisions.

GENDER

A child's **gender**—that is, whether the child is a boy or a girl—affects development. People tend to treat girls and boys differently from the moment of birth.

Boys and girls are different biologically. Most obviously, they have different sex organs. Also, boys tend to have a higher percentage of muscle by weight and more often excel in analytical

FIGURE 2-5   Some activities, such as cooking, have been mistakenly associated with one gender.

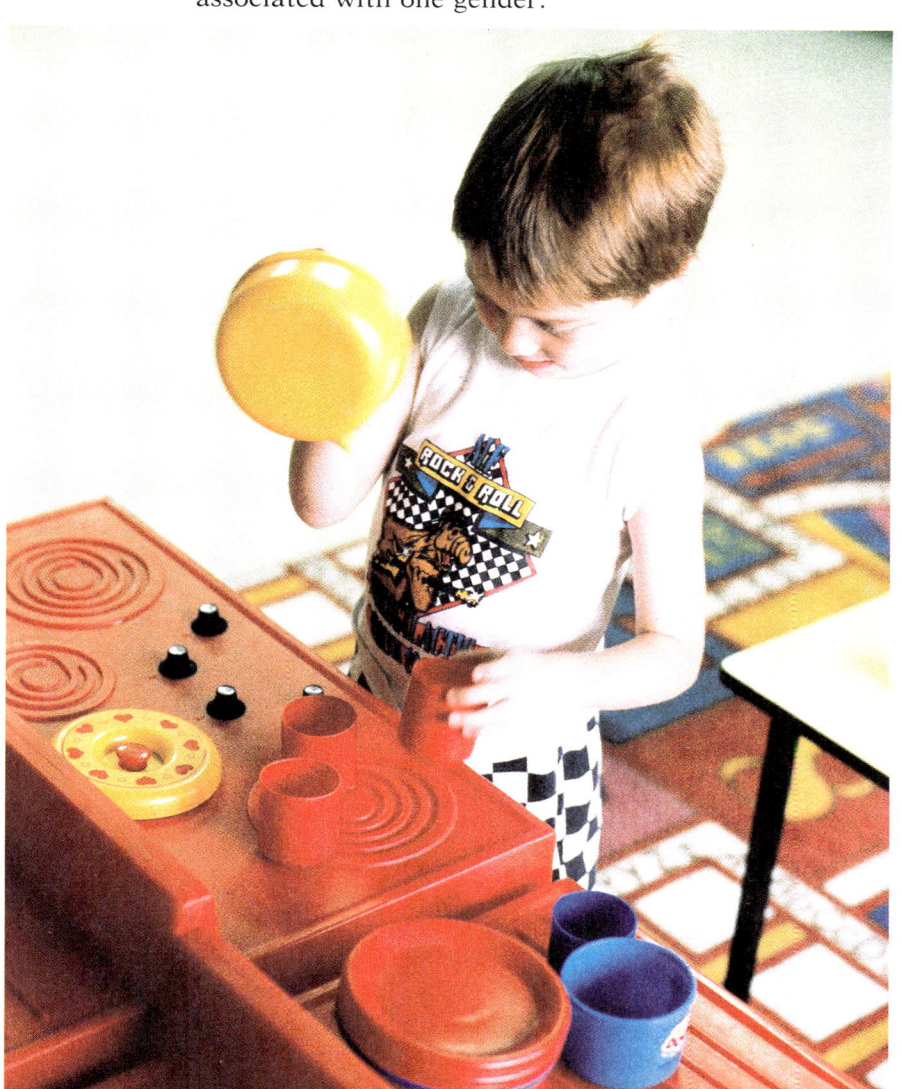

and mathematical tasks. While they are still in the mother's body, boys secrete a hormone that affects their brain development. The result is related to the kind of mental skills more frequently attributed to boys. Girls tend to have a higher percentage of fat by weight and more often excel in verbal tasks and work that requires attention to detail.

However, even though biological differences exist, many children are born with both male and female strengths and abilities. Certainly boys can be trained to do things that are more often done by girls, and girls can be trained to do things that are more often done by boys. Sometimes it is society, rather than genetics, that decides what boys or girls can do. Training a child to do something that is generally done only by the other sex is easier when that is the case.

Sometimes it is genetics and sometimes society that defines the roles of parents. Which parenting tasks typically assigned to men or to women do you think are related to biological strengths and which ones are not?

CHALLENGES FOR TEEN-PARENT FAMILIES

James and Vicki had not planned to become parents so young. They love Jimmy and wouldn't give him up for anything, but they know that life would have been easier for all three of them if they had waited. They experienced many of the problems of teenage parents. As they struggled to succeed in their marriage and parenthood, they learned many things, which they shared with their younger brothers and sisters at every opportunity.

The following are challenges teenage parents face:

- Teenage mothers are more likely to experience medical complications during pregnancy.

- Teenage parents have more emotional stress to deal with.

- Often teenage parents are isolated from friends and family.

- Teen-parent families are less stable and are more likely to break up.

- Divorce is more common among couples who marry as teenagers.

- Teenage parents have more babies, spaced closer, than couples who wait until their twenties to have their first baby.

- Many teenage parents are unable to finish school.

- Teenage parents have low and undependable incomes and are more likely to become dependent on welfare; they are often quite poor.

- Teenage parents who try to stay in school experience stress.

- Teenage parents often face a lifetime of lower paying, less satisfying jobs.

- Teenage parents are often obliged to give up their goals and dreams and take on adult responsibilities before they are really adults.

Babies of teenage parents can have special problems, too, as little Jimmy did. Some problems for babies of teenage parents include the following:

- A higher percentage of babies born to teenage mothers are premature or have a low birth weight.

- Babies of teenage mothers are at greater risk for illness and birth defects.

- Babies of teenage parents may have more learning problems in school.

- Babies of teenage parents tend to develop more behavior problems.

James and Vicki beat the odds against successful teen parenthood. They are in their early twenties now. Both have finished high school and are attending night school in order to reach their goals. Since they both work and go to school, they leave Jimmy in a child care center part of the time. They must manage their money carefully to pay for Jimmy's care and their own education.

Summary

Choosing parenthood involves being aware of the reasons for having a baby, determining readiness for parenthood, and calculating the cost of parenthood. Some people choose not to become parents.

Parents, siblings, and grandparents must make adjustments for the new family member and the changes in the family. Adoption can be a good alternative both for young parents who feel unable to raise a child yet and for childless couples who want to be parents.

Building a family requires parental leadership. Strong families show the characteristics of commitment, appreciation, communication, time together, spiritual wellness, and coping skills.

Children's development is influenced by heredity, physical environment, other people, history, culture, and the community. A child's temperament and gender and the choices he or she makes also affect development.

Teenage parents have difficulty making enough money, continuing their education, and filling the needs of young children. Children of teenage parents are more likely to have physical problems at birth and may later have some difficulty in learning.

Terms and Concepts

Postpartum blues	Appreciation
Siblings	Communication
Childlessness	Time together
Adoptive parents	Spiritual wellness
Birth parents	Coping skills
Open adoption	Heredity
Spontaneous abortion	Environment
Gynecologists	Temperament
Obstetricians	Stereotyping
Induced abortion	Gender
Commitment	

Checking Your Understanding

1. Write a paper describing positive and negative reasons for becoming a parent.

2. List and briefly describe the adjustments necessary when a baby joins a family.

3. Describe the benefits and problems of adoption for the birth parents, the adoptive parents, and the child.

4. What leadership responsibilities of parents can you think of? List them in order, beginning with the one you think is the most important and continuing to the least important.

5. List and briefly describe the characteristics of a strong family.

6. List the main influences on the development of children. Choose the one you think is the most powerful and write a paragraph describing how it affects children's lives.

7. Select one of the problems faced by teenage parents or their children and write a paragraph suggesting how it might be handled.

8. What kind of support do teenage parents need from their parents and other relatives in order to develop a strong family?

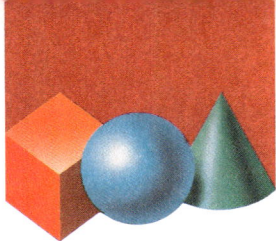

2 HANDS ON WITH CHILDREN

HELPING OLDER CHILDREN ADJUST TO A NEW BABY

Babies and young children have a very special place in the lives of most families. Because of their needs and their appealing appearance, children receive more attention than most of us.

When a new family member arrives who gets an extra amount of attention, older children can suffer a loss. Their own special position in the family often seems to them to fade as family members, particularly parents, welcome and care for the new baby.

What can be done to help older children have an easier time accepting new babies and feel less of a loss of their own importance?

■ Prepare the older child ahead of time for the arrival of the new baby by telling him or her about it.

■ Assure the older child that his or her own special place in your heart and in the family is assured—that no one can ever replace him or her.

■ Allow the older child to help make preparations for the new baby. If the baby will be sleeping in a crib the older child has been using, provide a "big-child" bed two or three months in advance. If possible, prepare a new or improved place for the older child. If the older child's needs are met well before the new baby arrives, he or she is less likely to feel "replaced."

■ Find ways of including older children in the care of the new baby. For example, toddlers can hand a diaper, help to fold over the corners of the baby's blanket, and sit in a parent's lap as they both hold the new baby. Older children can do more.

■ Find a few minutes each day to be alone with and do "grown-up" things with the older child.

■ Express appreciation to the older child for any help that is given.

CHAPTER 3
Challenges for Children and Parents

OBJECTIVES

When you have finished this chapter, you will be able to

- Identify some challenges of foster parenting
- Describe the special problems of single parents
- Explain the problems of blended families
- Point out the effects of separation on young children
- Suggest ways to help children handle divorce and death
- Point out some developmental indicators of handicaps in preschool children
- Tell how you might prepare a young child for a hospital stay

Brad and James were raised by their dad after their mom died, so they are well acquainted with the problems of single-parent families. Vicki was a member of a blended family, with several stepbrothers and stepsisters. Monica once spent six months living in a foster family. Although their family situations had been different, they all felt a strong sense of family membership.

FAMILIES WITH SPECIAL CHALLENGES

Family life is seldom easy. Some families have unique sets of problems because of their structure. Others face challenges because of circumstances.

Foster Families

Foster families provide full-time care for someone else's child for a designated period of time. Foster parents give the children placed with them special care and help them to feel like members of the family for the time they are there. They also help the children prepare for any changes that may occur in their lives and deal with any problems related to their own family. While they are providing love and acceptance, foster parents sometimes become attached to children. Even so, they are responsible for helping the children they are caring for to keep a positive attitude toward their own family. Usually some money is provided to foster parents by the state, although most of them report that it seldom covers the expenses.

Children placed in foster homes frequently come from troubled homes. Their parents may be unable to care for them because of serious problems and may have requested that the children be placed in foster care until those problems are solved. Sometimes the courts place children in foster homes. A few parents even abandon their children. Thus children going into foster homes may have special problems:

■ They may be confused and upset.

■ Those who have been abused may have health and emotional problems.

■ They may experience grief because they have been removed from their family.

■ They may have difficulty adjusting to the foster family's routines.

■ They may be worried about their parents and siblings.

■ They may have difficulty trusting and respecting members of the foster family.

■ They may find it difficult to learn to love the foster family and find a place in it.

Most states require that foster homes be approved by a state agency before any children are assigned to them. Approval generally includes meeting health, fire, and safety standards and obtaining references. A caseworker places children in homes and works with foster parents to ensure that children's needs are met.

Although foster parents must face many challenges, many people find foster parenting to be very rewarding. Certainly caring people are needed to help children who have this special need.

Single-Parent Families

An increasing number of children live in **single-parent families** for at least some part of their childhood. A parent can have sole responsibility for a family for any of a number of reasons. A single parent may be someone who never married and had or adopted a child. One parent may die, leaving his or her partner to raise a family alone. Sometimes a person must parent essentially alone because the other parent is absent for an extended period of military service or has a job that requires a lot of traveling. Most single parents, however, are separated or divorced.

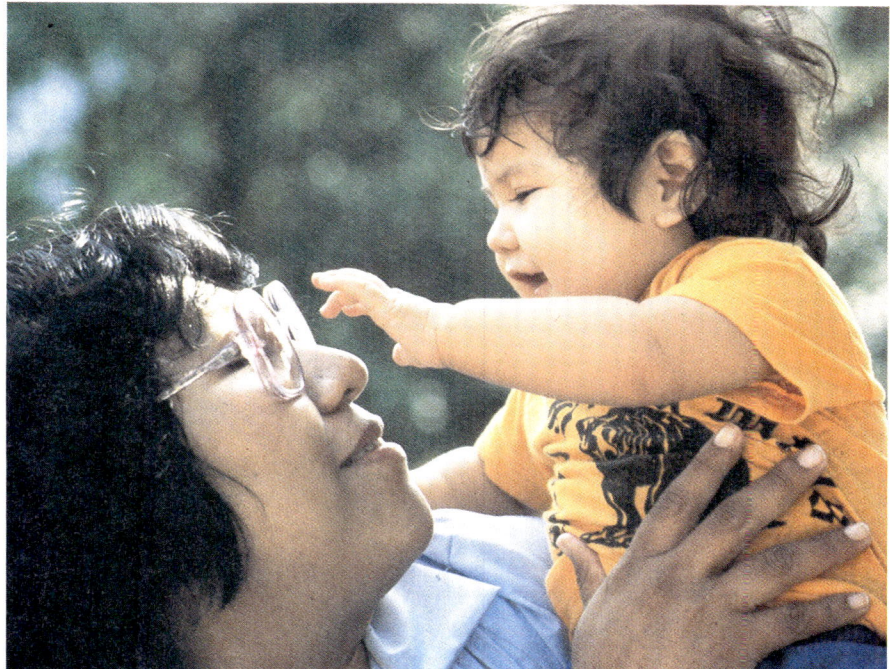

FIGURE 3-1   A single-parent family faces special challenges.
Source: USDA photo

Parents who must do the parenting tasks alone may face certain problems:

- Balancing a job with child rearing
- Making enough money to make ends meet
- Feeling lonely
- Dealing with grief (their own and their children's) when there has been a death or divorce

- Identifying personal needs and finding new avenues to meet them
- Securing adequate child care

Single-parent families need support from relatives and from the community. Community support can come from friends, churches, parent support groups, and service agencies. Older children in single-parent families who assist with parenting tasks add strength to the family. Successful single-parent families are usually those who are able to develop a strong network of support.

Blended Families

Blended families are those in which at least one parent brings children from a former marriage into the new family. Blended families are more complex than families made up of children and their birth parents.

- One parent may bring more children into the new family than the other. Each child requires more emotional energy and money and influences the new family's political structure.

- One or both parents may have varying custody arrangements concerning children from former marriages. They may have full custody, joint custody, or no custody at all.

- Children may come from more than one former marriage.

- New babies may be born into the blended family.

- There has been at least one loss due to divorce or death.

The grief resulting from a loss is always there in a blended family. Family members remember feelings from previous experiences and need to express their grief. Painful feelings can recur years later with similar intensity. Successful blended families learn to accept these feelings and allow members to work through them.

Children who have learned to deal with one family must learn to cope with a different one. In most cases children have had no voice in choosing their parent's new mate or the mate's children. Children in blended families must often contend with problems due to a divorce. Blended families must deal with family members who are not present from day to day. Problems can result from visitation rights or from the complete absence of one parent.

Families in Difficult Circumstances

Regardless of family structure, circumstances sometimes cause problems for parents and children. These may include the following:

- Loss of income or insufficient income to meet needs
- A family member in prison
- Serious illness of a family member
- Frequent moving
- Frequent job change
- Birth of a new baby
- Ongoing conflict among family members
- Absence of a parent due to job-related circumstances
- Serious conflicts with extended family or neighbors
- Alcohol or substance abuse by a family member
- Disruption of family structure by friends of family members
- Death of a family member
- Loss of home or property
- Extreme stress at work

Difficult situations can create crises in families, particularly when they happen too suddenly for a family to handle sufficiently. How can parents and caregivers help children whose families are in crisis?

HELPING CHILDREN HANDLE CRISES

A crisis can begin when a person is faced with a hard decision, a big change, or a serious problem. Crises can represent either happy events, such as marriage or birth, or unhappy events, such as loss of income or death. Crises hold both danger and opportunity. The danger is that the change will devastate the person or change life in an unacceptable way. The opportunity lies in the chance for a new beginning and for making something positive out of the experience.

Each of the difficult situations above can become a crisis for those involved, particularly if it happens suddenly. Crisis can

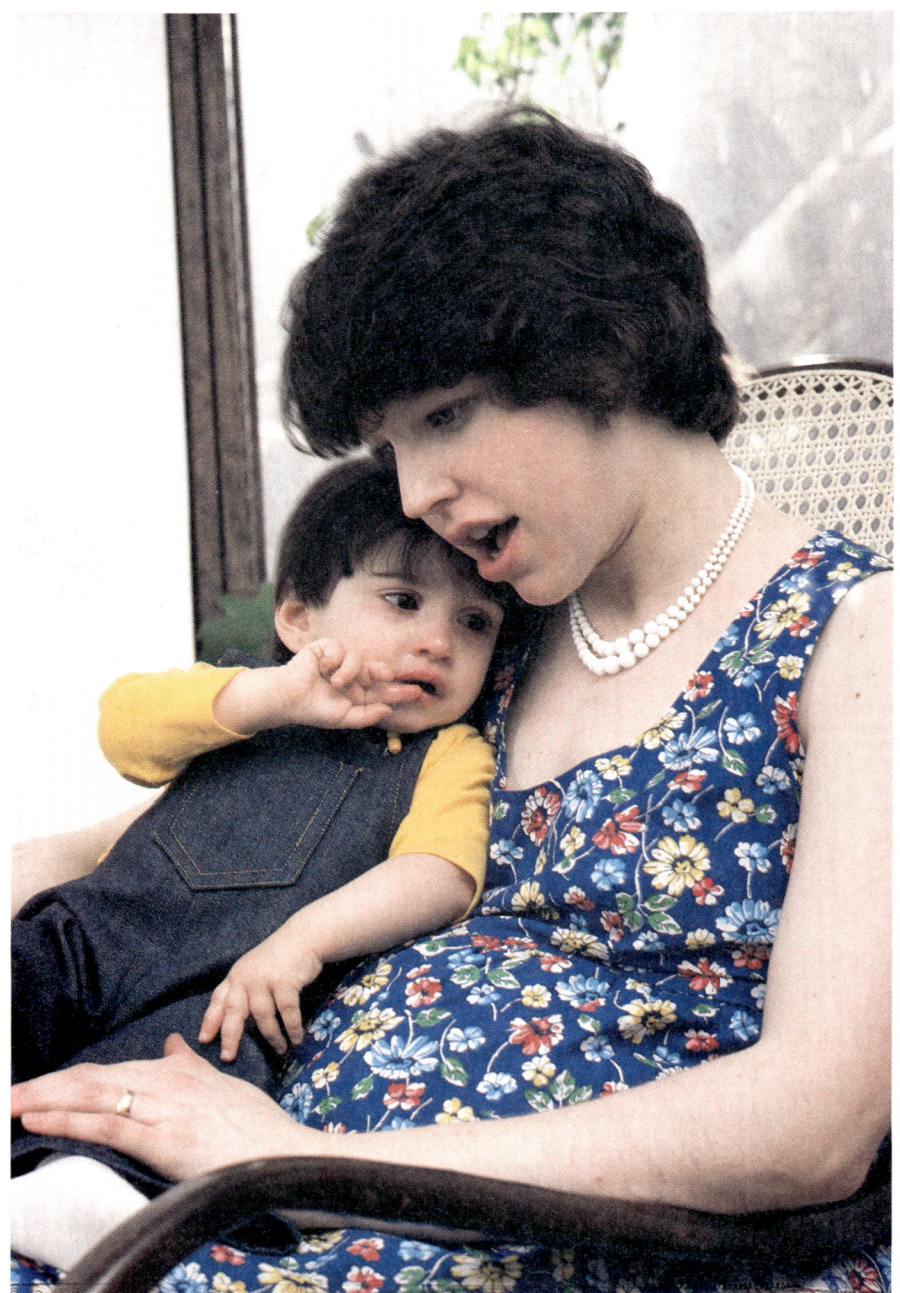

FIGURE 3-2 A child whose family is going through a period of crisis is likely to need extra reassurance and comforting.
Source: © *Erika Stone*

involve threatened loss, and many crises mean possible separation. How do separation and loss affect children?

Separation and Loss

For young children the effect of separation can be powerful. Children fear abandonment. When they are separated from parents for even short periods of time, they begin to grieve. Being separated from someone or something you care about involves loss. **Grief** is an emotional process people go through when they lose someone or something they love or care for very much.

HOW MUCH SEPARATION IS TOO MUCH?

For infants, simply a few hours apart from parents may activate a sense of separation. For toddlers, a whole day away from parents is quite a long time. Some preschoolers, but not all, are ready for an overnight stay with a close relative or friend. It is best if young children's visits away from parents are limited to two to three days.

EFFECTS OF SEPARATION

When parents are required to or choose to be away for a long time or become permanently separated from a child, the child grieves. When Sandra was 17 months old, her mother had a second child. Sandra's grandmother wanted to help out, so she took Sandra home with her for two weeks. The separation was too long for a toddler. When Sandra's parents went to get her, they were eager to see her. Sandra was excited about her little brother, but she backed away from her mother with hurt in her eyes. She was too young for such a long separation. The effects of feeling abandoned stayed in her memory for many years.

Sandra had grieved for her mother and had begun to accept the fact that her mother was gone. Like older people, children feel anger and sadness when they grieve. They often go through times of denying their feelings or of trying to manipulate a change before they accept a loss. As Sandra moved through these emotions of grief, the love that bonded her to her mother began to diminish, a process that allows the grieving person to go on with life. Grief serves as a reverse bonding process, in a sense an unbonding. Even though the feeling for the loved one remains, the sense of loss becomes a part of the relationship as well.

Divorce

Young children seldom understand the reasons why adults divorce. Preschool children sometimes blame themselves and are confused about what is happening. They may fear that they will be sent away, replaced, or abandoned. When one parent no longer sustains a relationship with the child, the child grieves for the loss of that parent.

Children's grief over the loss of a parent and the family unit is very real. Often it results in emotional and behavioral changes, which can include: intense anger, aggressive behavior, withdrawal (staying away from people), increased hyperactivity (loud, noisy activity that is related to being upset), feelings of frustration and confusion, and expressions of insecurity.

Children of divorcing parents need help to handle their grief and their concern about being unloved and unlovable. How can parents and caregivers help?

- Point out for them the normality in the event
- Encourage them to express their feelings of grief and to learn to live with the changes
- Offer hope and genuine support
- Provide structure and stability in the other areas of their lives
- Avoid exposing them to custody issues whenever possible

Parents and caregivers are in the best position to provide children with the kind of help they need during and after a divorce. Caregivers in day care and preschool centers may be the best source of structure and stability. What do children need to know when they are hurting after a divorce? These are some things they may need to hear:

- Your parents still love you.
- It is all right to feel hurt and sad.
- The divorce is not your fault.
- Children from divorced families are normal people.
- What you want to believe or want to happen may not be real or possible. (This helps children separate reality and fantasy.)
- You are valuable and important.

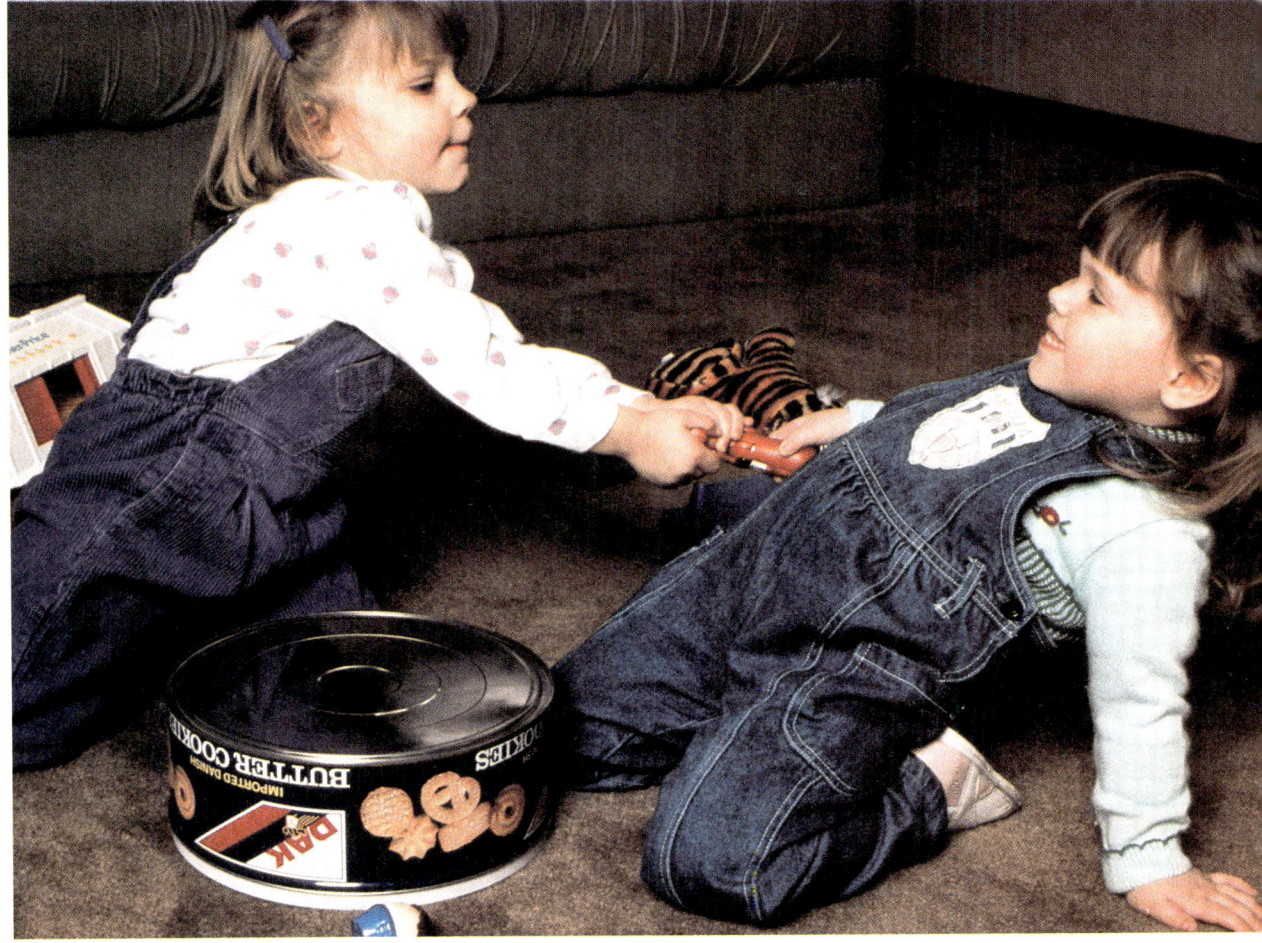

FIGURE 3-3   One of the ways a child may show grief over the divorce of his or her parents is by an increase in aggressive behavior.
Source: © Laura Dwight

■ Parents divorce each other—not their children.

■ Decisions sometimes have long-term consequences.

■ Parents feel hurt, too.

Adults cannot afford to overlook children's misbehavior during a divorce. Understanding that children are having a tough time can put such behavior into perspective, however, and make the situation easier to manage. Children who are hurting need extra support and patient guidance from adults. Often those best equipped to help children handle problems that arise from a divorce are their caregivers and teachers. Since they are familiar with the child's routine behavior, they can see changes. Also, they are not closely involved with the problems, so they can offer objective help.

Death

When someone you love dies, you hurt. Children experience this feeling, too. They have formed human bonds from their earliest days. Once bonds are formed the child experiences loss when a person dies.

Robbie was only ten months old when her twin sister Bonnie died, and throughout her life Robbie yearned for Bonnie. She named one of her own children after her twin, kept a picture of herself and Bonnie with their mother, and spoke often of how she missed her twin. Although she was too young to remember Bonnie consciously, she still felt a loss.

How can adults help children to manage the death of someone they love? There are two important ways: prepare them for the experience and give them support when it occurs.

PREPARING CHILDREN TO DEAL WITH DEATH

Children as young as 18 months old comment about dead bugs and birds. Toddlers recognize these are different from living things, even though most cannot put this difference into words. When they ask you to explain, it is important to be truthful but not excessively emotional about the event. You might say something like "The bird is dead, which means no eating, no chirping, no breathing, and no flying."

Another way of preparing children to deal with death is to monitor carefully what they are allowed to watch on television and in films. Some things that are portrayed might cause problems. For example, an actor who is "killed" on one show may turn up alive on a later show. Children may fail to realize that death is permanent. Horror movies play on fears. Children can be terrorized by watching movies that may intensify their own fears. Violence, particularly if it includes a great deal of blood and gore, unnecessarily stimulates children. They may decide that dying always involves mutilation. Cartoons often present incorrect information about death. It is a mistake to assume that everything that is animated is acceptable for children.

Most parents who have religious faith instruct children in basic beliefs. This builds a foundation for dealing with death that can be helpful. It is important to avoid using death to frighten children into a particular type of behavior. Threats and bribes usually backfire. People who teach concepts of faith to children seldom recommend these tactics.

GIVING SUPPORT TO CHILDREN WHEN A DEATH OCCURS

Like all people, very young children need to be touched, held, and comforted when they experience a loss. They need someone who understands their sadness.

Children cope best with death when they understand the concrete reality of it. Death means no moving, no sleeping, no eating, no pain—no life. Children want to know what happened and why. They need to have their questions answered clearly and honestly, but they may be spared unnecessary details, particularly when there has been a great deal of suffering. It is better to be direct, better to tell a child "Grandmother died last night" than to say "Grandmother passed away last night," or "Grandmother is just sleeping."

Children need to express their feelings of sadness and anger. They should be allowed to offer their own explanations and should be listened to with understanding. An adult may need to take the encouraging first step by expressing feelings of sadness. Children who have short and manageable separations from parents and important others will gain strength for dealing with death.

Should children be allowed to go to funerals? It depends on their age and what their needs are. By the time they are four or five years old, most of them can make a choice if given the simple facts. Open caskets and long services are usually difficult for children, however. If a child wants to view the body briefly, it is probably best to do this before the service. Funerals are a way of saying good-bye to a loved person. They help all of us—children included—to grieve and then to get on with life. What is important is that children be included in the family activities and be allowed to talk and ask questions, and even to help with simple activities surrounding the funeral.

Young children basically ask three main questions about death:

What is dead?

Can I die?

Will it happen to other members of my family?

Are you prepared to help children answer these questions? What would you say? If your own child or a child you were caring for were seriously ill, how would you answer these questions?

CHILDREN WITH SERIOUS PROBLEMS

When most people think of young children, they think of small beings who run, play, smile, and make messes. Children represent hope for older people, who picture them as having a long lifetime ahead of them. There are many children, however, who may not live to become adults, and others who have major obstacles to overcome if they do.

Handicapped Children

Children who have difficulty adjusting or responding to people, objects, and events around them because of physical, mental, or emotional problems are identified as **handicapped children.** A large majority of handicaps begin before birth.

Part of the pain of being handicapped is that affected children are often not able to do the things other children do. It is quite important to children that they be accepted by other children.

Sometimes people laugh and say cruel things. For significant people surrounding a child to respond positively and with acceptance is important. **Significant people** are those who are important to a child emotionally and who have influence in his or her life. Parents' attitude with regard to a child's handicap is probably the most important. It is best if parents can love their handicapped children for who they are while striving to help them develop their potential.

The cause of some handicapping conditions is known and is specific. Others may have multiple causes, and some are not completely understood.

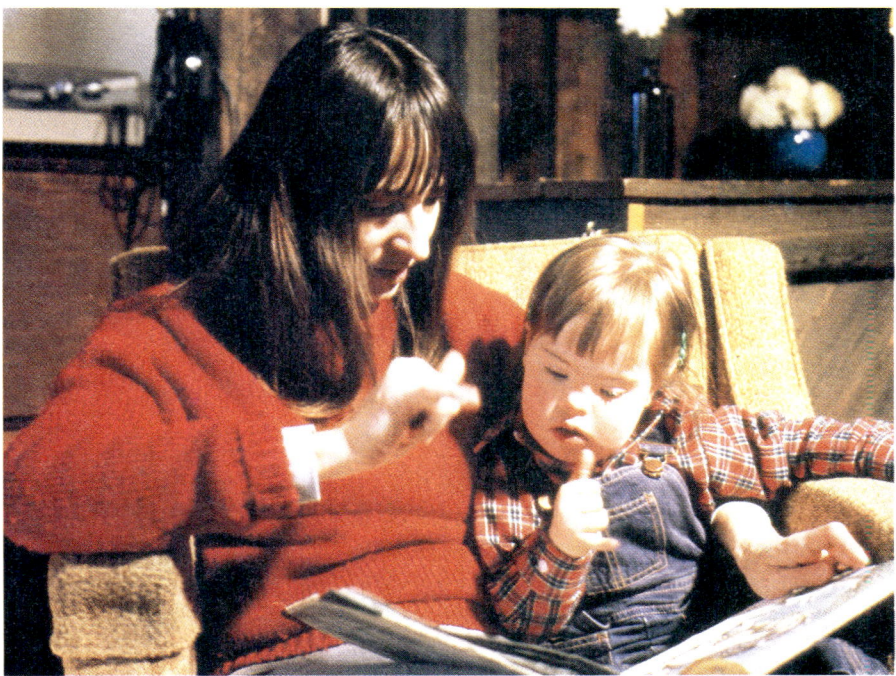

FIGURE 3-4   Providing handicapped children with opportunities similar to those given other children helps them to learn as much as they can and to feel accepted.
Source: March of Dimes Birth Defects Foundation

BIOLOGICAL CAUSES OF HANDICAPS

Abnormalities in genes and chromosomes are the **biological causes of handicaps.** Some birth defects can be avoided through genetic counseling. A few can be corrected. There are many, however, that simply have to be lived with, for a lifetime.

ENVIRONMENTAL CAUSES OF HANDICAPS

Factors in a person's surroundings, or environment, are the **environmental causes of handicaps.** The first and most crucial environment is the uterus. Many handicapping conditions are developed during the prenatal period. One of these that is totally preventable is the mental retardation that can result from fetal alcohol syndrome. It occurs only in children whose mothers consume alcohol during pregnancy.

Accidents after birth can result in handicaps. What conditions in the home or preschool center might cause accidents?

Children who are poor are more likely to be handicapped because there is less money for prenatal care and for other health concerns. Who is responsible to help children who are poor, homeless, or handicapped? The Something to Think About feature considers this issue.

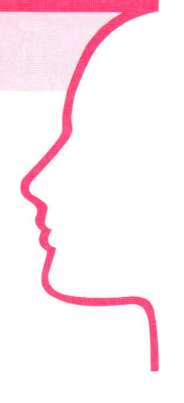

Something to Think About

Who Helps the Children?

Young children whose families are poor or homeless are victims of their circumstances. No matter what the reason for the difficulty, children suffer along with and sometimes more than adults.

Children who are poor are more likely to have certain problems, and their families have less ability to cope. Poor children have

- More sickness but less medical care
- More handicaps but less help in coping with them
- Less quality time with their parents but more needs to be met in that time
- Less nutritious food available but more need for health-giving food because health is poorer
- Less of the other basic necessities of life but more need for them because of other problems

What are some other special needs of poor children?

Homeless children have all the problems of poor children, but even more severely. The lack of a home obviously has a great effect. In addition to giving basic protection from the weather, a home provides a sense of security and identity that is seriously endangered when a family is homeless.

Who is responsible to see that poor and homeless children are helped? Some would respond that it is the responsibility of government to provide what parents do not. Others would say that providing money for poor families does not solve the problem in the long run—that children who live on welfare learn how to be welfare adults.

Some would respond that filling these children's needs is the responsibility of the community of faith—that what parents do not provide the church or synagogue should. It is true that during much of history religious organizations have been the main source of help to the poor. Is it possible for the community of faith to handle the needs of these children today? If this is the way to meet the needs of those who need help, do people who do not belong to a religious organization have no responsibility of this type?

Some would respond that children's needs are solely the responsibility of parents and families—that if a couple brings children into the world, it is their job to take care of them. Is this always possible? What happens when parents become ill, die, or lose their jobs? How should society respond to parents who do not take adequate care of their children? When children are handicapped or are seriously ill and the expense of their care goes beyond the family's ability to pay, who then is responsible?

As the number of people increases, the number of children who need help also increases. Seeing that children's needs are met will be a growing challenge to future generations. What do you think should be done to try to meet that challenge?

IDENTIFYING HANDICAPS IN PRESCHOOL CHILDREN

There are more handicapped children among us than most of us see. When all types of handicaps are considered, about one out of every ten children is affected. Since 1965, a series of laws have been passed that provide money to give handicapped preschool children help in the form of free public education and experimental preschools that might develop programs that work better for handicapped children. Funds have also been made available for demonstration programs that involve parents and provide information to communities, inclusion of handicapped children in Head Start programs, and identification of eligible children and offering of services to those identified.

Children who are handicapped make more progress if they get help when they are very young. Thus teachers and caregivers of preschool children need to be alert to possible symptoms of handicapping conditions. Identifying these in young children can be difficult. Tests for identifying handicapped children do not always accurately predict the handicapping condition, and some handicaps are not easy to identify early in life. Children may be kept at home and thus out of reach of those people who know how to help them. Caregivers and parents may not be aware of what can be done to help.

For preschool children, handicaps can often be identified because of developmental lags. A **developmental lag** means that a child is significantly behind other children of the same age in some aspect of development. (Chapter 5 contains a brief overview of normal development for children under six.) Handicapped children do not function the way most children at that age level do. Development may be delayed or may not occur at all in any of the following areas: mental, language, motor (muscle), and social development. **Multi-handicapped children** have conditions that affect more than one, or even all, of these developmental areas.

Mental development. Young children develop mentally mostly through their senses, but also through their own activities or experimenting. As they grow, they build on early experiences to solve problems and develop concepts. Indications that a child might be mentally retarded include the following:

- Being much slower than other children of the same age to learn concepts

- Injuring himself or herself intentionally

- Being aggressive toward people or property

- Behaving in ways that are meaningless in a given situation (waving or smiling)

- Stealing things or eating nonedible objects to get attention

Mentally retarded children learn concepts more slowly—sometimes much more slowly—than other children. Some never learn them. Some mentally handicapped children can memorize ideas and apply them in one situation but can't transfer them to another.

Sometimes slow learning is a result of a deficiency in hearing or sight. Such conditions are known as **sensory disorders.** The child's brain may work well, but the amount of information that can be absorbed may be limited because he or she does not hear or see well. Sometimes children with emotional handicaps have slowed mental development.

Language development. Infants communicate first only by

crying. Later they coo and babble and then use words. Toddlers combine words to make simple sentences. Children with language problems may do one or more of the following:

- They may not talk by the time other children of the same age are talking well.

- They may use noticeably shorter sentences than do other children of the same age.

- Their speech may be difficult to understand.

- The voice may sound different from other children's. (It may not change pitch, or it may sound very hoarse.)

- They may stutter.

- They may not be accepted by other children because their language is different.

Slow language development may indicate deafness, or it may accompany other disabilities. It may also be an indication that the child simply does not have anyone who talks with him or her. Poor speech development is the language disorder most commonly diagnosed among preschool children. Teachers and caregivers can help by listening.

Language disabilities are sometimes tied to learning disabilities. Children who have otherwise normal intelligence sometimes have great difficulty learning in a particular area, such as reading or math. This kind of problem may not be apparent until the child begins school.

Social development. Social development begins in the delivery room as soon as parents and babies meet. Babies make eye contact with parents, vocalize in response to parents' speech, and show delight in their presence. Infants who do not make eye contact or respond to adults' repeated attempts at socialization may have a social development problem. Infants who cry in place of all other forms of communication after three months of age may have such a problem.

Toddlers and preschoolers who do not play alongside or with other children may be having problems with social development. Other possible indications of these problems are when preschoolers will not exchange or share playthings or do not imitate other people or pretend.

Social development is often delayed when children have other types of handicaps. What kinds of problems in making friends and getting along with others might be experienced by children who are blind, or hearing impaired, or physically unable to run and play?

Motor development. In children under six months old, large muscles work together in response to reflexes. As children grow, they learn to use specific muscles for specific purposes. They crawl, stand, walk, climb, dance, and run. Children may be slow to do any of these movements and yet not have a significant problem. However, slow motor development may indicate the presence of specific handicaps. Generally speaking, the more profoundly retarded a child is, the less capable he or she is of using muscles effectively.

Sensory disorders can produce slow motor development. Hearing problems that affect the inner ear may cause problems with balance. Blind children may also show reduced motor skills.

Children who have motor-related problems may exhibit poor coordination. They may have difficulty in limiting or controlling movement, in making their bodies respond to their impulses. They often learn motor skills much later than do other children.

Another form of physical handicap is related to a child's general health. Children with some genetic diseases, such as cystic fibrosis, may have problems breathing. Children with diabetes and epilepsy may have seizures if their activity or excitement level gets too high.

Children who are handicapped often have problems with self-help skills. **Self-help skills** are those that children must master in order to care for themselves. They include washing hands, brushing teeth, toileting, dressing, and bathing. Handicapped children require more specific help, more steps, in learning to help themselves.

HELPING HANDICAPPED CHILDREN

Handicapped children need understanding and acceptance. For children whose handicaps have not been identified, careful teamwork from caring adults is needed to assist them in getting the help they need. There are many specific ways caregivers and teachers of young children can help handicapped children. Some of these are as follows:

▪ Accepting handicapped children into preschool programs if it is at all possible to work with them

Leadership at a Glance

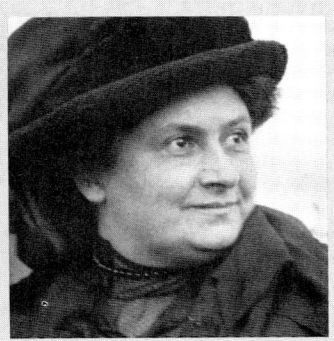

Source: *UPI/BETTMANN NEWSPHOTOS*

Maria Montessori

Maria Montessori (1870–1952) was the first woman to complete a medical education in Italy. At the time there was such strong prejudice against a woman's becoming a doctor that she had to work alone at night in the medical school labs at the University of Rome.

After she graduated, she became concerned with the problems of what were known in Italy as "deficient" children. She developed a method for teaching them to do basic things, and even in some cases to read, write, and do simple math problems. Because of the success she had with these children, she was able to apply her approach, now called the Montessori method, to teaching children in general.

Today, Montessori's methods are frequently used in both special education and regular classrooms. Teachers using the Montessori method need special training. You can get more information concerning Maria Montessori and teaching in Montessori schools by writing to either of the following organizations:

American Montessori Society
150 Fifth Avenue
New York, NY 10011

Association Montessori Internationale
2119 S Street, N.W.
Washington, DC 20008

- ▪ Seeing handicapped children as persons, with the same needs as other children plus special needs of their own
- ▪ Learning to identify developmental delays and working with colleagues and parents to obtain needed help
- ▪ Adapting the preschool environment to make it possible for handicapped children to do as much as possible for themselves

- Helping handicapped children acquire as much independence as possible by teaching self-help skills and by allowing extra time for tasks

- Working with therapists to help children to overcome or to live more effectively with handicapping conditions

- Referring children they cannot help to a center or service agency that can provide help

Therapists are an important part of the handicapped child's caregiving team. Caregivers and parents are frequently asked to help children with various activities prescribed by a therapist to help correct a physical handicap. **Physical therapists** are skilled professionals who train children to use muscles that do not work well. **Occupational therapists** train children to perform tasks and gain skills. For example, a physical therapist helps a child to exercise a "lazy" muscle, and an occupational therapist helps a child learn to throw a ball or to carry a glass of water without spilling. **Speech therapists** help children to correct problems they have with learning to speak well.

Seriously Ill Children

Seriously ill children may be handicapped, or they may have a life-threatening illness. Some face long-term hospital stays or even death.

FACING HOSPITALIZATION

When a child must be hospitalized for any procedure or condition, it is helpful to prepare him or her in advance. A visit to the pediatrics or surgical unit a day or two before the scheduled admission can usually be arranged. Meeting the people involved and becoming familiar with the hospital surroundings make the new experience of being hospitalized go more smoothly.

FACING DEATH

Should children be told if they are going to die? Usually families consult with their physicians to make decisions of this nature. Most feel that simple honesty is best.

Children, like parents, need hope, encouragement, and support when faced with difficult situations. Teachers and caregivers, however, need to work with parents rather than talking to children on their own. If a child initiates a conversation with a caregiver or teacher about a serious illness, it is best just to listen without comment, then discuss the child's concerns privately with the parent. It is important to remember that it is the role of caregivers and teachers to assist parents, not to take their place.

BUILDING A SUPPORT SYSTEM

When a child is seriously ill, parents and caregivers can generally find help in the medical community. Pediatric nurses and

FIGURE 3-5 When a child has to spend time in a hospital, preparing him or her for the experience ahead of time helps to lessen fears.
Source: Children's Hospital Medical Center

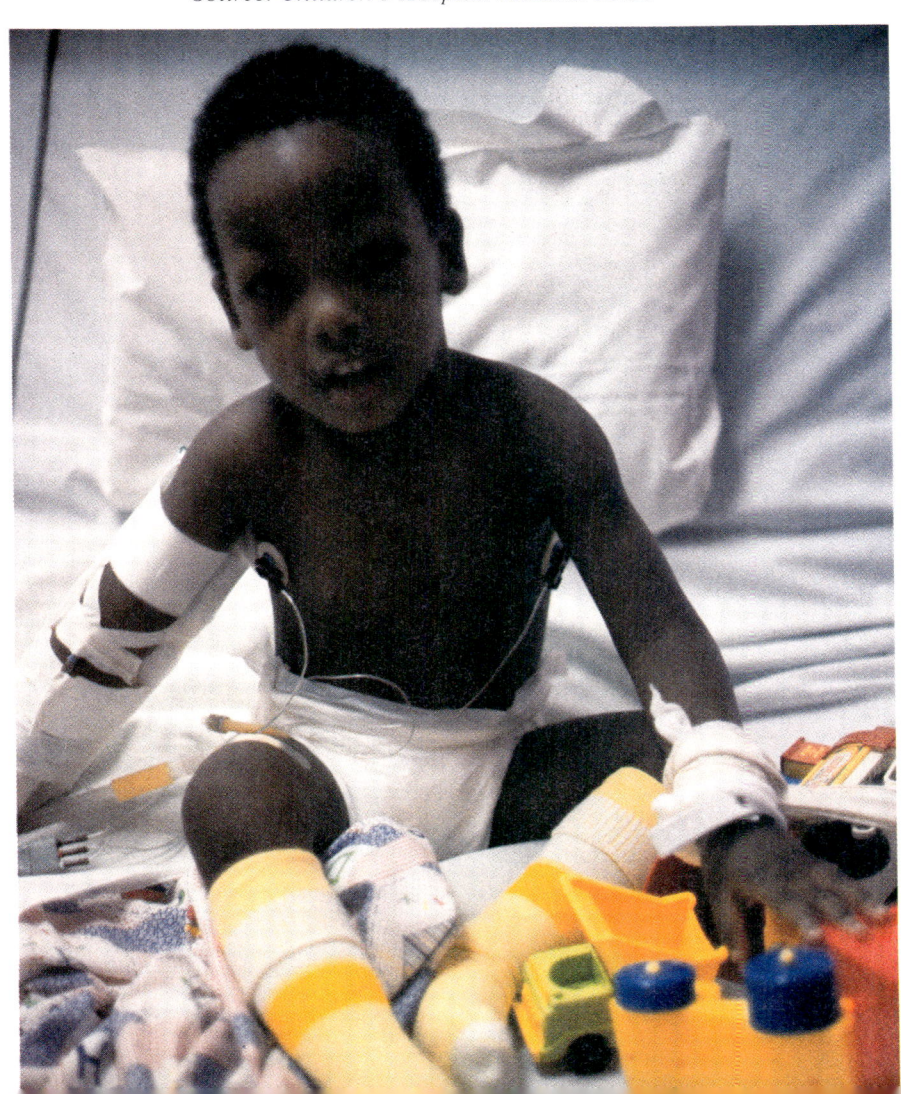

pediatricians are trained to help children and families cope with hospitalizations and the illnesses. These professionals can also provide information about special services or agencies that can give help.

Ronald McDonald houses and similar organizations provide low-cost temporary housing for families whose children are in a hospital a distance from their home. For most handicapping conditions and serious illnesses, organizations have been formed. Literature, emotional support, and sometimes financial help can be obtained from these groups.

Parents need support when their children are seriously ill or handicapped. These difficult situations drain parents physically and emotionally. Getting to know and relating to other parents who have faced similar situations helps. Support groups that help parents cope can be found in many communities.

Other family members may have problems dealing with the situation, too. The added strain can cause families to break up. In many communities counseling services are available to help families to work through their problems. Families can also get support from their community of faith.

Brad and Monica and James and Vicki were fortunate. Their children had no serious problems. Some of their friends' children, however, were not so well off. And they knew that Sarah and Jimmy would have friends at school who would need understanding. As parents, they determined that they would help their children to have compassion for handicapped children and understanding of their needs.

Summary

Families faced with extra challenges include foster families, single-parent families, and blended families. Foster families provide temporary homes for children who have special problems. Single-parent families have ony one adult to do the job of two. Single parents sometimes have a difficult time meeting their own needs as well as those of their children. In blended families, at least one member has previously experienced a loss. These families' problems can be very complex because of the many needs of both parents and children. Any family can be faced with difficult circumstances that cause problems for its members.

Parents and caregivers are important to children who are in a crisis situation. Most crises for children are a result of separation from those they love and depend on. Children experience real grief when they are separated from those they love. A limited amount of separation can strengthen children and help them prepare for loss as they grow; too much can cause serious difficulty.

Divorce often causes problems for children. Wise parents and caregivers can help children to handle changes in their families. Children also experience death. Parents can help children understand death and give them support when the occasion arises.

Children's handicaps can be caused biologically or environmentally. Adults can identify handicaps in young children by being alert to delays in the developmental areas. They can help children deal with such handicaps by being an active part of a caregiving team.

Children who are seriously ill need to be prepared in advance for difficult situations when possible. At such times they and their parents need extra support from those around them.

Terms and Concepts

Foster families

Single-parent families

Blended families

Grief

Handicapped children

Significant people

Biological causes of handicaps

Environmental causes of handicaps

Developmental lag

Multi-handicapped children

Sensory disorders

Self-help skills

Physical therapists

Occupational therapists

Speech therapists

Checking Your Understanding

1. Describe the kind of people you think would make suitable foster parents.

2. List some of the challenges that are unique to the blended family. How would you suggest that parents help children

to develop a sense of family membership in a blended family?

3. Select one of the difficult circumstances for families and write a paragraph describing how it might affect children.

4. Discuss the effects of separation on young children.

5. Write a paragraph describing how children feel when their parents divorce.

6. Why is it important for children to be able to express their grief?

7. How can you help young children prepare for and cope with the death of someone they care about?

8. List some of the causes of handicaps in young children.

9. Name two ways to identify possible handicaps in each of the following developmental areas: mental, language, social, and motor.

10. Suggest how you might help a child prepare for hospitalization.

11. Where can families whose children have special problems find support and help?

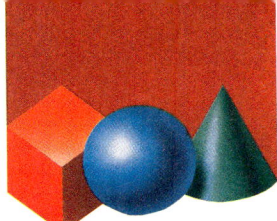

CLOTHING FOR HANDICAPPED CHILDREN

Standards for clothing for handicapped children are similar to those for children's clothing in general. These standards, however, are essential for handicapped children's clothes.

Handicapped children want to look nice, to look like other children. Besides appearance, there are other considerations that apply to their clothing. First, its fabric should be

- Sturdy enough to wear well

- Made from cotton or other nonirritating and absorbent fiber

- Lightweight, flexible, and nonclinging so children can move easily, without feeling burdened

- Washable and wrinkle-resistant for easy care

Clothing should be well-made so it will withstand the extra stress handicapped children may place on it. Construction features should include:

- Easy-to-use fasteners, such as large buttons or snaps or Velcro

- Well-constructed buttonholes

- Generous seam allowances that are finished on woven fabrics

- Flat seams that are double-stitched to withstand strain

- Even and securely stitched hems

Clothing should be flattering to the child and comfortable. It should be styled in keeping with the child's handicap.

- Selections should be based on the movements that are characteristic of the child's disability.

- Neck openings and sleeves should be easy to get into.

- Fasteners should be in the front of the garment where the child can operate them easily.

- Zippers should have pulls on them to allow easy opening.

- Buttons should be of at least medium size and attached with a shank.

Clothing should be safe for the child to wear. Aspects of safety include these considerations:

- Fabric should be flame-retardant.

- Extra fullness should be avoided because children may become tangled in fabric or clothes may get caught in doors or on furniture.

- Fabrics with looped threads that can catch on surfaces should be avoided (an example is terrycloth).

CHAPTER 4
Pregnancy, Birth, and the Newborn

OBJECTIVES

When you have finished this chapter, you will be able to

- Define terms associated with conception and pregnancy
- Describe the growth and development of an unborn baby
- Discuss ways a baby's health is related to the mother's health and habits
- Describe the labor process, using the stages of labor
- Describe the abilities of newborns

Carlos and Maria had wanted a baby for a long time. They planned carefully so that they would be able to nurture and provide for the baby. Maria did all she could to stay in good health.

Once Maria became pregnant, Carlos insisted that she begin to have medical care immediately. Although Maria didn't smoke, Carlos did. He decided to give up smoking so that Maria would not have to breathe his cigarette smoke during the pregnancy. When they were invited to parties, they let friends know that they would be drinking nonalcoholic beverages. They were careful to avoid contact with people who had contagious illnesses. Maria ate a balanced diet and avoided foods that had a great deal of salt, sugar, caffeine, or fat.

During the pregnancy Maria and Carlos prepared a space for the baby to live, decided on names, and observed the baby's movements inside Maria's body. Even before being born, the baby was a dominant part of their lives. The day Jesse was born was one of high excitement and expectation.

Carlos was at work when Maria called to say she was in labor. They had attended childbirth classes, and Carlos was confident he could participate in Maria's labor and delivery. Carlos hoped that Maria would have a safe delivery and that the baby would be healthy. However, for a brief moment he was not sure that he wanted to become a father at all.

Carlos called his mother and asked her to take Maria to the hospital, promising to meet them there. Maria had already called her doctor and the hospital to tell them she was on her way. Maria and Carlos had registered ahead of time and had paid part of the hospital bill in advance. The hospital admitted her at once and quickly began preparations for delivery.

CONCEPTION

The **sperm** and the **ovum** are the reproductive cells. A baby begins biologically when the father's sperm fertilizes the mother's ovum. Most often this occurs in the mother's Fallopian tube shortly after ovulation. **Ovulation** is the expulsion of an ovum from the mother's ovary, as shown in Illustration 4-1.

Ovulation normally occurs midway between menstrual periods. As a result, a woman is mostly likely to become pregnant about halfway between the first day of one menstrual period and the first day of the next. Since the day the next period begins

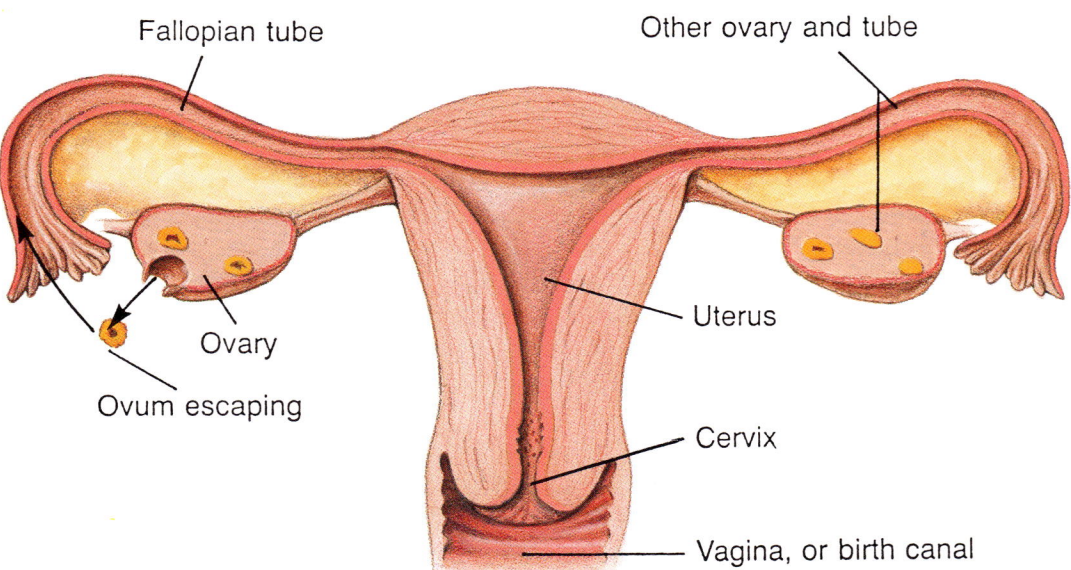

Fallopian tube

Other ovary and tube

Uterus

Ovary

Ovum escaping

Cervix

Vagina, or birth canal

ILLUSTRATION 4-1 An ovum (egg) is expelled from the ovary and travels through the Fallopian tube. The most common site of fertilization (joining of the sperm and egg) is in the Fallopian tube shortly after the egg is released from the ovary.

cannot be predicted exactly, it can be difficult to pinpoint ovulation. However, at ovulation a woman's body temperature goes up about six-tenths of a degree Fahrenheit in preparation for a possible pregnancy. Women who consistently keep track of their body temperature can determine when they ovulate.

Fertilization

Normally, only one sperm fertilizes an ovum. Once the sperm moves into the ovum, the surface of the ovum resists other sperm. The center, or nucleus, of the sperm and that of the ovum move toward one another and fuse. Another term for fertilization is **conception.**

Birth Control

Couples who are not ready to have children or who want to space their children a certain number of years apart can use some method of birth control. Some methods must be prescribed by doctors; others can be purchased without a prescription. Sterilization is a method that requires surgery. Natural birth control is based on the timing of the woman's menstrual cycle and ovulation.

A method of birth control is reliable only when it is used exactly as intended. Many babies are born each year to people who have not used methods correctly. Homemade methods of birth control are not reliable and may be dangerous.

DOCTOR-PRESCRIBED METHODS

Methods of birth control that require a doctor's prescription are oral contraceptives (the pill), the diaphragm, and the intra-uterine device (IUD). (**Contraceptives** are means of preventing conception, that is, birth control devices.) A woman is given a **pelvic examination,** a procedure in which the doctor examines her reproductive organs. Also, her general health is checked to be certain the best method is prescribed. Having a physical examination of this type annually is recommended whether contraceptives are prescribed or not. Doctor-prescribed methods of birth control are generally preferred for long-term use. They are more reliable if the woman consults regularly with a physician and follows his or her advice.

OVER-THE-COUNTER METHODS

Some birth control methods involve the use of contraceptive devices that can be purchased without a doctor's prescription. These include the condom, vaginal foam, and the sponge. These birth control methods work well for short-term use and are reliable as long as they are used exactly as the package instructions direct. Both the man and the woman need to use contraceptives when over-the-counter methods are chosen.

VOLUNTARY STERILIZATION

Sterilization involves a surgical procedure to close the passages that allow the sperm and the ovum to come together. For a man, this type of surgery is called a **vasectomy.** For a woman, it is called a **tubal ligation.** Either type of operation is almost always permanent. Usually only people who intend to have no children or no more children choose sterilization.

NATURAL BIRTH CONTROL

Couples who use **natural birth control** abstain from sexual intercourse until after the woman's fertile period, which is around the time she ovulates. From two or three days after ovulation until the next menstrual period is a woman's most infertile time. The occurrence of this time can be estimated by observing changes in body temperature, discharge of mucus, and the cervix. Training and commitment to the method by both partners in a stable and faithful relationship are necessary.

ABSTINENCE

A method of birth control that is always safe is **abstinence,** or not having sex. It can be a workable choice for teenagers but is reliable only for those who are completely committed to it. Anyone relying on abstinence must be absolutely determined that it is his or her method of choice, no matter what.

Abstinence before marriage is encouraged by many religious groups and most parents. Abstinence is also the *only 100% effective method of birth control.* Furthermore, it will protect one from getting the AIDS (Acquired Immune Deficiency Syndrome) virus and most other sexually transmitted diseases. Worldwide, AIDS is passed by heterosexual contact more often than in any other way. Abstinence is also an effective way for homosexuals to avoid getting AIDS. (AIDS is discussed further in Chapter 7.)

Signs of Pregnancy

How does a woman know when she is pregnant? There are several signs. The most familiar is that she misses her menstrual period. Since there are reasons besides pregnancy for missing a period, a woman needs to check for other signs. These include swollen or tender breasts, frequent urination, nausea, and changes in appetite. A woman who thinks she may be pregnant can obtain a home pregnancy test at a drugstore. Some of these tests can give results within one or two weeks after the first missed or late menstrual period. Pregnancy should be confirmed by a doctor by the time a woman misses a second period. Also, prenatal care should begin by that time.

When will the baby be born? The usual length of pregnancy is 280 days, which is about nine calendar months or ten lunar months (28 days each). The approximate delivery date can be calculated by identifying the first day of the mother's last menstrual period, subtracting three months, and then adding seven days. For example, if the mother's last menstrual period began on January 1 of the current year, subtracting three months would give October 1. Then adding seven days would give October 8. The baby would be due to be born on October 8 of the current year.

Pregnancy affects many lives—those of the mother, the father, the unborn baby, other family members, and sometimes friends. It is best to delay pregnancy until a couple is prepared to accept the responsibility of parenthood. What method of preventing pregnancy is preferable? The Something to Think About feature deals with preventing pregnancy.

PRENATAL DEVELOPMENT

The term of a pregnancy can be divided into three time periods called **trimesters.** A trimester is about three months long. The first trimester is from conception through the end of the third month. The second trimester consists of the fourth through the sixth months. And the third trimester begins with the seventh month and lasts until birth.

The First Trimester

The first trimester begins with conception and ends three months from then. At the end of this time, the unborn baby is

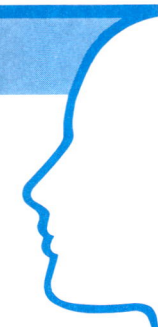

Something to Think About

Preventing an Unwanted Pregnancy

There are two main ways to prevent an unwanted pregnancy: proper use of birth control and saying no.

Birth control allows people to participate in sexual intercourse with a lessened chance of pregnancy. (The basic methods of birth control are discussed in this chapter.) Birth control is used by many people who feel it is better to use contraceptives than to bring an unwanted child into the world, one they may not be able to care for or raise to adulthood. For these people sexual freedom means being able to engage in sex without becoming pregnant.

Other people choose abstinence—and not just because it prevents pregnancy. These people feel that having sex alters a relationship—that the relationship with the partner is forever changed once sexual intercourse is chosen. They see sexual freedom as being free to choose not to have sex—to say no when a sexual relationship is not a wise personal choice.

Some people regard sex outside of marriage to be damaging to those involved. Coleen Kelley Mast, author of the *Sex Respect* program, asserts that there is no way to have premarital sex without someone getting hurt. Ms. Mast also suggests that being assertive is the ability to set and keep limits—to be in control of your life.

Risks associated with having sex tend to be greater outside of marriage than for marriage partners who are faithful to one another. There are several kinds of risks associated with sex outside of marriage. Physical risks include increased chances of getting venereal diseases (such as herpes II, chlamydia, and syphilis), AIDS, or cancer of the cervix (for women with multiple partners). Psychological risks include fear, disappointment, guilt, and doubt. An emotional risk is that premarital sex may prevent the growth of one's personal identity. Thinking risks include being fooled into marrying the wrong person or hanging onto a relationship that is not really satisfactory. Other thinking risks are the risks that one may believe a relationship is deeper than it really is and that sex may be used to avoid rather than to express true closeness.

Benefits of waiting to have sex include the following:

- Freedom to grow and mature
- Freedom to develop confidence and strong character
- Freedom to make choices that might not be open if sexual activity is a preoccupation
- Increased ability to use communication skills rather than sexual intimacy to express feelings

Preventing unwanted pregnancy is important. If you have been lucky so far, it is time to stop taking chances and to make choices. What you do with your life from now on is what counts. How will you choose to prevent pregnancy?

about the size of a peach seed and has features that are recognizably human.

PERIOD OF THE OVUM

The **period of the ovum** begins as soon as conception takes place. The first cell of the new baby, the **zygote**, begins to make more cells. It becomes two cells, then four, then eight. By the ninth day the cells have formed a hollow ball called the **blastocyst.** The blastocyst draws nourishment from the ovum. Small hairlike structures called cilia inside the Fallopian tube brush against the blastocyst, moving it toward the uterus. Also, the Fallopian tube gently pulses. The **uterus** is where the baby develops until birth. The trip down the Fallopian tube takes 10 to 14 days.

By the time the blastocyst has reached the uterus, the cells in the cluster have already begun to specialize; some will become the baby, some the placenta, some the umbilical cord, and some the amniotic sac. The **placenta** is the connection between the mother and the baby through which oxygen and carbon dioxide and food and waste are exchanged. The **umbilical cord** contains two arteries and one vein to carry the unborn baby's blood back and forth to the placenta. The **amniotic sac** surrounds the baby and becomes filled with amniotic fluid. The **amniotic fluid** is essentially water. It keeps the baby's body temperature even, protects the baby from injury by acting like a shock absorber, and helps the baby to slip out of the mother's body during delivery.

The final event of the period of the ovum occurs when the blastocyst becomes attached to the lining of the uterus. This is somewhat like planting the roots of a small plant in the soil and is called **implantation**. Illustration 4-2 shows the movement of the blastocyst down the Fallopian tube and its implantation.

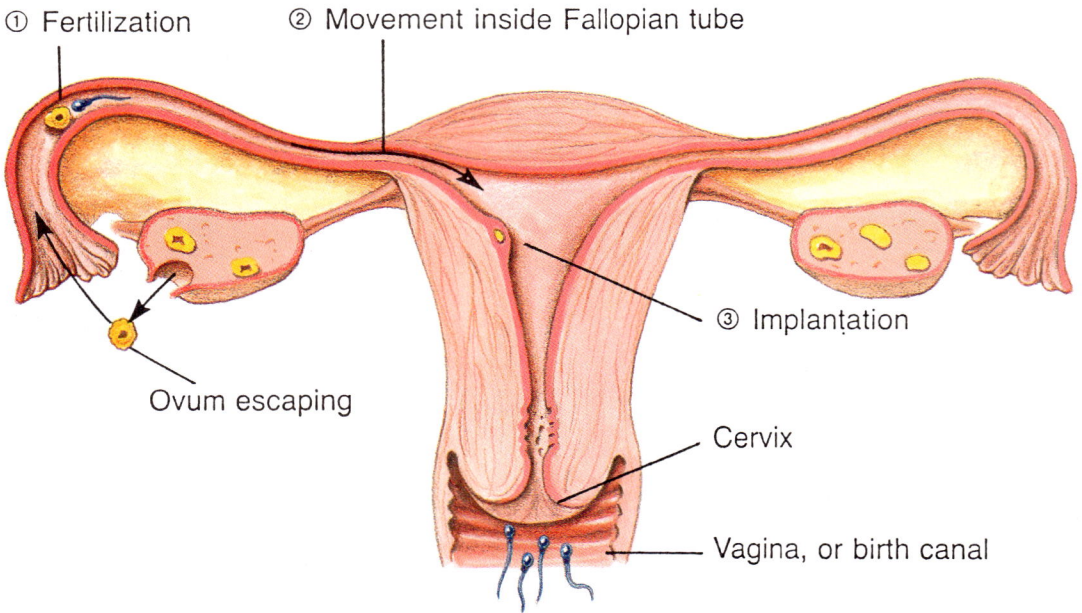

① Fertilization   ② Movement inside Fallopian tube

③ Implantation

Ovum escaping

Cervix

Vagina, or birth canal

ILLUSTRATION 4-2

① Conception takes place high in the Fallopian tube near the ovary. ② The fertilized egg is propelled by fine hairlike structures and a gentle motion of the Fallopian tube toward the uterus, in the direction shown by the arrows. The cell multiplies many times while traveling. ③ Ten to fourteen days after conception, the blastocyst adheres to the uterine lining. This is called implantation.

PERIOD OF THE EMBRYO

From implantation until about the eighth week of pregnancy is the **period of the embryo.** The developing baby is called the

embryo during this period. The brain, liver, genitals, and heart are formed. About the twenty-fourth day after conception, the heart begins to pulse. Before the eighth week, the muscles are developed enough that the baby begins to move very slightly. It will be several weeks before the mother is able to feel the baby's movement. By the end of the period of the embryo, the face has developed its basic structure; the baby is recognizably human.

PERIOD OF THE FETUS

From the eighth week of pregnancy until birth, an unborn baby is called a **fetus.** When the **period of the fetus** begins, the baby weighs only about an ounce. By the end of this period, at birth, the baby usually weighs between 6 and $8\frac{1}{2}$ pounds and is 19 to 22 inches long.

During the third month, hard structures such as bones, teeth, and fingernails are formed. Blood begins to form, the kidneys take shape and the genitals become recognizably male or female.

The Second Trimester

At the beginning of the second trimester, the doctor can hear the baby's heartbeat through a standard stethoscope. **Lanugo,** or soft downy hair, begins to form on the baby's head. Blood vessels become visible through the skin, and muscle movements become more active. In the fourth month, the mother begins to feel this movement, called **quickening.** Lanugo begins to cover the baby's shoulders, and the skin becomes less transparent.

During the fifth month, the eyebrows and eyelashes become defined. The skin is wrinkled. A waxy substance called **vernix caseosa** that protects the baby's skin before and after birth begins to form.

By the sixth month the baby weighs about $2\frac{1}{2}$ pounds and is about 15 inches long. The skin is red, wrinkled, and covered with vernix caseosa, so the baby looks like a little old person. Membranes that have covered the eyes disappear, but they remain open. If the baby is born during or after the sixth month, there is a chance for survival with good medical care.

The Third Trimester

From the seventh through the ninth month, the baby gains most of the birth weight. A layer of fat forms under the skin to help regulate body temperature after birth. The baby's nervous

FIGURE 4-1   Near the beginning of the period of the fetus, the unborn baby begins to become recognizably human.
Source: © *Superstock International Inc.*

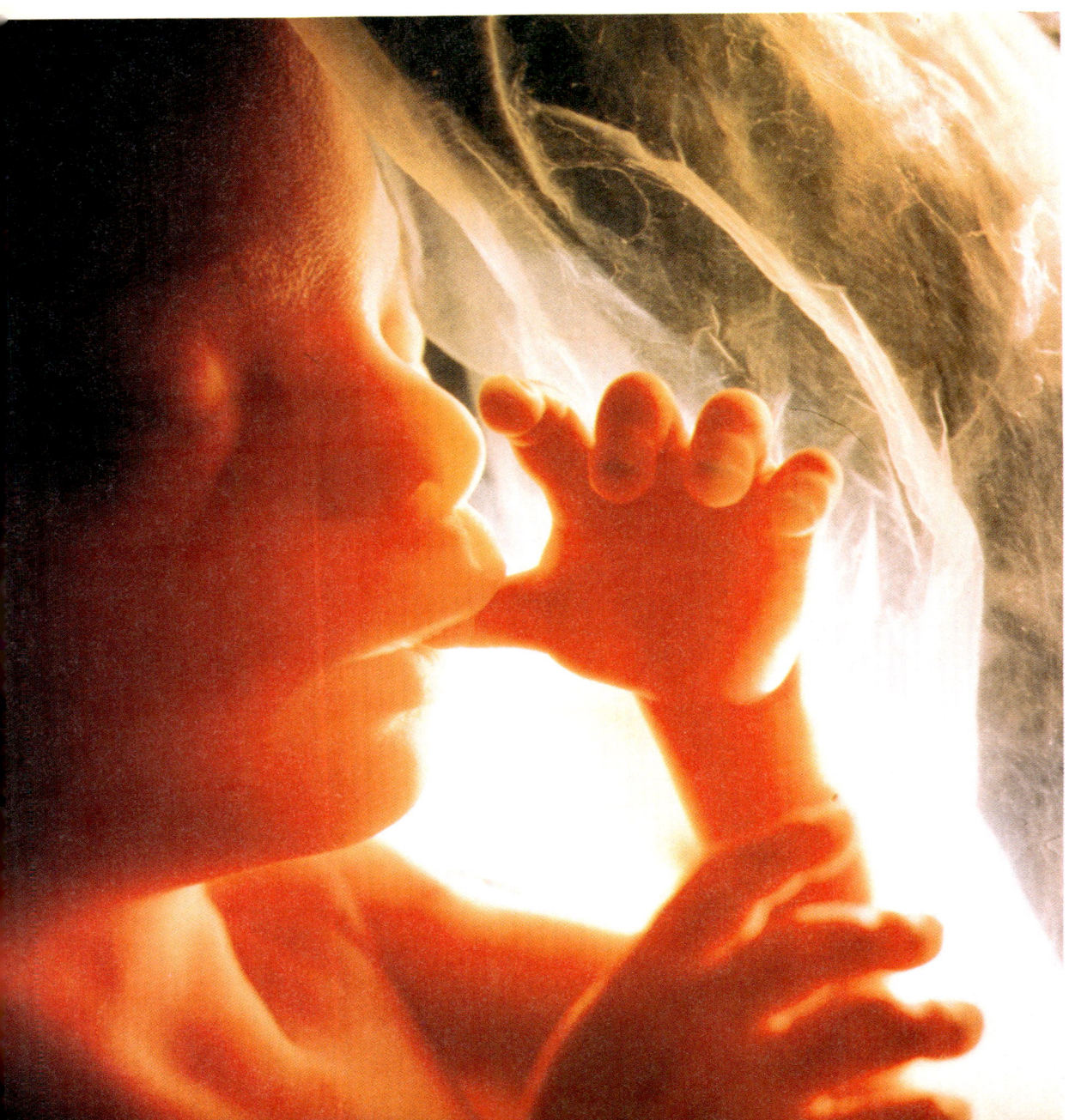

system develops rapidly. The digestive system and the lungs become ready to function outside the uterus.

Finally, as the birth approaches, the baby moves into position for delivery. The most usual position is head down. The heartbeat increases as the time of birth approaches. Illustration 4-3 shows a fully developed baby inside the uterus before labor begins.

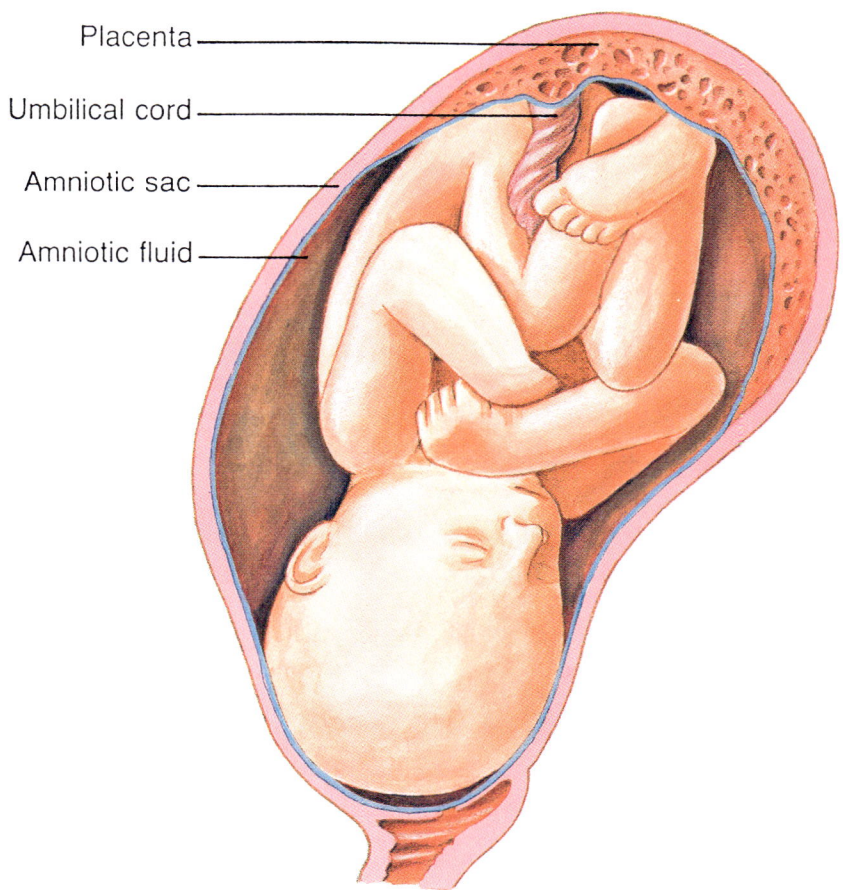

Placenta

Umbilical cord

Amniotic sac

Amniotic fluid

ILLUSTRATION 4-3
The placenta connects the unborn baby to the mother. Oxygen and food are passed through it to the baby, and carbon dioxide and waste are returned to the mother. The umbilical cord carries the baby's blood back and forth to the placenta and is attached to the baby at the navel. The amniotic sac is filled with amniotic fluid and surrounds the baby and placenta.

Environmental Problems During Prenatal Development

The mother's body is the first environment for a baby. Because physical structure and strength are largely established before birth, the prenatal environment is very important. When it is good, the baby thrives. However, problems during the prenatal period can cause the baby to be formed incorrectly, to become sick, or even to die.

Pollutants and radiation in a pregnant woman's environment can have damaging effects on her body and thus on her unborn baby, too. Conditions inside a woman's body that can cause serious damage to her baby are caused by poor nutrition, poor health or disease, or the Rh factor. If the mother consumes alcohol, takes drugs that have not been prescribed by her doctor, or smokes cigarettes, the baby may be seriously harmed. A pregnant woman can give her baby the best chance to be born healthy by taking good care of herself during pregnancy, eating a balanced diet, getting enough rest, and exercising moderately and appropriately.

LABOR AND BIRTH

Labor is the process of physically separating the infant from the mother's body. Labor usually takes 12 to 15 hours for a first baby and less time for later babies. About a week before birth, the baby usually settles into its birth position. This is called **lightening,** because the woman feels lighter even though she may look larger. Sometime within the 24 hours before labor begins, the mucous plug comes loose from the cervix. The **cervix** is the opening of the uterus through which the baby must pass.

Stage 1: Dilation and Effacement

The mother's uterus is basically a large bag of muscle with a tightly closed opening (the cervix). When it is time for the baby to be born, the uterine muscles begin to contract, or shorten. **Contractions** are regularly spaced in true labor. When contractions begin, they usually last only a few seconds and are several minutes apart. As labor progresses, they last longer and become stronger and closer together.

The contractions of the uterine muscles gently push the baby's head against the cervix. The cervix begins to thin out. This is called **effacement.** (See Illustration 4-4.) As the cervix effaces, it

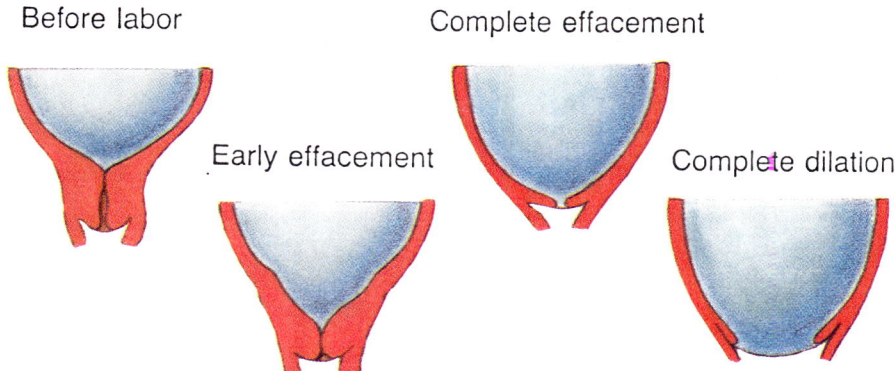

Before labor   Complete effacement

Early effacement   Complete dilation

ILLUSTRATION 4-4   During the first stage of labor, the cervix thins out (effaces) and opens up (dilates). The opening of the cervix begins at less than 1 centimeter and must reach 10 centimeters before the baby can be born.

also dilates. **Dilation** is the opening up of the cervix. During the first stage of labor, the opening in the cervix must increase in diameter from 1 centimeter to 10 centimeters (about 4 inches). The opening must be large enough for the baby to pass through.

The first stage of labor requires a lot of patience, which can become difficult to maintain as labor progresses. When labor begins, women feel first excited, then apprehensive. Most remain at home until the contractions are about five minutes apart. By this time the contractions have usually become rather uncomfortable. The woman's mood usually changes to impatience, and she can become quite irritable.

When a woman in labor arrives at the hospital, she is admitted to the labor room and is prepared for delivery. This is a time when a supportive partner is most helpful. Many hospitals attach a fetal monitor during labor so the staff can observe the condition and the progress of both the mother and the baby. The **fetal monitor** keeps track of the mother's contractions and the baby's heartbeat.

At some point during the first stage of labor, the amniotic sac breaks or is ruptured by a doctor or nurse. Toward the end of the first stage of labor, the hospital staff will move the mother to the delivery room to prepare for delivery. Most of the total labor time is taken up by the first stage.

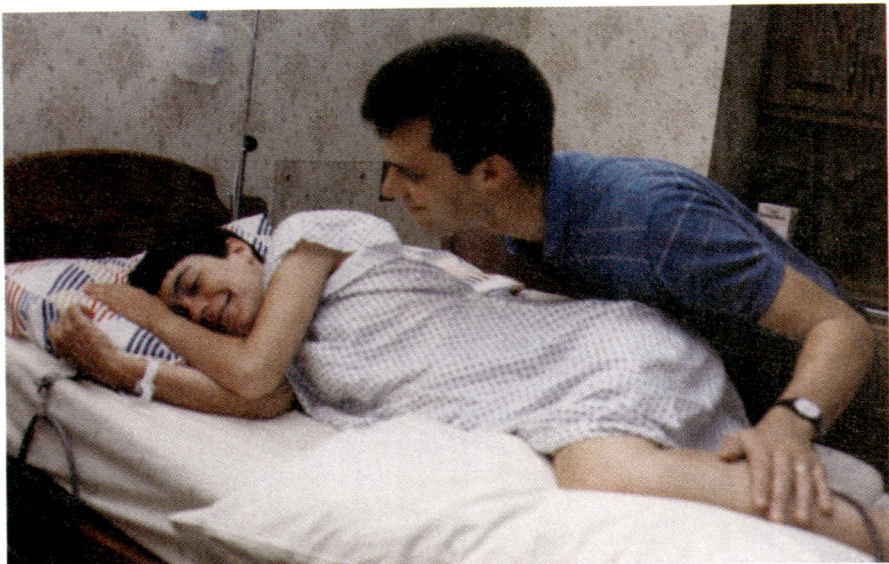

FIGURE 4-2 A husband—especially one who has taken classes to learn about childbirth—is a welcome support to a woman during labor.
Source: Courtesy of Husband-Coached Natural Childbirth Association

Stage 2: Birth

Once the cervix is completely open, the mother assists in the delivery of the baby by pushing as contractions occur. This helps the baby pass through the birth canal. The **birth canal** is the passageway between the cervix and the outside of the woman's body. Illustration 4-5 shows the second stage of labor.

Most babies are born head first. If another part of the baby comes through the birth canal first, the birth is called a **breech delivery.**

Immediately after the baby is born, the doctor suctions mucous from the baby's nose and mouth so that breathing can begin. Once the baby is breathing, the umbilical cord stops pulsing. The doctor then places two clamps on the umbilical cord near the baby and cuts between the two clamps. There is no pain for either the mother or the baby because there are no nerves in the umbilical cord.

A nurse tags the baby with an identifying arm or ankle band that matches the mother's and then checks to be sure the baby

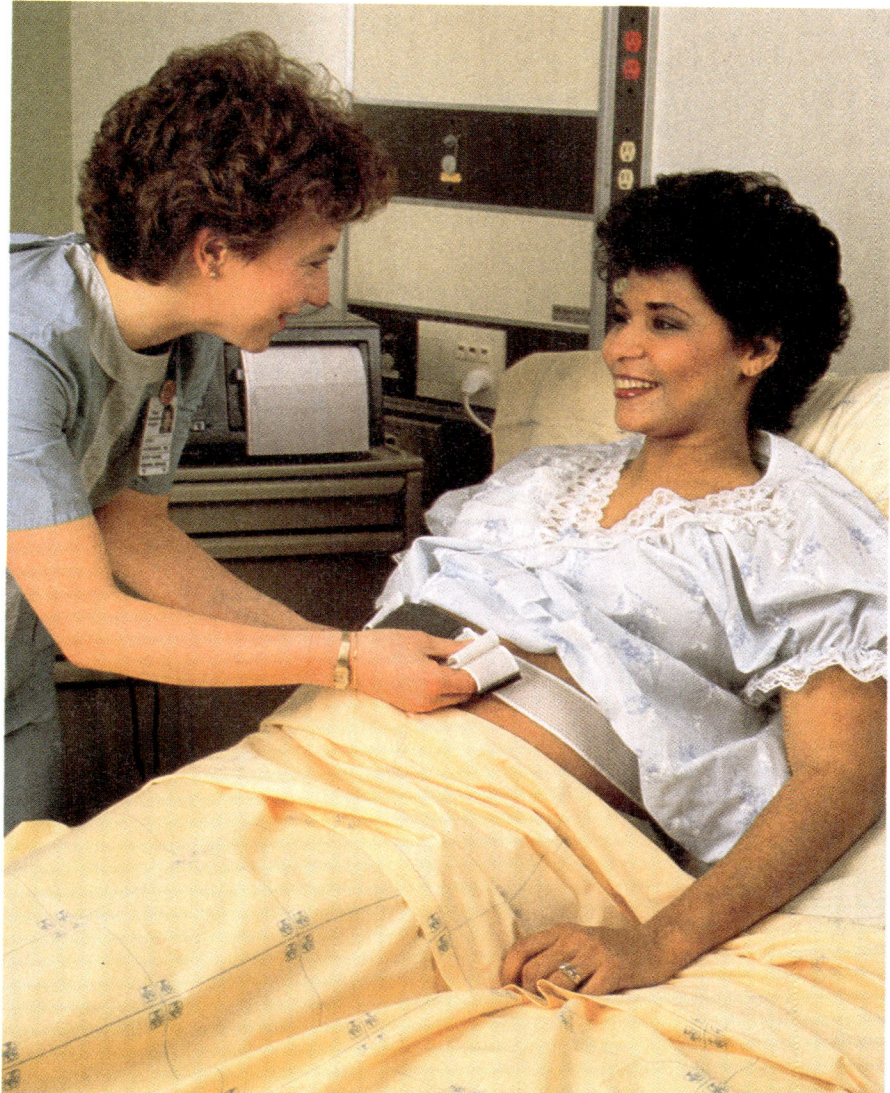

FIGURE 4-3 A fetal monitor allows nurses or doctors to check regularly on the baby's condition during labor.
Source: Good Samaritan Hospital

is functioning properly. This test used in many hospitals is the **Apgar test,** which shows how well the baby is doing at one minute and at five minutes after birth. (See Table 4-1.) If the baby needs any special help in getting a healthy start, the Apgar test usually shows what needs to be done. The nurse examines the baby and

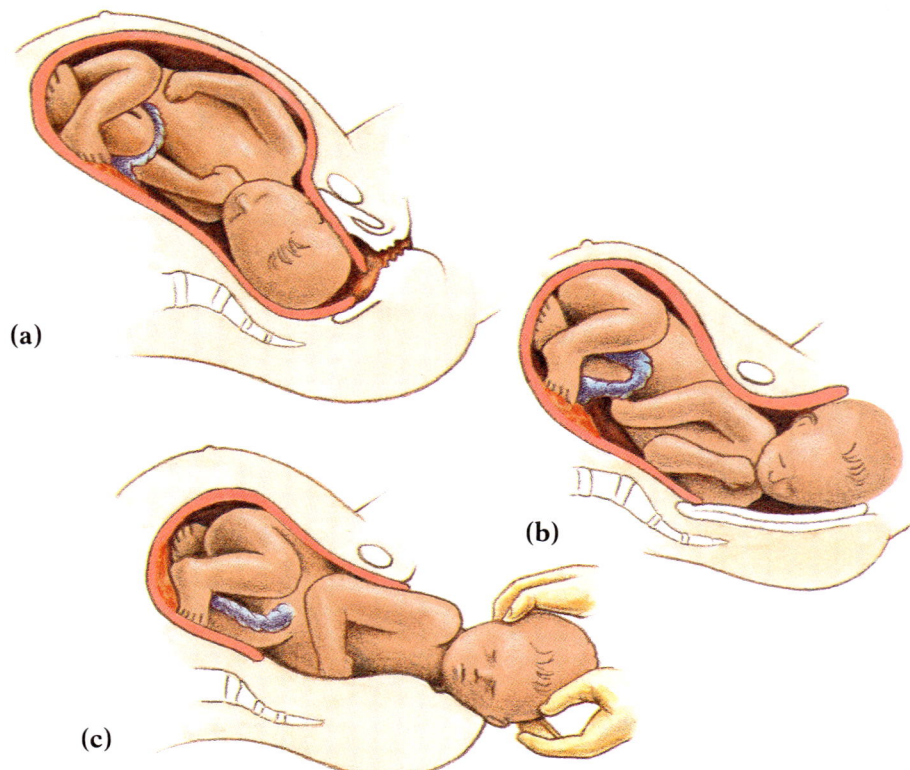

(a)

(b)

(c)

ILLUSTRATION 4-5 (a) The cervix is completely dilated, and the baby starts through the birth canal. (b) The baby's head is born. The face is usually down. (c) The baby turns so the face is toward the mother's leg. The shoulders come out, and the rest of the body follows quickly.

gives a score of 0, 1, or 2 in each of five categories, for a possible total of 10 points. Heart rate, breathing (respiratory effort), reflexes, muscle tone, and color are the five things checked.

Stage 3: Delivery of the Afterbirth

During the third stage of labor, the afterbirth is delivered from the mother. The **afterbirth** consists of the placenta and the amniotic sac. These are no longer needed because they are formed with each new baby. The doctor then stitches up the episiotomy. The **episiotomy** is a surgical cut sometimes made during delivery

TABLE 4-1   Apgar Scoring System for Newborns

Sign	Score 0 if:	Score 1 if:	Score 2 if:
1. Heart rate	Not detectable	Below 100	Above 100
2. Respiratory effort	Absent	Slow, irregular	Good, crying
3. Muscle tone	Flaccid, limp	Some flexion of extremities	Active motion
4. Reflex irritability[a]	No response	Grimace	Cough, sneeze
5. Color[b]	Blue, pale	Extremities blue, body pink	Completely pink

[a]When stimulated by suction in nose
[b]If the natural skin color of the child is dark, other tests for color are applied.

Source: Reprinted with permission from the International Anesthesia Research Society from "Proposal for a New Method of Evaluating the Newborn Infant," by V. Apgar, Anesthesia and Analgesia, vol. 32, pp. 260–267.

to increase the size of the opening of the birth canal and prevent the mother's tissues from tearing.

Recovery

When delivery procedures are complete, the mother rests and is cared for closely by nurses for a short period of time. The baby is cleaned and examined more thoroughly. If the delivery has occurred in a delivery suite rather than an L-D-R room, the infant is usually taken to the hospital's nursery. The mother is moved to a recovery area for about an hour; then she is taken to her room.

NEWBORN BABIES

As soon as Jesse was born, the doctor laid him on Maria's stomach until the umbilical cord was cut. The doctor then encouraged Carlos to wrap Jesse in a blanket and hand him to the nurse for Apgar scoring and cleaning up. Jesse was only a few minutes old when the nurse told Carlos he could carry the baby back to Maria. Being together in the L-D-R room gave Maria and Carlos a chance to look at Jesse closely and for as long as they wanted.

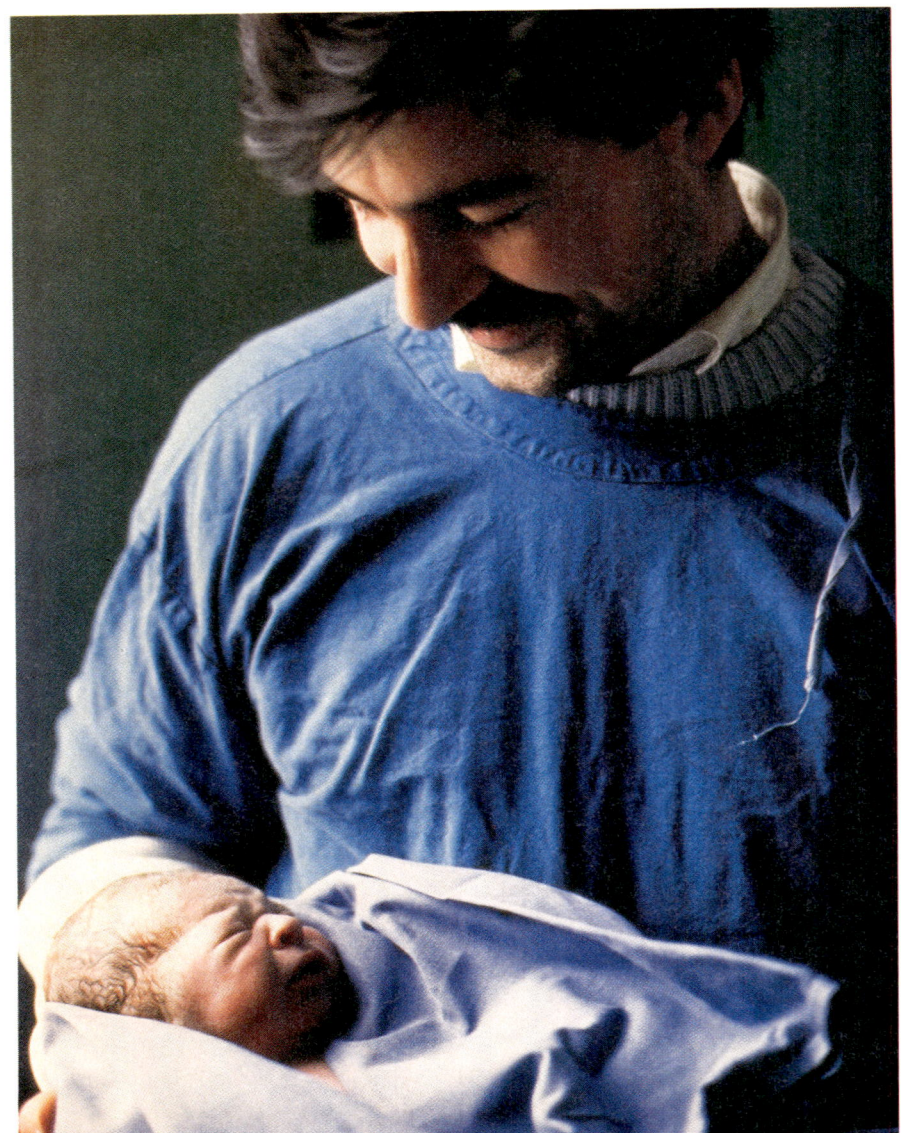

FIGURE 4-4   Being present in the delivery room allows a new father
to get acquainted with his child minutes after birth.
Source: © Jerry Cooke/Photo Researchers, Inc.

"He has so much hair. I can't believe it!" Maria said. "Look how tiny his fingers are." Maria ran her finger softly over Jesse's fingers, then gently across his arm.

Carlos loosened Jesse's blanket and looked at his legs and feet. Just above his diaper the stub of the umbilical cord was still held by the clamp. "How long will he have that?" Carlos asked the nurse.

"About a week or ten days," the nurse replied. "You need to clean it each day with alcohol. Don't give him a tub bath until the stub falls off on its own and the navel is completely healed."

Maria wrapped the blanket around her son and laid him against her knees so she and Carlos could look at his face. His eyes were closed tightly and were still a bit puffy. A few red and purple blemishes remained from the delivery.

Jesse stretched, arching his back. He opened his eyes and looked straight at his mom.

"Hi, Jesse," Maria said gently, raising the pitch of her voice. She brought Jesse's face closer and turned him so that his eyes met hers. Quietly they looked at each other for some time. Then Maria drew Jesse close to her own body and wrapped her arms around him. For the first time, Maria began to feel that Jesse was really theirs.

Carlos, too, was beginning to feel that Jesse was his son. He lifted the baby gently from Maria's arms and cradled him in his left arm. Carlos touched the end of Jesse's nose and said, "Hey Jesse! I'm your dad."

Bonding and Attachment

When parents have their first opportunity to look at, touch, and talk to their baby, a special feeling begins to develop. This feeling of belonging to one another is called **bonding.** It is very important for newborn babies to be with each of their parents within a few hours after birth so that the bonding process can begin. Fathers and mothers need to share this bonding process as parents. Through this process parents and children begin to feel like a family unit. Bonding helps parents feel that they want very much to take good care of this new small person, and it helps babies begin to rely on their parents to take care of them.

Sometimes new babies and parents do not get an early chance to be together. When a baby or mother has problems during delivery and needs extra medical care, it may be a few days before the bonding process can begin. When that happens, special care and determination are necessary to help the feeling of being a family to develop.

As parents care for newborns and meet their needs in a helpful and consistent manner, the babies start to feel secure. By the eighth month most feel safe enough to explore their environment if their parents are nearby. This secure feeling is called **attachment.** Babies whose parents do not meet their needs consistently or accurately may be confused about their parents' dependability. Such babies spend less time exploring and learning.

Reflexes

When babies are born, they have built-in actions called **reflexes.** Reflexes are a person's automatic responses to stimuli in the environment. For example, when you turn on a bright light, a baby's eyes will close. Many reflexes are designed to help the baby survive. These include the rooting, sucking, and startle reflexes. Some reflexes are related to using the hands and feet. These include the grasping, stepping, and Babinski reflexes, which are automatic at birth but disappear later. Once they are gone, the baby learns to make the movements intentionally.

Abilities of Newborns

Like most new parents, Carlos and Maria wondered about Jesse's capabilities. Could he see well enough to tell the difference between them and other people? When they talked to him, did he understand what they said? Could he smell? How did it affect him when they touched him?

A baby's five senses all work very well. For the first year or so, nearly everything they learn comes through their five senses and their motor activity. **Motor activity** is a term used to describe the way muscles and nerves work together to make movement.

Dr. Berry Brazelton, a well-known pediatrician, has identified many abilities of newborns. He developed a testing procedure called the **Brazelton Neonatal Assessment Scale.** It is used by some hospitals to show parents how their infants respond as individuals to various actions. Nurses or doctors can show parents how infants' reflexes work, how they can follow objects moving slowly a few inches from their face, and how they often copy what an adult does (such as sticking out the tongue).

The purpose of the Brazelton Neonatal Assessment Scale is to help parents understand their baby as a new person and see how complex he or she is. A newborn baby is a person, and it is important to respect him or her as such. The assessment also allows nurses or doctors to detect problems the baby may have in de-

Leadership at a Glance

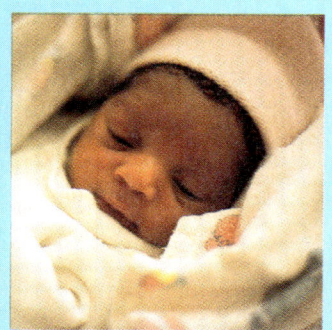

Source: Bob Ohr for The Christ Hospital

T. Berry Brazelton, M.D.

Dr. Berry Brazelton has been known as a leader in both pediatrics and child development for many years. He has taught at Harvard Medical School and is currently a professor at Brown University.

Dr. Brazelton's interest in child development led him to found the Child Development Unit at Children's Hospital in Boston. Much of his study has centered around the behavior of newborn babies—how their behavior affects the way they get along with parents and how they become attached to parents during their early months. He has used what he learned to recommend ways to help parents do a better job in early infancy.

Dr. Brazelton writes articles and books on child development for both parents and professionals. His best-known work is probably his book *Infants and Mothers,* but he has written more than twenty other books and videotapes for parents.

Among medical professionals, Dr. Brazelton is best known for developing the Brazelton Neonatal Assessment Scale, a set of guidelines for nurses and doctors to use in checking the abilities of newborns. The results of the assessment are used to help identify problems and to teach parents about the many abilities of their infants.

Dr. Brazelton has also worked to support national child care legislation and is a co-sponsor of a national organization called Parent Action.

velopment. Watching this assessment of their baby helps parents appreciate his or her special abilities. All studies show that this can enhance their sensitivity to the baby and increase their self-confidence as parents.

SIGHT

Newborn babies see very clearly for the first hour or so after birth. After that, their eyes focus best on objects that are between 9 and 16 inches from their faces. Fold your arms and look down at your elbow. Your eyes should be 9 to 16 inches from where a baby's eyes would be if you were holding one in your arms.

Babies prefer to look at a human face. By the time they are two weeks of age, they will look longer at their mother's face than at the face of another person, if the mother has been the main caregiver.

As mentioned earlier, newborn babies will follow an object with their eyes if it is moved slowly at the right distance to allow focusing on it. This ability is called **tracking.**

SMELL

Babies can sense smells very well shortly after birth. They make a face if someone places an object having an unpleasant odor near the nose. They can identify the smell of their mother by the time they are two weeks old.

TASTE

Unborn babies have been photographed sucking inside the uterus when something sweet was placed near them in the amniotic fluid. Soon after birth babies give clear indications that they enjoy certain tastes.

HEARING

During the third trimester of pregnancy, unborn babies respond to sounds outside the mother by moving more or less than they were before. Newborns sleep readily listening to a recording of their mother's body sounds. They are able to tell the difference between sounds that come from people and those such as music that come from other sources.

You may have observed that when people talk to babies they often raise the pitch of their voices. Babies tend to turn toward a high-pitched voice. Father's voices are important, too. Babies will usually remember their fathers' voice if they have heard it shortly after birth.

FIGURE 4-5   Newborns can focus on a nearby face very well, and mutual eye contact between parent and child is very important just after birth.
Source: Courtesy of Husband-Coached Natural Childbirth Association

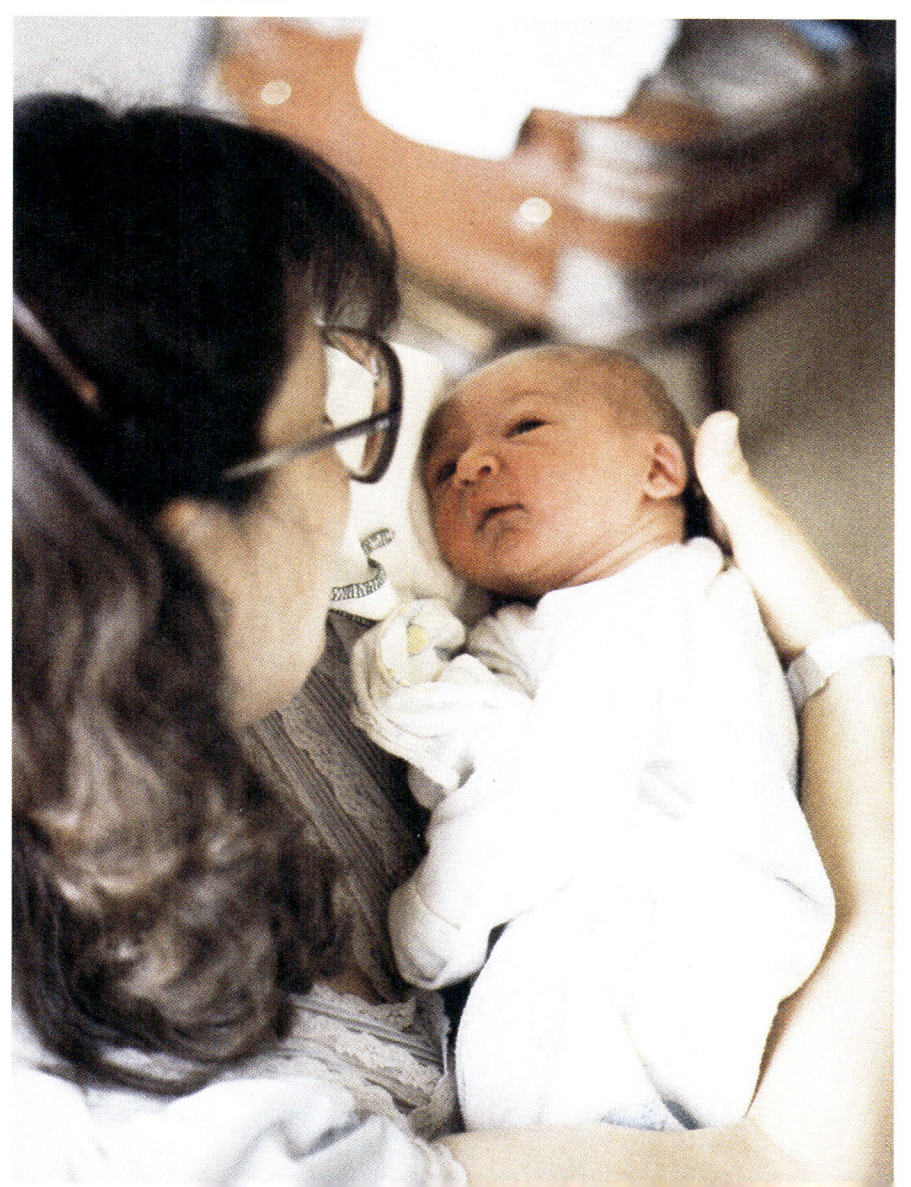

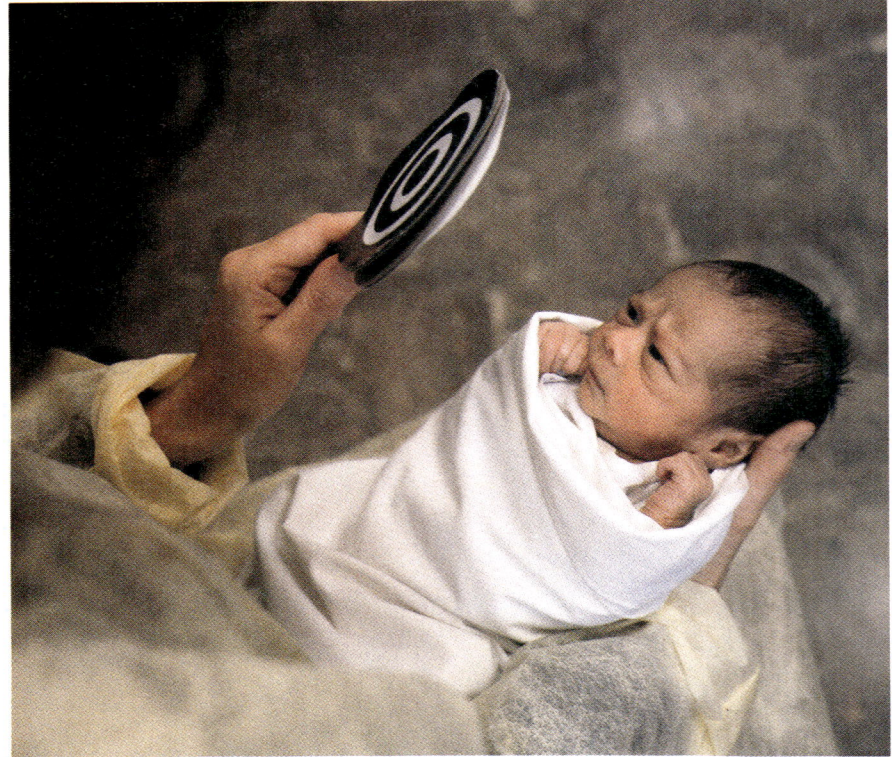

FIGURE 4-6   A newborn's eyes will follow a slowly moving object that is a few inches from his or her face.
Source: © Guy Gillette 1982/Photo Researchers, Inc.

TOUCH

Babies are very sensitive to touch. Many of their reflexes are stimulated by touch. They sense whether a parent is tense or relaxed by the way the parent holds and touches them. When parents are nervous, babies are more likely to become upset; when parents are relaxed, babies tend to relax.

Summary

Kinds of birth control methods include prescription methods, nonprescription methods, rhythm, and abstinence. Women can determine whether they are pregnant by interpreting various signs and can estimate the date on which the baby will be born.

Conception takes place when an ovum and a sperm fuse, usually in a Fallopian tube. Pregnancy is divided into three trimesters. During the first trimester the baby grows from ovum to embryo to fetus. All the vital organs develop and begin to function during this time. During the second trimester details of the baby's body become clear, and the mother begins to feel movement. The baby is getting ready to begin life outside the uterus during the third trimester.

The prenatal environment can cause problems for a baby if there are harmful elements in the mother's environment, if the condition of the mother's body is not healthy, or if the mother takes drugs or alcohol or smokes cigarettes during pregnancy. To prevent problems, an expectant mother needs to eat properly, take care of herself, and have regular medical care.

Labor involves three stages: (1) dilation and effacement, (2) birth, and (3) delivery of the afterbirth. Once the baby is born, the parents begin to get to know their child. This is called bonding. As they care for the baby, the baby begins to feel secure, or attached to the parents.

A healthy baby is born with a number of reflexes. Newborn babies have the abilities to see, smell, taste, hear, and feel touches at birth.

Terms and Concepts

Sperm	Period of the ovum
Ovum	Zygote
Ovulation	Blastocyst
Conception	Uterus
Contraceptives	Placenta
Pelvic examination	Umbilical cord
Vasectomy	Amniotic sac
Tubal ligation	Amniotic fluid
Natural birth control	Implantation
Abstinence	Period of the embryo
Trimesters	Embryo

Fetus

Period of the fetus

Lanugo

Quickening

Vernix caseosa

Labor

Lightening

Cervix

Contractions

Effacement

Dilation

Fetal monitor

Birth canal

Breech delivery

Apgar test

Afterbirth

Episiotomy

Bonding

Attachment

Reflexes

Motor activity

Brazelton Neonatal Assessment Scale

Tracking

Checking Your Understanding

1. List the dangers to an unborn baby that can arise in the uterine environment.

2. Write a short paper defending abstinence as a method of birth control and a way to protect health.

3. Describe the unborn baby's development during the period of the ovum, the period of the embryo, and the period of the fetus.

4. List the three stages of labor and briefly describe what happens during each.

5. How does holding and touching a baby soon after birth help parents feel that the baby really belongs to them?

6. List the sensory abilities of newborns. How do you think knowing what a baby can do would affect how new parents treat the baby?

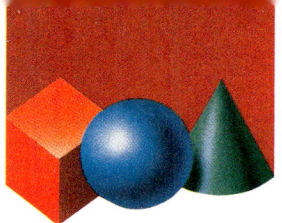

4 HANDS ON WITH CHILDREN

BATHING A BABY

Step 1   Gather supplies and prepare bath water. The room should be pleasantly warm—at least 75° F. The bath water should feel comfortably warm to the wrist but not hot enough to sting. Supplies may include the following:

- Tub or lined sink containing warm water
- Padded area for washing and dressing baby
- Cotton balls
- Sterile water
- Cotton-covered swabs
- Mild soap (not a detergent)
- Mild shampoo (should not sting baby's eyes)
- Baby oil and hairbrush
- Clean towel and washcloth
- Two clean diapers (one may become soiled during dressing)
- Clean clothes and receiving blanket

Step 2   Clean the baby's eyes.

- Use a fresh cotton ball for each eye.
- Dip cotton ball in clean water.
- Wipe the eye area gently, beginning with the corner near the baby's nose and moving outward. Throw away the cotton ball.
- Repeat for the other eye using a clean cotton ball.

Step 3   Clean the baby's outer ear area.

- Use a fresh cotton-covered swab.
- Dip both ends in sterile water.

115

- Using one end of the swab, gently remove lint and dirt from the outer creases of the ear. Do *not* push swab into the ear hole, even if you can see wax.

- Clean the other ear using the other end of the swab.

- Throw away the used swab.

Step 4   Clean the baby's nose.

- Use a fresh cotton-covered swab.

- Dip both ends in sterile water.

- Gently remove lint and dirt from the opening of one nostril by twirling one end of the swab just under the baby's nose. Do *not* stick the end of the swab up into the baby's nostril. Any mucus ready to be released will be caught by the cotton.

- Use the other end of the swab to clean the other nostril.

- Throw away the used swab.

Step 5   Clean the baby's face.

- Use clear warm water to wet a folded washcloth and squeeze out the excess water.

- Beginning on the baby's forehead, make an S motion by moving the washcloth across the forehead, back across the top of the nose, down one cheek, and back under the baby's chin.

- Rinse the washcloth.

- Beginning on the other side of the baby's forehead, make a reverse S motion by moving the washcloth in the opposite direction across the forehead, over the baby's nose, down the other cheek, and under the chin.

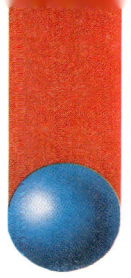

Step 6 Clean the baby's scalp (and hair, if any).

- Hold baby over tub or sink, cradling him or her in your arm with the head in the crook of your elbow. Gently wet the scalp using handfuls of water. Talk to the baby during this time and move slowly to prevent upsetting him or her.

- With the free hand, place a small amount of mild shampoo on baby's scalp. Set the shampoo bottle down.

- Rub the entire scalp slowly and gently with the fingertips. Do *not* use fingernails.

- Rinse the baby's scalp thoroughly, using handfuls of warm water. Rinse again.

- Dry the baby's hair and scalp with a towel, using a blotting motion.

Step 7 Undress the baby.

- Remove the baby's clothing slowly, being careful to pull the clothes away from the baby rather than pulling the baby away from the clothes.

- If the baby's diaper is soiled, clean the diaper area as you would for any diaper change before placing the baby in the bath water

Step 8 Bathe the baby's body.

- Test the water once more to make sure it is warm but not too hot. Only two to three inches of water in a small tub are necessary.

- Just before putting the baby into the water, pour a handful of water over the foot. This keeps the water from being a surprise.

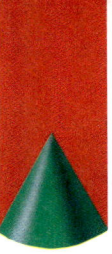

- Hold the baby, getting a firm grip on the far leg or arm, and lower the baby slowly into the water.

- Soap the baby with a mild soap.

- Be certain to wash the folds of the baby's skin where lint and bacteria can collect.

- Rinse the baby thoroughly so that no soap is left to cause skin irritation.

- Wrap the baby in a clean soft towel as soon as possible to prevent chilling.

- Blot the baby dry by pressing the towel gently over the skin. Rubbing will irritate the skin and may upset the baby.

Step 9   Put lotions, diaper, and clothing on baby.

- Oil scalp lightly with baby oil and brush all over scalp to remove any loose dry skin.

- Put lotion (or powder—not both) on the baby's body. Place the lotion or powder in your hand before transferring it to the baby.

- Diaper and dress the baby.

Never leave a baby alone during bathing—not even for a second. If you must look away from what you are doing for even a moment, place your hand firmly on the stomach so the baby cannot roll off the counter or table. Older babies may reach for objects around the bath area to play with. Parents need to be very alert to prevent injury.

Bath time can upset babies at first. Parents who move and talk gently to the baby during the bath reassure the baby and help bathing to be a pleasant time for both parents and the child.

CHAPTER 5
Growth and Development in Children Under Six

OBJECTIVES

When you have finished this chapter, you will be able to

- Identify examples of the principles of growth and development
- Explain how a child's relationship with people changes from birth until age six
- Describe the theories of personality, moral, and cognitive development
- Point out the differences in the development of infants, toddlers, and preschoolers
- Compile the changes in each kind of development to show how a child progresses
- Compare mental development with the changes in a child's curiosity

Jesse grew faster than Carlos and Maria had expected. It seemed as though every day he could do something new, and his parents found this exciting. Maria took lots of pictures so she could remember him as he was at each stage of his development. Carlos wondered what Jesse would be like as a schoolchild, an adolescent, and an adult. Maria and Carlos began to see that their parenting during the first six years would lay the foundation for Jesse's continued growth and development. What would the important accomplishments of this period be?

GROWTH AND DEVELOPMENT

Growth refers to increasing in size and becoming stronger. Development takes place as a result of growth and involves bringing together and advancing physical abilities, improving skills, and defining a personality. In other words, development refers to the processes involved in forming a unique person, an individual.

Principles of Growth and Development

Although each child is different, children's growth and development tend to follow patterns. The ways in which these patterns operate can be summarized as **principles of growth and development.**

GROWTH PROCEEDS FROM HEAD TO TAIL

The head and spinal area of each person develop before the arms, hands, legs, and feet. Note in Illustration 5-1 that the head of a newborn is about a fourth of the length of the body and the head of an adult is only about an eighth of the length of the body. A term sometimes used to describe growth that begins at the head and moves to the tail is **cephalocaudal development.**

GROWTH PROCEEDS FROM NEAR TO FAR

The principle that growth proceeds from near to far means that parts of the body in the torso or trunk area grow and begin to work before the extremities do. Another term for this pattern

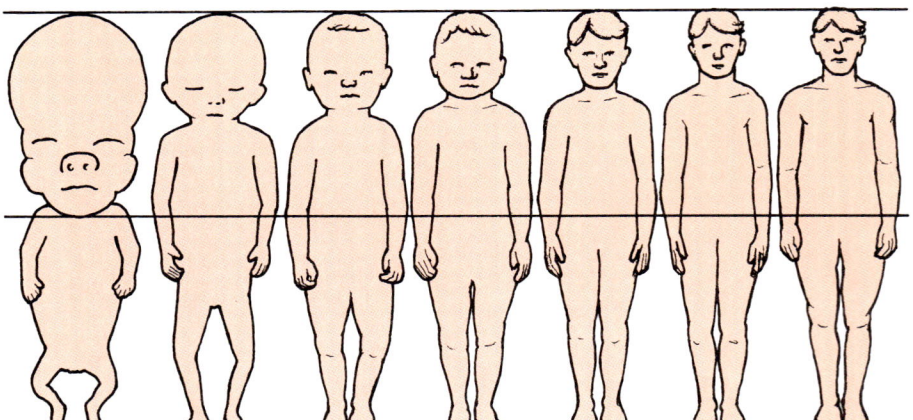

2 months   5 months   At birth   2 years   6 years   12 years   25 years
(fetus)   (fetus)

ILLUSTRATION 5-1   The change in body proportions from infancy to adulthood illustrates how growth begins in the head area and later proceeds through the rest of the body.

←— P R O X I M O D I S T A L —→

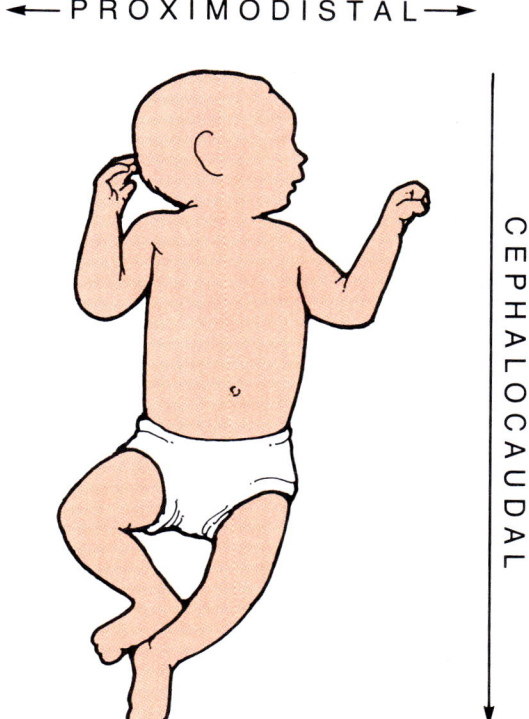

C E P H A L O C A U D A L

ILLUSTRATION 5-2
Cephalocaudal development proceeds from head to tail. Development of the head (cephalo) occurs before that of the rest of the body. The torso develops next, and finally the tail (caudal) area. Proximodistal development proceeds outwardly from the centerline of the body. Development occurs in the internal organs and trunk first and then in the extremities. Control of motor activity follows the proximodistal direction of development. The baby learns to twist the torso, then develops skills in the arm and leg muscles (gross motor areas) and finally in the fingers (fine motor area).

of growth is **proximodistal development.** Babies are able to use the large muscles in their legs and arms before they can use the small muscles in their hands. Illustration 5-2 shows the directions of cephalocaudal and proximodistal development.

GROWTH IS CONTINUOUS AND ORDERLY

The principle of **continuous and orderly growth** means, first, that growth is going on all the time, even though it may sometimes be difficult to perceive. Also, growth progresses in an orderly manner, which means that children will usually learn to do things in a particular sequence. In addition, growth is gradual. Children do not move from one stage to another suddenly.

During the first year most babies achieve physical milestones in the following order:

- Hold head up for a moment at first, then for longer periods
- Roll from side to back
- Roll from stomach to back
- Roll from back to stomach
- Sit with support
- Sit without support
- Crawl
- Pull to standing position
- Walk while hanging on to objects
- Crawl up (but not down) stairs or other objects
- Stand alone
- Walk

DEVELOPMENT PROCEEDS FROM SIMPLE TO COMPLEX

An example of **simple to complex development** involves the use of hands. At first babies are only able to wrap their fingers around objects. By the time they are about a year old, they can begin to hold objects in their hands and to use those objects to do something. For example, a one-year-old can scoop sand or bring food that has already been speared on a fork to his or her mouth.

By eighteen months most children can hold a marker or pencil and make marks on a surface. By age three these marks become dots, lines, and circles. Shortly thereafter, they begin to combine these basic forms into recognizable shapes, usually human-looking. By age five many children can draw simple pictures of objects around them.

Thus the child builds on his or her own physical growth and maturity in a progression. Developing increasingly complex abil-

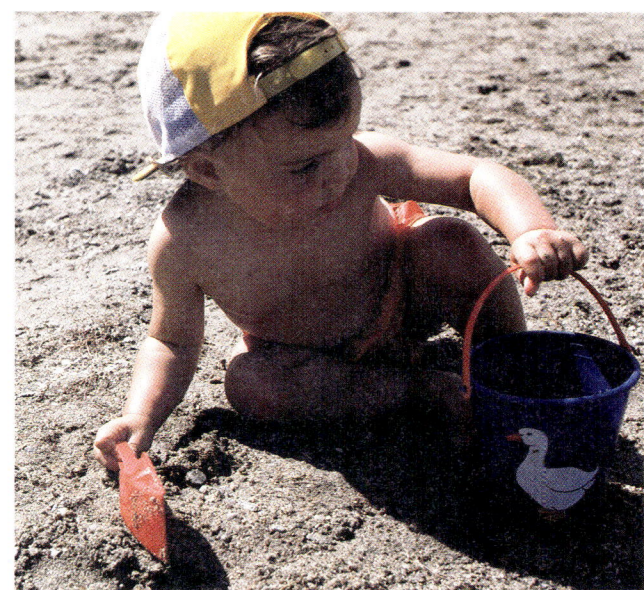

(a)

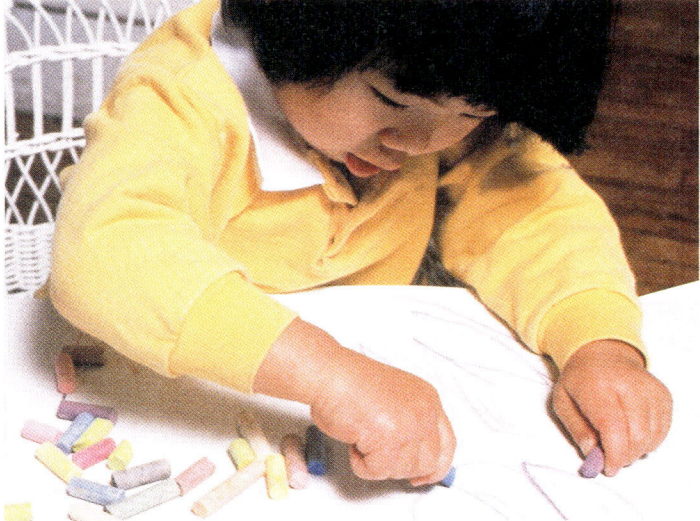

(b)

FIGURE 5-1 (a) A one-year-old can use his or her hands to do simple actions such as scooping sand with a toy shovel. (b) A three-year-old can use his or her hands to do more complex actions such as drawing lines and circles with chalk or crayons. This kind of sequence is an example of how development progresses from simple to complex.
Source: (a) © Erika Stone 1986   (b) © Laura Dwight

ities requires practice and patience. As children develop, parents observe their abilities becoming more complex.

KINDS OF DEVELOPMENT WORK TOGETHER

Early development affects later development. For example, a child needs to experience being wet before learning about how to talk about water. A child needs to feel the security of parental love before developing the courage to reach out to other people. Early development, then, is a foundation for later development.

The various types of development include the following:

- **Physical development** is reflected in changes in the body, in motor (muscle) abilities, and in coordination. This kind of development is usually what is meant when people refer to growth because physical changes are easily seen.

- **Emotional development** is reflected in children's feelings, especially feelings about themselves and their relationships with other people.

- **Social development** refers to learning to care for and to love people. It includes learning ways of getting along with others, such as discovering how and when to cooperate or compete.

- **Moral development** involves learning a sense of right and wrong.

- **Language and speech development** involves learning to communicate with other people.

- **Mental development,** or cognitive development, concerns how the child's mind moves from simple and partial ways of learning and solving problems to more complex and complete ways. Early thinking is tied to contact with the senses or the body's movements. This kind of thinking is called **sensorimotor thinking.** As a child matures, thinking that is not tied to the senses or movement takes place. This is called **abstract thinking.**

- **Spiritual development** means developing an awareness of life's meanings and gaining the personal strength necessary to live consistently with one's beliefs.

Each type of development affects the others. For example, children who are well developed physically tend to like themselves better. A positive self-concept aids emotional development.

Children who like themselves tend to be liked by other children, and their social development progresses well. Children who get along well with other children have people their own age to talk with, so they acquire more language skills and learn how society expects them to behave.

Although strong language skills help children learn other skills more easily, the reverse is also true. Children who do not have good language skills may not be able to make friends easily and so they may have poorer social skills and lower self-esteem. Children who have poor language skills may find difficulty in the areas of learning that are tied to the use of words.

As you can see, all forms of development are somewhat interdependent; that is, they affect one another and work together. Separating them in order to look more closely at each one is mainly done in order to get a clearer understanding of their total effect.

DEVELOPMENT REPEATS ITSELF

The tasks of development are faced in similar ways at various times in life but with different challenges. An example of a repeating and changing challenge is that of becoming independent. Toddlers assert themselves with their parents and insist on doing things for themselves. Another strong surge of independence comes in the early teens when children insist on beginning to make their own decisions. Young adults take another strong step in independence when they become more emotionally independent of their parents. Thus, developing independence occurs at many stages in life, but each time in a unique way and with different tasks to accomplish.

Nature versus Nurture

Do parents and other caregivers need to help development along, or do children progress well enough if they are just left alone? People who think children need encouragement to reach their full potential believe that nurturing is more important. Those who believe children develop best if adults do not interfere too much think that nature is more important. The Something to Think About feature deals with this issue.

Theories of Development

When people who study children look at growth and development, they sometimes try to define how children change with

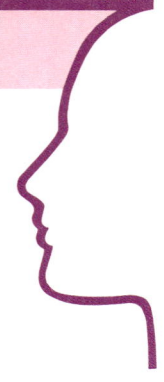

Something to Think About

Should Parents and Caregivers Intervene in Children's Development?

Intervening in a child's development involves providing the child with every possible opportunity to reach his or her potential. Some people believe children have much more potential than is usually developed at home or even in school. They believe that the role of caring adults is to step in and intercede in each child's behalf. They believe that concentrating effort on helping children develop will enable them to move ahead faster and be more competitive. Intervening centers on a child's performance. Some parents and caregivers can push children too much. Putting pressure on children can result in serious problems.

Allowing a young child to grow in whatever way he or she chooses and to enjoy casually whatever play seems appealing is the opposite of intervening. People who follow this approach see intervening as interfering with children's lives and intruding on their development. They believe that children can find the best way for themselves. This approach can also be carried too far—when children are ignored or not given guidance when they need it.

Is some intervening good for children, giving them useful assistance in their development? Does too much intervening pressure children into feeling tense? Does intervening overlook children's individual personalities by trying to make all develop in a certain way? To what extent should parents and caregivers intervene? What do you think?

age. These professionals are usually interested in describing a particular type of development. Often they establish **stages of development** to describe the characteristics of different age groups. They may produce a **theory of development,** a statement or set of statements intended to explain how a particular type of development progresses.

PERSONALITY DEVELOPMENT

It may take most of your life to develop a clear understanding of who you are as an individual. Erik Erikson maintained that developing a personal identity was one of the most important tasks of a human being.[1] He proposed that people go through eight stages during a lifetime as they attempt to discover and establish a personal identity. Each stage represents a crisis necessary to the development of a healthy personality. When one crisis is successfully handled, the person is better able to face the next. If a person does not successfully meet the challenge of one crisis, moving on to the next will be more difficult.

MORAL DEVELOPMENT

Learning about rules and how to treat other people in relation to those rules is the focus of Lawrence Kohlberg's theory of moral development.[2] During early childhood, understanding of what is right and wrong is mainly based on whether the child expects to be rewarded or punished for a given behavior. Older children begin to develop a concept of fairness. Both of these stages are part of Kohlberg's preconventional period of moral development.

COGNITIVE DEVELOPMENT

The recognized leader in the study of children's mental development was Jean Piaget, who is the subject of this chapter's Leadership at a Glance feature.

Piaget proposed four stages of cognitive development. (Cognitive refers to the way people take in and process information, or think.) These stages are summarized in Table 5-1.

Ages and Stages

Do all children go through the same stages of development at exactly the same age? The answer is no. Children tend to follow the same order, or sequence, of development. They do not, however, develop at the same speed; that is, they do not have the same **rate of development.** What developmental characteristics, then, do children have in common if they are all developing differently?

Children under six are usually grouped into three general categories: infants, toddlers, and preschoolers. **Infants** are babies

---

[1]Erik H. Erikson, *Childhood and Society* (New York, NY: W. W. Norton, 1986).

[2]Lawrence Kohlberg, *The Psychology of Moral Development* (New York, NY: Harper & Row, 1984).

Leadership at a Glance

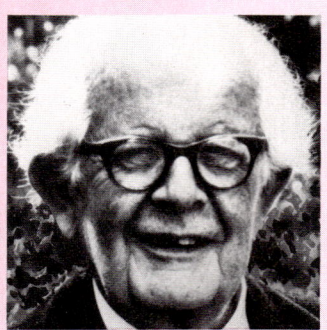

Source: The Bettmann Archive

Jean Piaget

Jean Piaget was born in 1896 in Switzerland and died there in 1980. He is now appreciated throughout the world for developing a theory about how children's thinking develops. Although he was trained in psychology, he considered himself to be more of a philosopher. He founded a school in Geneva, Switzerland, where scholars from different disciplines could work together and exchange ideas.

Piaget developed experimental games that were designed to find out what children know and how they think. He spent many hours observing his own children. As they grew, he observed that the way they used their minds changed. He expanded his study to include many other children and later developed his theory of cognitive development.

It is difficult for most Americans to read Piaget's original writings because he wrote in French. However, many books interpreting his work have been written. College students who study education or psychology learn a great deal about what Piaget thought. His work has had a great deal of influence on early childhood education.

from birth until they are nearly able to walk, which usually occurs around age one. **Toddlers** are young children who are just beginning to walk. Toddlerhood ends when children can walk and talk fairly well, usually at about age three. Children from three to about six years old are called **preschoolers**.

■ INFANTS

People grow more and change faster during the first year of life than at any other time. Healthy babies triple their birth weight during the first year. They proceed from being totally helpless to being able to get into everything in sight. When life

TABLE 5-1 Piaget's Four Stages of Cognitive Development

Stage (Age)	Definition	Characteristics
1. Sensorimotor (0–2 years)	Children process information mostly through their senses and their own movements.	Children learn they can make things happen by their movements. They discover that objects do not cease to exist when they can no longer see them. They learn that some objects and people can be controlled. They imitate actions of caregivers.
2. Preoperational (2–7 years)	Children are making a transition from thinking based on senses and movements to logical thinking.	Children find it difficult to see situations from another's viewpoint. They find it difficult to understand that something that has changed can again be like it was before the change. They sometimes draw conclusions after seeing only the details and not the whole picture. They have difficulty understanding how things change, especially in understanding what happens in the midst of a transition.
3. Concrete operations (7–11 years)	Children begin to think logically.	Children do not have the limitations of the preschool child. They can think about how objects are related to each other. They can classify items into groups, deciding which should be included and which should not. They know the number of objects stays the same when arranged differently. They can count items and arrange them in order in a series. They can shift from their own viewpoint to another person's and back to their own. They become aware of their own thinking process and see themselves and others as thinkers.
4. Formal operations (11 + years)	Children can think about ideas and events they have not directly experienced.	Children think about their own thoughts. They compare real things to possible things or ideas. They think about possibilities for the future and plan. They follow logic of an argument even when they do not agree.

Source: H. Ginsburg and S. Opper, Piaget's Theory of Intellectual Development, 2nd ed. (Englewood Cliffs, NJ: Prentice-Hall, 1979).

goes well, they develop a secure attachment to their parents. They figure out that when something disappears from sight, it has not actually ceased to exist.

Parents and other interested adults usually spend a great deal of time watching babies learn to do new things, cheering them on, and comparing one baby with another. It is important to remember that normal, healthy babies learn at their own rate, when their muscles and nervous systems are ready. **Maturation** is the term that describes the process of development in which the child's muscles and nervous system get ready to learn. The state of being ready to learn is called **readiness.**

A baby may do things either much earlier or much later than other babies and still be normal. Although it is important to encourage babies and to give them opportunities to learn something new, it is unfair to push them or to compare them to other children. Also, when parents take too much credit for what babies do, the parents' needs are being put ahead of the baby's needs.

Birth Through the Third Month

The first three months are a period of adjustment, as the child makes the transition from life in the uterus to an independent life outside the mother.

PHYSICAL ABILITIES

Full-term newborn babies begin life weighing between 6 and 9 pounds and measuring 19 to 22 inches in length. They clench their fists tightly and sneeze and cough readily. Their arm and leg movements are somewhat jerky and their jaws may tremble. Breathing is shallow and irregular. They cry when they have needs.

Shortly after birth, healthy babies are able to hold their heads up for only a moment. By the end of the third month, they have learned to hold their heads up steadily and move them in a controlled manner. Their hands are mostly open, and they spend a lot of time simply watching their own hands move. They have greater strength than they did at birth.

LANGUAGE

A baby's first language is crying. Babies between birth and three months of age become quiet when they hear rhythmic

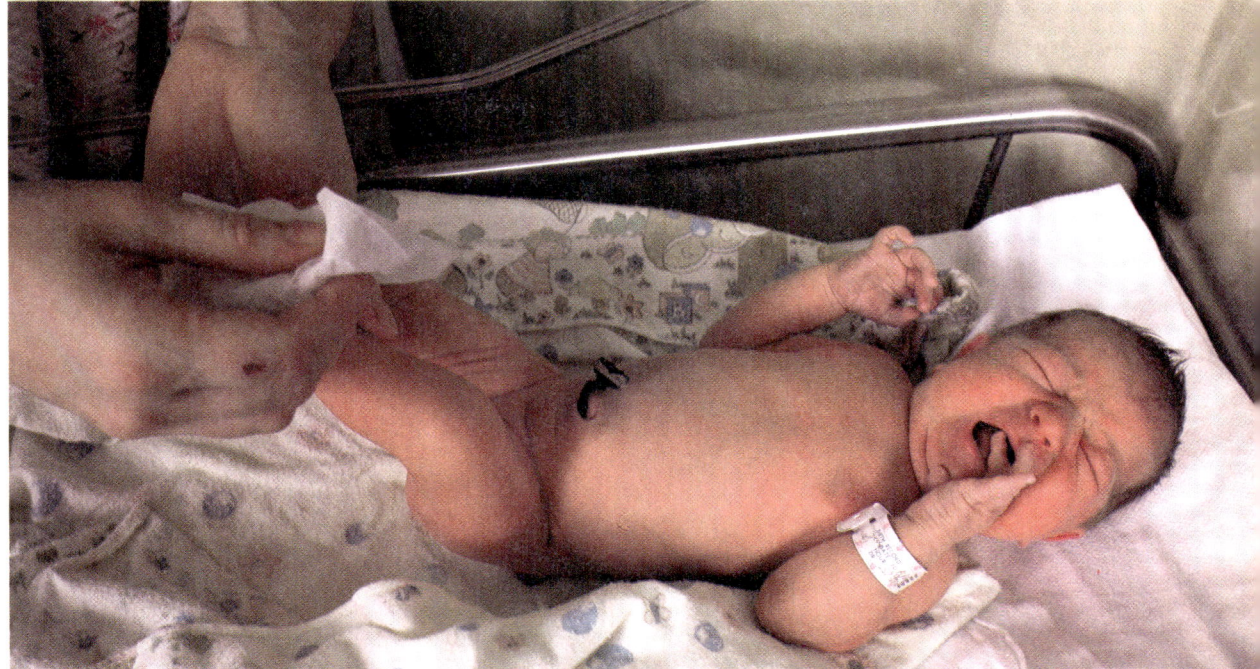

FIGURE 5-2   A newborn cries to express needs and may move arms and legs jerkily.
Source: © Larry Mulvehill/Photo Researchers, Inc.

sounds. By three months they become quiet when they hear someone approaching. During this period infants pay attention to voices. Crying has different meanings—it may tell the parents that the baby is tired, hungry, angry, or lonely.

By the end of the third month, infants begin to coo. **Cooing** is made up of sounds that are mostly vowels or vowel-sounding utterances. An **utterance** is something a baby "says"—a sound or group of sounds that may or may not resemble words. Examples of cooing sounds are "o-o-h," "a-a-h," and "u-u-h." When a baby is spoken to, he or she listens and tries to make a sound in return. By the third month many babies engage in regular and expressive conversations with caregivers.

MENTAL DEVELOPMENT

By three months most babies show an interest in objects, reach for things, and react to the disappearance of a face.

RELATIONSHIPS WITH PEOPLE

Babies up to three months old not only recognize their parents, they watch them as they move about the room. They usually respond in a special way to their mothers. By the end of the third month, they smile almost anytime someone smiles at or speaks to them.

When babies start to "talk," they want caregivers to stop and listen. When they stop vocalizing and look at the other person, they are ready for that person to begin talking. Talking with babies helps them learn to interact and is a necessary beginning for their own language development. **Interacting** means taking turns listening and talking to one another, while giving special attention to the other person.

The Fourth Through the Sixth Month

During the fourth, fifth, and sixth months, babies gain even more strength and show a variety of developmental changes.

PHYSICAL ABILITIES

Four-month-old babies are waving their arms, usually together. They move legs alternately with a great deal of energy. They figure out how to roll over—first from side to stomach, then from stomach to back, and finally from back to stomach. They

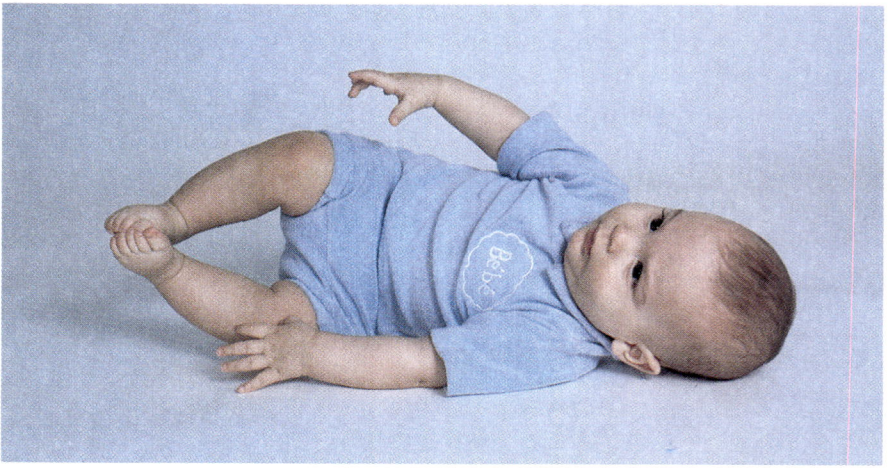

FIGURE 5-3 At about four months of age, babies begin to roll over.
Source: © Erika Stone 1980

learn to sit up with support, but most will not sit up independently until later.

LANGUAGE

From four to six months of age, babies begin to respond to the sound of their own name, and they react to tone of voice. Their vocalizing changes from cooing to **babbling.** Babbling is similar to cooing except that the sounds usually begin with consonants. Examples are "pa," "ta," and "de."

MENTAL DEVELOPMENT

Four-month-old babies can identify strangers. They love to play peek-a-boo and enjoy play that involves movement. However, it is important not to frighten the baby or to play too rough. Shaking and tossing can cause serious injury and can lead to mental retardation or even death.

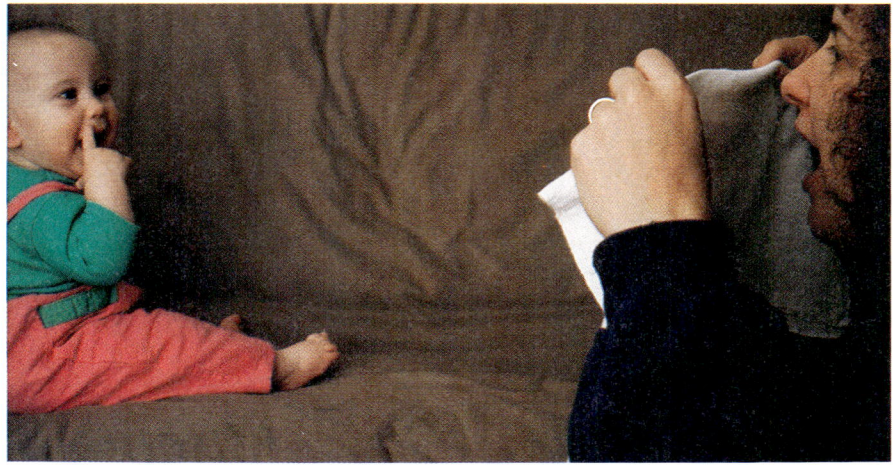

FIGURE 5-4   Peek-a-boo is a favorite game of many infants between four and six months old.
Source: © Laura Dwight

RELATIONSHIPS WITH PEOPLE

Babies of this age are usually very friendly and like to be with people. They show a clear preference for their parents, but most will allow others to hold them for a time without fussing. They giggle and laugh aloud. When placed in front of a mirror, they touch their fingers to the image. By six months they usually smile at and vocalize with their mirror image.

The Seventh Through the Ninth Month

Babies between seven and nine months old are going through a period of expansion and attachment. They learn to crawl, imitate sounds, and discover they can make things happen.

FIGURE 5-5   From about six months on, babies interact with their images in mirrors.
Source: © Ken Horii/International Stock Photography

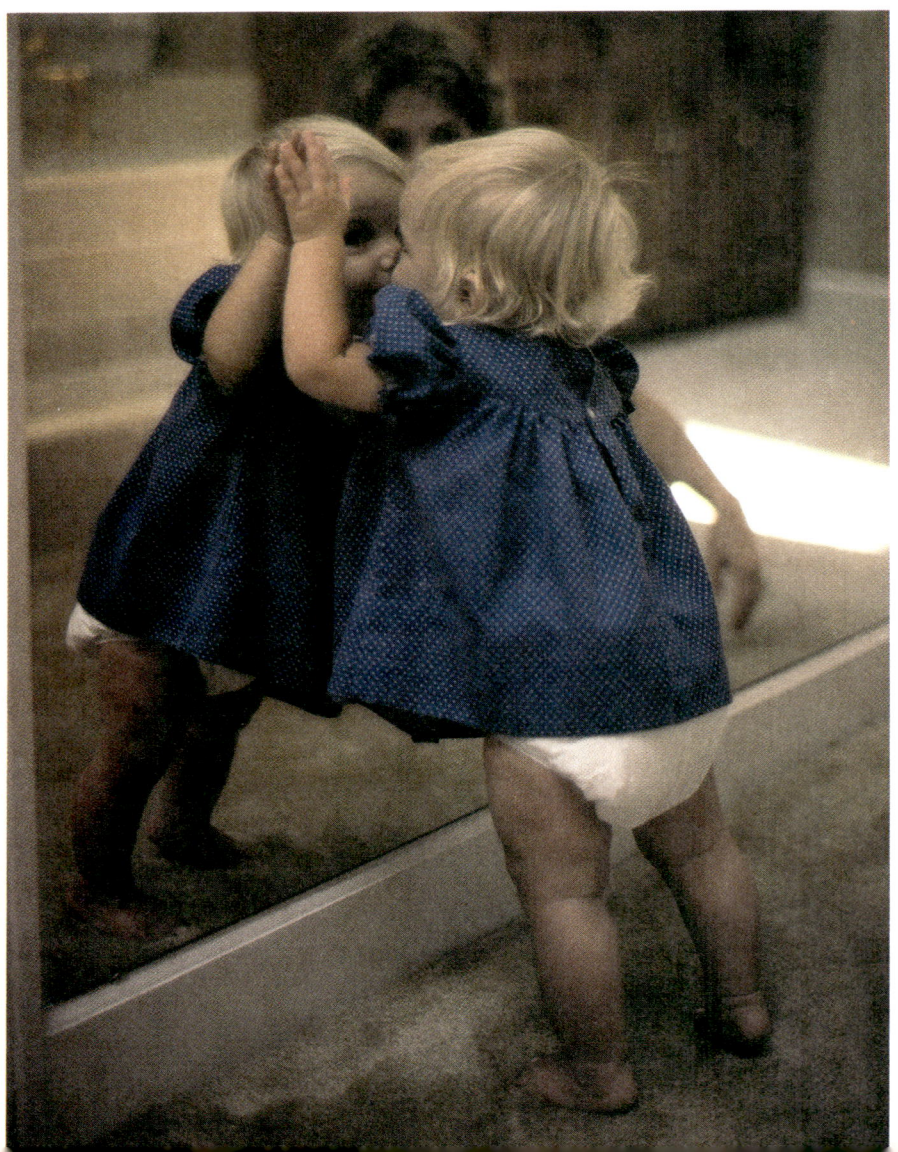

PHYSICAL ABILITIES

Sometime between the seventh and ninth month, babies begin to move around fairly well on their own. They are able to sit without support for several minutes at a time, and they have learned to crawl, which greatly expands their world by giving them more ability to explore it. They are both excited and anxious about this newfound ability. During this period babies also learn to pull themselves into a standing position and may walk by holding onto furniture or other convenient objects.

LANGUAGE

Between the seventh and the ninth month, babies begin to point to and pick up objects and show them. They are preoccupied

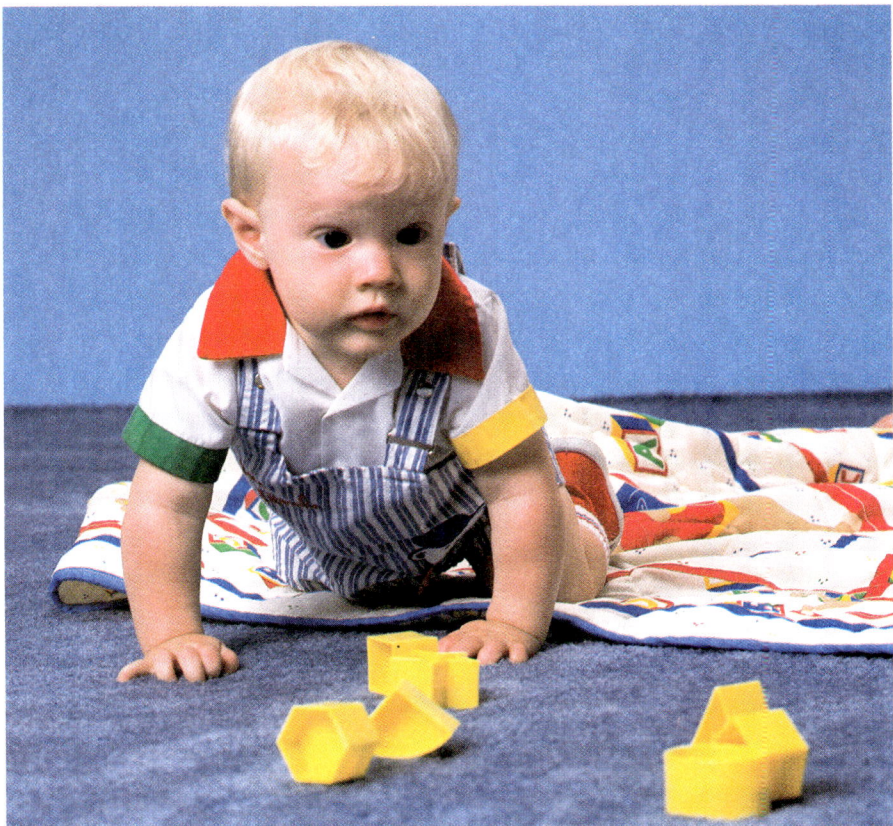

FIGURE 5-6   Seven-month-olds usually love to explore their surroundings by crawling, but may feel a bit anxious about doing this.

with sounds and try to imitate speech sounds. This imitation is called **echolalia.** Their speech develops a languagelike sound. As they babble and imitate sounds, their tone sounds conversational even though their words are not recognizable. They respond to some words spoken by adults. When children understand speech, they have developed **receptive language.** Most babies utter their first recognizable word in the eighth or ninth month. Surprisingly, it is often a word for father, such as "pa-pa" or "da-da." Soon other familiar words are added, such as "ma-ma," "baby," and "bye." They respond to the word "no." When babies form words purposefully, they have developed **productive language.**

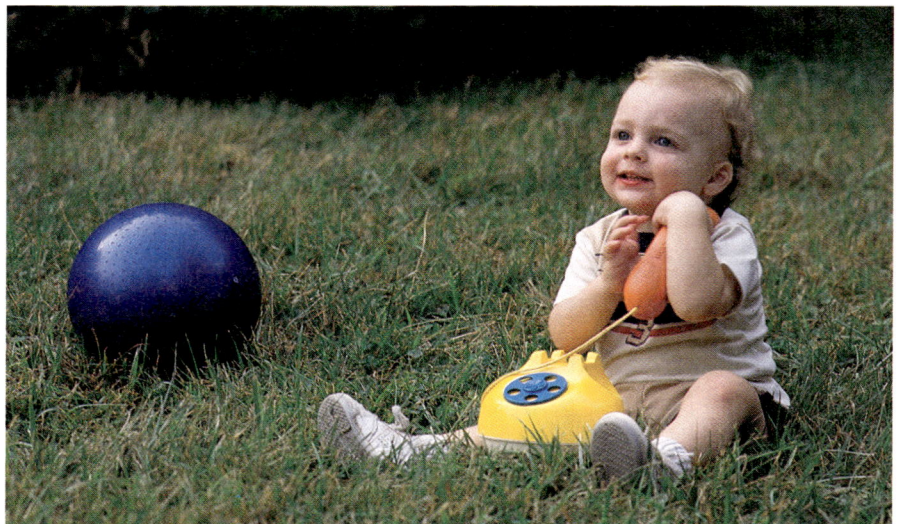

FIGURE 5-7   Most young children start to say recognizable words when they are about eight or nine months old.

MENTAL DEVELOPMENT

Babies between six and nine months old figure out that they can cause things to happen. A favorite game might be called "Drop the Toy." As soon as the toy hits the floor, the baby gestures for the adult to retrieve it. Then the baby drops it again. This sequence may be repeated again and again and again.

RELATIONSHIPS WITH PEOPLE

By the eighth month, most babies have become securely attached to their primary caregiver, usually their mother. This secure attachment enables them to feel comfortable exploring their environment when the caregiver is close by.

A baby can be attached to more than one person but will have preferences for one over another. For example, when a grandparent picks up an infant at a child care center, the infant cheerfully waves good-bye to the caregiver, although he or she has stuck close to that person during the day. Then, when grandparent and child get home and the baby sees mom or dad, only one of them will do. A baby's preferences can change, but there is always one adult, usually a parent, to whom the infant is most securely attached.

Along with their secure attachment, at this age babies develop **stranger anxiety.** They frequently react with displeasure to people they do not know and cling to more familiar people. This reaction to strangers can be quite strong and sometimes even includes grandparents. Some children continue reacting negatively to strangers until they are three or even older.

The Tenth Through the Twelfth Month

Babies between ten and twelve months old begin to move about on their feet rather than on their hands and knees. They generally start saying a few important words.

PHYSICAL ABILITIES

Babies between ten and twelve months old learn to climb—usually well before they can walk. They can climb high enough to hurt themselves if they fall, so they must be watched *all the time.* Many babies will learn to walk during this period—first with someone holding both their hands, then with someone holding one hand, then alone.

LANGUAGE

At this age babies begin to add words to their vocabulary. First words are those that represent something that means a great deal to the baby, such as "bye-bye," "go," and "mine."

MENTAL DEVELOPMENT

Babies this age have an insatiable **curiosity,** or desire to know. They are eager to learn, and their new power to move about drives them to explore. Parents have to learn to exercise enough discipline to establish their authority and keep the baby safe while at the same time allowing them to learn by satisfying their curiosity.

RELATIONSHIPS WITH PEOPLE

By this age babies usually have clear preferences for some people. They usually don't like anyone other than family members

FIGURE 5-8   Clinging to one's mother when faced with an unfamiliar person is common behavior in one-year-olds.

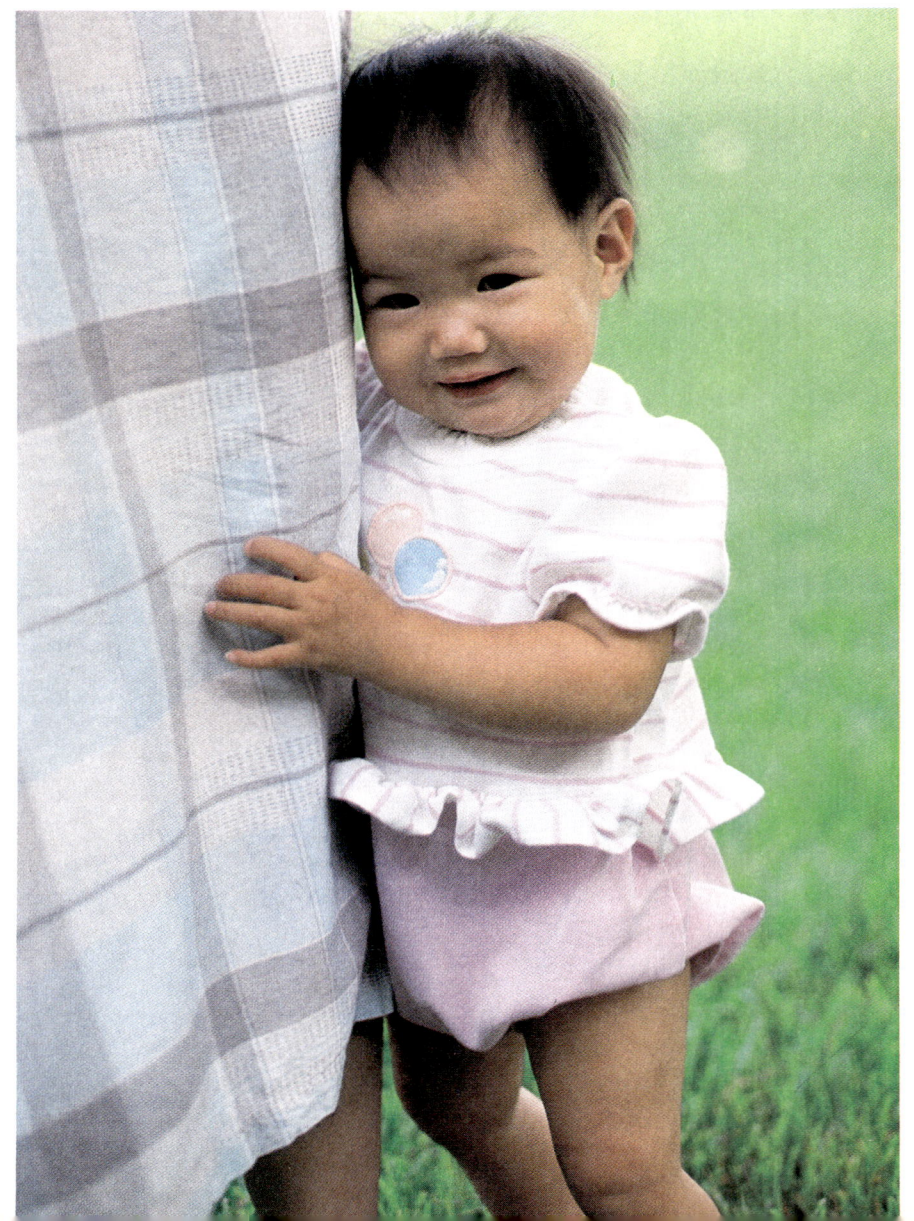

and regular caregivers. Even among those persons they have and express preferences—sometimes for their fathers over their mothers, or vice versa. Usually this is temporary. Parents who are patient and available usually find that their child's preference will shift from one parent to the other over time.

TODDLERS

Toddlers are children between one and three years of age. During this period there are incredible changes in children's physical abilities, language skills, thinking, and relationships with people.

Dr. Burton White has spent a great deal of time studying toddlers. He emphasizes the importance of toddlers' growing curiosity.[3] Curiosity is what makes them want to learn. One-year-olds are very excited about a world new to them and filled with things to explore. They are not aware of many dangers and explore just to learn. They are like small sponges soaking up every possible piece of information. These children are interested in their parents and in small objects. They touch everything and bring things to their mouths if they can. They love water and will play in it for as long as they are permitted.

Children between 14 and 24 months old begin to manipulate objects to see what they can make them do. This period is one of exploration for the sake of gaining information and is marked by trial and error. Toddlers are frustrated by abilities they have not yet mastered, yet they have an intense desire to do things for themselves. The danger is that discipline will be either severe enough to destroy the toddler's curiosity or inadequate.

Children need adult help to learn self-control. They need an authority figure. If there is not enough discipline, they lack direction and can become overstimulated. Achieving a balance between encouraging curiosity and providing discipline is one of the most difficult tasks of parenthood, yet such a balance needs to be successfully established during the child's second year of life.

Toddlers between 24 and 36 months old are often referred to as **twos.** During this time curiosity causes the child to investigate

---

[3]From notes taken on lectures by Burton White at University of Northern Colorado, Greeley, June 1982 and at Parenting Infants and Toddlers Conference, Houston, February 1983.

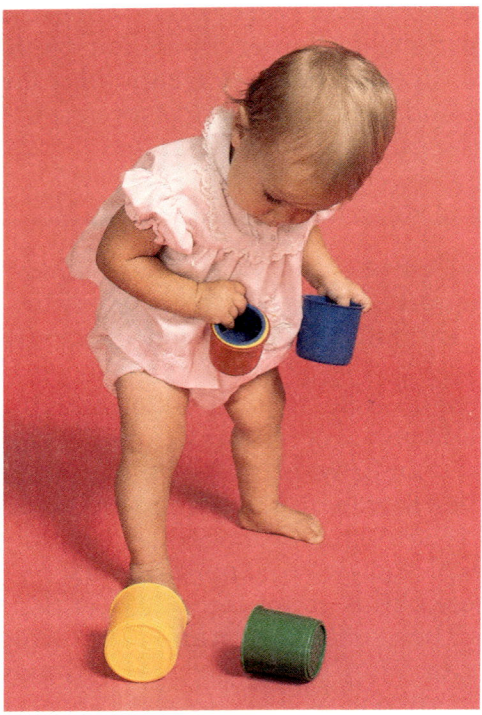

FIGURE 5-9
Manipulating objects to see what can be done with them is one of the ways toddlers explore their environment.
Source: © Erika Stone 1986

more complex parts of the world. Twos begin to construct and create from what they learn through imitating during play.

Physical Abilities

Toddlers begin as babies who can barely walk. By the time they are three they are running, jumping, and climbing everywhere. At one year old they use the muscles in the hand well enough to pick up small objects between finger and thumb. By three they can hold a pencil and use it. At one year of age they are quite clumsy. By three they are well coordinated enough to manage fairly complicated activities, such as pouring, throwing, catching, and changing directions abruptly while running.

During their second year (between the first and second birthdays), toddlers gain the strength and coordination to walk and climb successfully. They develop enough control in their hands to work simple puzzles and stack a few blocks.

During their third year (between the second and third birthdays), toddlers gain enough coordination to run, throw, catch, and jump. They can control their hands well enough to draw lines, dots, and circles.

Language

One-year-old toddlers speak only a few words. They understand more than they can say. Their language focuses on what is going on around them in the present. They rarely talk about people or things that are not in sight. By age three toddlers can

FIGURE 5-10 Three-year-olds are good at and enjoy climbing.
Source: © Erika Stone 1989

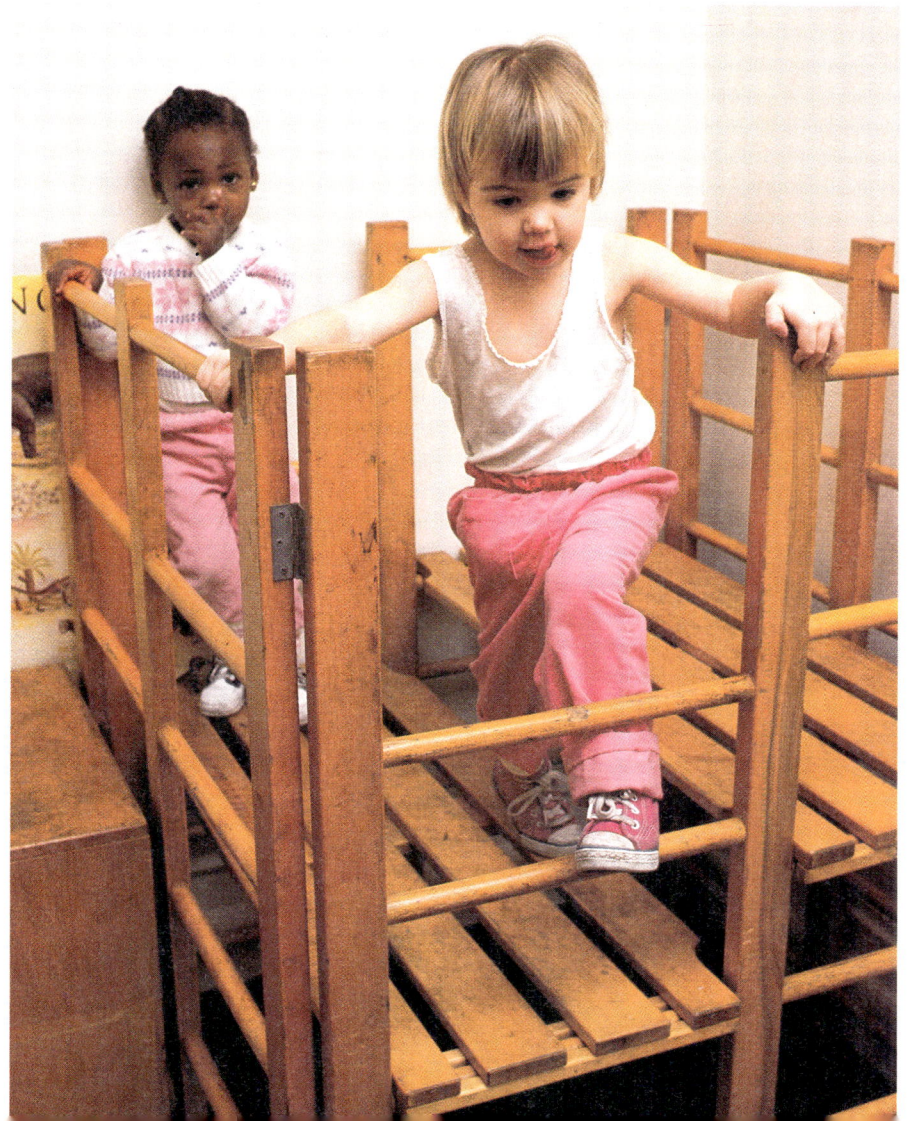

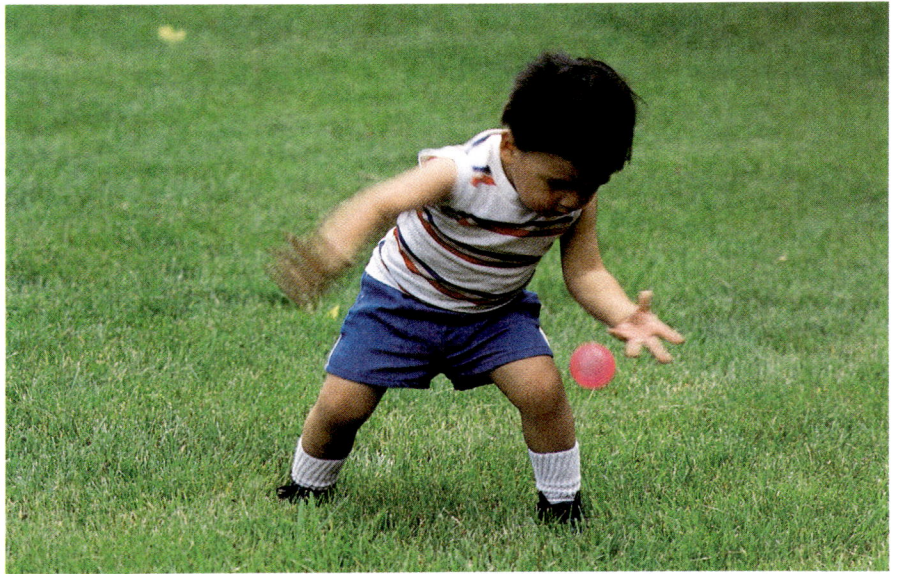

FIGURE 5-11   A toddler may be able to catch a ball by age three.

speak in understandable sentences and comprehend most of the words they hear. They can talk in simple terms about past events or people who are not present. They also have begun to understand that some recognizable signs always mean the same thing. For example, they may recognize labels on favorite food products or signs over places they enjoy.

During their second year toddlers begin to express opinions, make requests, and indicate desires. They speak in simple sentences.

By the end of the third year, most toddlers can speak clearly enough to be understood most of the time. Older toddlers take part in conversations and begin to talk about the world around them. Their vocabulary builds to about a thousand words. They begin to recognize some letters of the alphabet, especially those in their own name or other familiar words.

Mental Development

Piaget's work suggests that during the toddler years children grow a great deal mentally. Toddlers progress from simply attacking barriers to experimenting to find solutions. This process is called **trial-and-error learning.** Eventually the toddler learns to utilize solutions to old problems by applying them to new ones.

Before babies are a year old they will look for objects that have disappeared. By fifteen months they can find something that has disappeared if they have watched it being hidden. By two years most can find it even when they haven't seen it being hidden if they are given a clue.

Toddlers are also extremely interested in cause and effect. Very small babies repeat actions on purpose. For example, they notice the noise made by a rattle and shake it again to get the same result.

By the time they begin the toddler years, children are playing simple games that allow them to experience cause and effect. They sometimes learn how to manipulate their parents to do things for them. By the time they are two, they begin to think about possible consequences before doing something. This suggests that they understand that an action causes a result and that they are able to do some simple thinking.

Toddlers become experts at imitating. When they are only a year old, they often copy what others are doing right in front of them. They learn a great deal by imitating, and by age three they sometimes imitate behavior observed a day or two earlier. Imitation can be very detailed and accurate by age three.

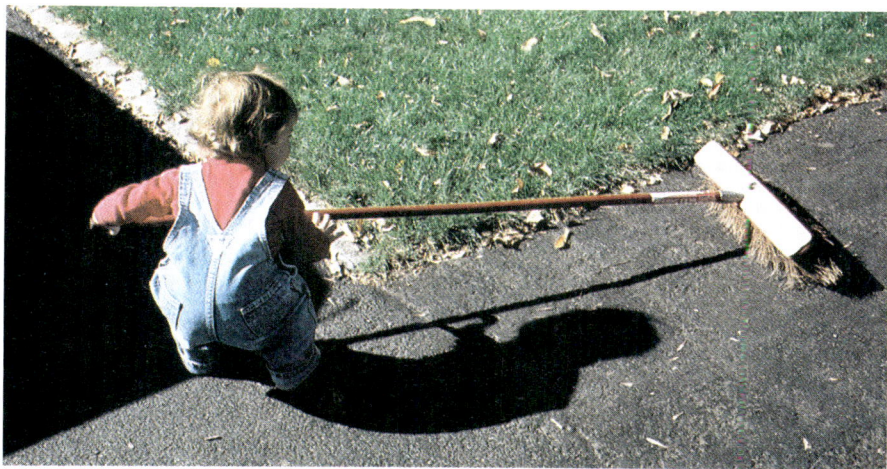

FIGURE 5-12   Toddlers learn a great deal by trying to imitate things adults do, such as sweeping.
Source: © Laura Dwight

Toddlers also register their opinions and show preferences. They can say sentences like "I want a cookie." They draw attention to themselves or to an object by pointing to or showing the object. A favorite gesture is shaking the head negatively; they learn to say "no" and may use the word often. They begin to make requests with gestures and then with words.

Most one-year-olds will do the following:

- Solve simple problems
- Understand that some actions cause other actions
- Imitate other people
- Explore everything and show very powerful curiosity
- Learn by trial and error and enjoy experimenting

Two-year-olds will generally do the following:

- Solve more complicated problems
- Build simple structures from blocks
- Begin simple role play
- Imitate actions seen earlier

Relationships with People

Toddlers rely a great deal on their caregivers. They use these familiar adults as a secure base from which to explore. They look to them as consultants to answer their questions and to guide their behavior. Toddlers alternately hang on to and push away from the important adults in their lives. They seem to be trying to make up their minds about whether they want to be dependent and protected like infants or independent and self-directed like older children.

By 30 months ($2\frac{1}{2}$ years) toddlers have gained more confidence and usually have become more relaxed around other people. They start to become interested in other children.

During their second year toddlers continue to develop a more secure relationship with their parents, while avoiding contact with strangers. During their third year they become more at ease with people outside the family. They may take on a role in which they express opinions, protest, and exert their own personality.

Sense of Self

Toddlers are also developing a sense of self. They have a strong desire to control themselves and everything around them, including their parents. Although it is important for parents to use the word "no," as little as possible, those who cannot say it to a toddler when necessary may find that the child has trouble developing self-control.

The toddler years are a time of learning to do simple self-care tasks. Small children become afraid and confused when they tackle more than they can handle. When toddlers can't make things work the way they want them to, they sometimes become frustrated and angry. The result is a temper tantrum. **A temper tantrum** is an outburst of emotion, sometimes spontaneous and sometimes intentional, in which a child may cry expressively, kick, throw things, bite, or bang his or her head against something.

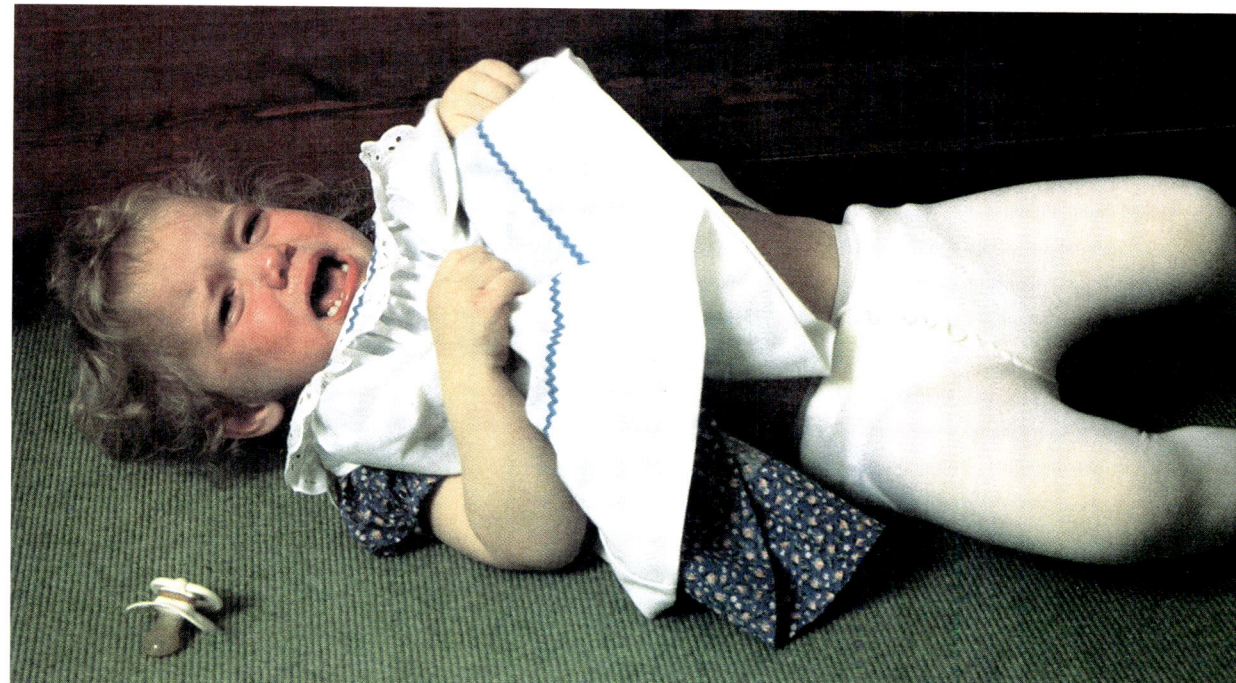

FIGURE 5-13   Temper tantrums are most often caused by toddlers' feelings of frustration because they can't do something they want to do.
Source: © Mimi Cotter/International Stock Photography

During the second year the child's growing sense of self is demonstrated in these ways:

■ The child assists in self-care tasks, such as washing hands.

■ He or she feeds self with a spoon.

■ He or she begins toileting (bowel and bladder control).

During the third year the child's sense of self exhibits its growing strength in further ways:

■ The child feeds self with a fork.

■ He or she does simple self-care tasks such as hand washing alone.

■ He or she understands some familiar signs.

■ He or she follows a set of simple directions.

■ He or she helps an adult to pick up toys.

PRESCHOOLERS

Preschoolers are children between the ages of three and six. During this period they are busy building physical skills, developing their imaginations, and learning the basics of living with other people.

Physical Abilities

Growth slows down during the preschool years. The breathing rate and the heartbeat become slower and steadier. Physically, preschoolers grow from about 32 to about 45 pounds and may add 10 to 12 inches to their height. At age three children average just over three feet in height; by age six they may be four feet tall. When children are about five, their nerve fibers become coated with a fatty substance that helps them react faster and more accurately.

Time spent in play helps preschoolers to improve coordination and to gain physical skills. Gaining these skills helps children develop a good feeling about themselves and get ready for the elementary years.

Three-year-olds have these physical abilities:

- They can run smoothly, speeding up and slowing down.
- They can turn curves easily.
- They can alternate feet when going up and down stairs.
- They begin to give up the daytime nap and sleep longer at night.
- They carry containers without spilling.
- They can ride a tricycle.

Four-year-olds add several more abilities:

- They can throw a ball.
- They are able to hop, skip, and stand on one foot.
- They pour from one container to another.

Five-year-olds can generally do these things:

- They show greater control over motor activity.
- They use skates, sleds, wagons, and scooters.

Language

During the preschool years language becomes very important. Vocabulary increases rapidly. Preschoolers talk not only about what they are doing at the moment but also about events that happened somewhere else or people who are not present. By age six most children can pronounce most of the sounds used in their own language. Most are familiar enough with letters to identify them by name.

A three-year-old is usually able to do the following:

- Listen to a story
- Tell a simple story
- Sing simple songs and recite nursery rhymes
- Learn his or her name, address, and telephone number
- Use new words, including verbs and pronouns

A four-year-old is generally able to do the following:

- Use a vocabulary of about two thousand words
- Use and justify direct requests such as "Stop! That hurts."
- Learn that words have power and perhaps use words of which adults do not approve
- Experiment with rhythms and rhymes
- Use all parts of speech

Most five-year-olds can do the following:

- Print first name without help
- Define simple words

Curiosity

When parents and other caregivers do a good job of balancing discipline and curiosity during the toddler years, children's curiosity continues to motivate them to learn. Three-year-olds can ask two or three hundred questions every day. Sometimes they ask the same question over and over. Preschoolers are eager to learn. They are particularly interested in language and can readily learn a second language during these years.

Mental Development

Preschool children can think well enough to be logical in parts but not in a whole solution. Piaget called this the preoperational period of mental development. (Preoperational means prelogical.) Most of their thinking centers around their own thoughts about their world. They cannot understand how other people think about things. Yet their own thinking becomes rapidly more developed.

A three-year-old will usually do these things:

- Construct simple objects from blocks
- Draw lines, circles, and dots (An early drawing is often of the head. Arms, legs, and a body are added with experience. By the end of the fourth year some objects may be recognizable.)
- May begin to print a few capital letters
- Begin to cut with scissors

A four-year-old is generally able to do the following:

- Begin to know the difference between real and pretend
- Exercise his or her imagination
- Draw a person with two or three parts and a house
- May copy letters or simple words

FIGURE 5-14 A five- or six-year-old may be able to print his or her first name.

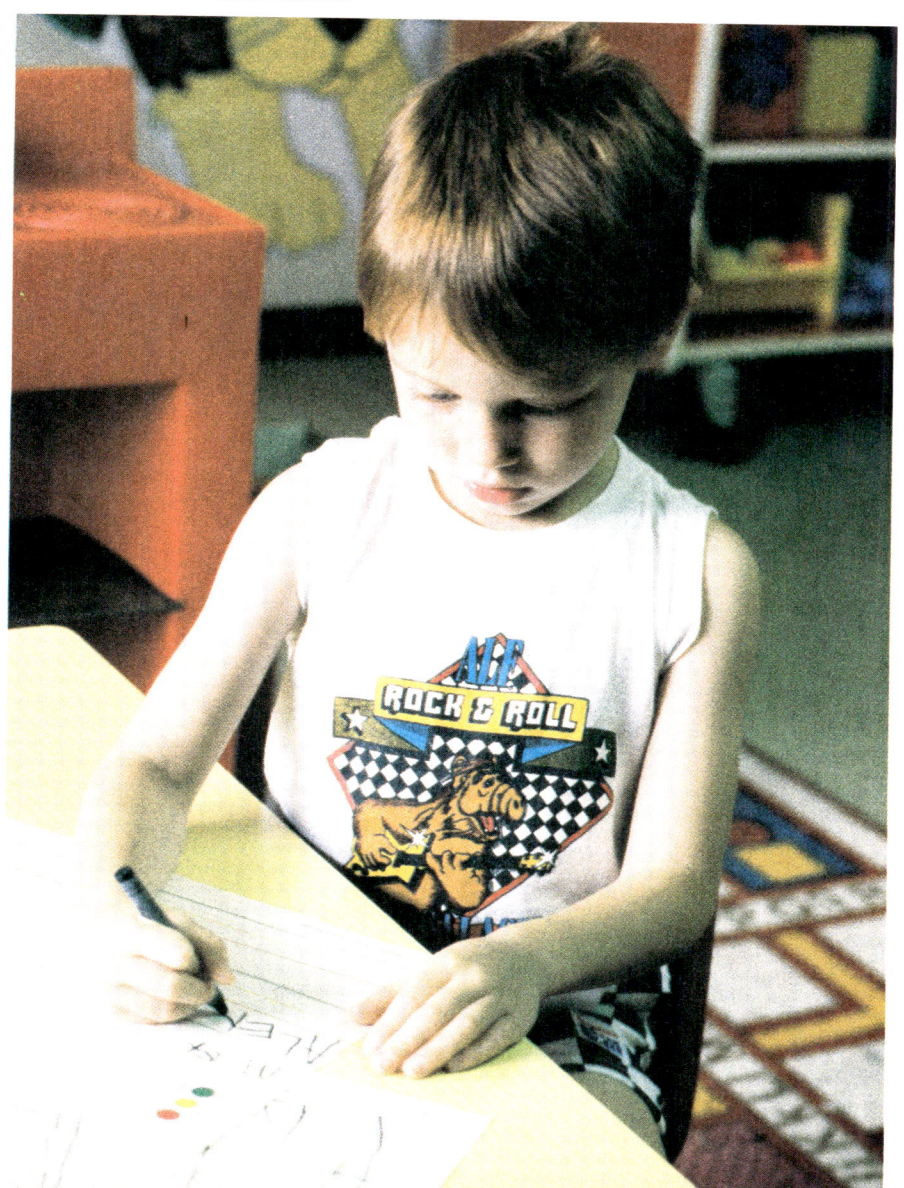

A five-year-old can often do these things:

- Figure out some problems independently
- Begin to develop judgment
- Draw recognizable person with head, trunk, legs, arms, and facial features and a simple house with doors, windows, roof, and chimney
- May print first name in recognizable large letters. (The letters may be reversed.)

Relationships with People

Preschoolers learn to enjoy **peers,** other children their own age. For a while their attention is often focused on the parent of the opposite sex.

Children begin to get an idea about why they are disciplined and what behavior receives adults' approval. For these years children's beliefs about right and wrong are based mostly on their idea of what adults approve and disapprove.

Most three-year-olds will

- Identify and appreciate their own gender
- Warn and tease and may threaten others
- Gain approval from adults
- Follow complex set of directions
- Begin to learn to take turns
- Take part in family activities
- Play with, rather than simply beside, other children
- Have conversations with other people

Four-year-olds are generally able to

- Develop an appropriate relationship with the parent of the opposite sex
- Play cooperatively with other children

Most five-year-olds can

- Understand privacy and modesty
- Begin to understand property rights
- Learn the meaning of family rules
- Begin to learn basic good manners
- Begin to develop a sense of fair play

Sense of Self

During the preschool years children develop an idea about themselves. The child's **self-concept** begins to form. If children like themselves, they tend to be encouraged to keep trying to accomplish a task. If they do not like themselves, they easily become discouraged. It is very important for them to like who they are. Preschoolers become aware of their gender. **Gender** means being a boy or a girl.

Things that a three-year-old will do include the following:

- Feed self with a fork
- Establish handedness (begin to use right or left hand for many tasks)
- Remove clothes and begin to put on shoes
- Brush teeth and wash hands
- Take some responsibility for regular tasks such as putting away clothes and toys
- Play well alone

Some things that four-year-olds are able to do include the following:

- Work buttons and tie shoelaces
- Learn to finish what is begun
- Wash hands and face
- Clean up after playing
- Help parents with household jobs
- Deal with fear, particularly fear of the dark
- Learn simple health rules

A five-year-old is likely to be able to do the following:

- Develop some ability to earn and spend small amounts of money
- Carry out simple tasks without encouragement
- Perform simple household tasks
- Learn to obey simple safety precautions

As Maria and Carlos watched Jesse develop, they delighted in each new skill. They learned to encourage him and to present him with new challenges. They were eager to keep him safe but also to give him every opportunity to become the best he could be—to give him a really good foundation for future growth.

Summary

Principles of growth and development are ideas based on predictable patterns that children tend to follow. They explain how children change as they grow. Researchers who study infants and children often develop theories, or explanations, about growth and development.

Infants grow rapidly. They change and learn new skills every day. By the time babies are one year old, they walk or will soon be able to. They can say a few words and understand more than they can express. They are eager and ready to learn.

Toddlers change from being babies to being children. They gain the ability to talk fairly well and can run, climb, and jump. After being very attached to parents and afraid of strangers, they begin to be more friendly with people outside the family. They begin to help with self-care and simple household tasks. They are very curious. At the close of the toddler years they are eager to learn and to meet the challenges of the preschool years.

Preschoolers grow nearly a foot in height in a couple of years and develop some thinking skills. They spend a lot of time polishing their language skills and learning to play with and get along with other children. They begin to develop a sense of right and wrong. They also are able to handle most self-care tasks and to pick up their own clothes and toys. Developing imagination and creativity are important tasks of the preschool years.

Terms and Concepts

Principles of growth and development

Cephalocaudal development

Proximodistal development

Continuous and orderly growth

Simple to complex development

Physical development

Emotional development

Social development

Moral development

Language and speech development

Mental development

Sensorimotor thinking

Abstract thinking

Spiritual development

Stages of development

Theory of development

Rate of development

Infants

Toddlers

Preschoolers

Maturation

Readiness

Cooing

Utterance

Interacting

Babbling

Echolalia

Receptive language

Productive language

Stranger anxiety

Curiosity

Twos

Trial-and-error learning

Temper tantrum

Peers

Self-concept

Gender

Checking Your Understanding

1. Give an example from your own experience that illustrates one of the principles of growth and one of the principles of development.

2. List the six types of development and describe each.

3. Write a paragraph explaining how infants change physically during their first year.

4. Write a short paper comparing the curiosity of a toddler with the curiosity of a preschooler.

5. Summarize the language development of children from birth through age six.

6. Explain how a child's relationships with people change from birth until age six.

7. How might a secure attachment to a caregiver make it easier for a baby to learn?

8. Explain how a child's curiosity is related to learning.

9. Design a plan for teaching children self-help skills.

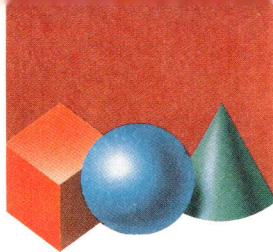

5 HANDS ON WITH CHILDREN

GETTING TO KNOW SMALL CHILDREN

How do you get acquainted with small children? It is much like getting to know anyone else, with a little extra understanding of young children mixed in.

Beginning at around six months, most babies develop stranger anxiety, a shyness with strangers that lasts until about 30 months (2½ years). They prefer to be with their parents or favorite caregiver. By age four most children are eager to make new friends, but some still want to approach new people slowly.

The following suggestions may help you to be accepted when you meet young children.

Step 1   Enter the room quietly.

Step 2   Stand back away from the child you are meeting until he or she has time to become accustomed to your presence (3 to 5 minutes is usually long enough).

Step 3   Approach the child slowly.

Step 4   As you approach, make eye contact. Say the child's name. Stay about three or four feet from the child for a minute or two.

Step 5   Position yourself at the child's eye level. If he or she is on the floor, sit or stoop to that level. Smile, and with a pleasant tone speak the child's name again. Tell the child who you are and wait for her or him to respond.

Step 6   When the child seems to accept you, extend your hand, palm up, and allow the child to touch you if he or she wants to.

Step 7   If the child responds, place both hands out toward the child, palms up, and allow the child to choose whether to come closer or to wait.

Step 8   If the child hangs back, acts shy, or refuses to respond, give her or him time for adjustment. Some children take longer to warm to an adult.

If the parents are leaving their child with you, ask them to hand the child to you rather than taking the child from their arms. Even if a child cries and pushes away from you when parents leave, invite them to say "good-bye" to the child and assure the child they will be back later. If children are distracted so that parents can leave without saying "good-bye," their trust in their parents is diminished and their fear of the child care situation will be greater.

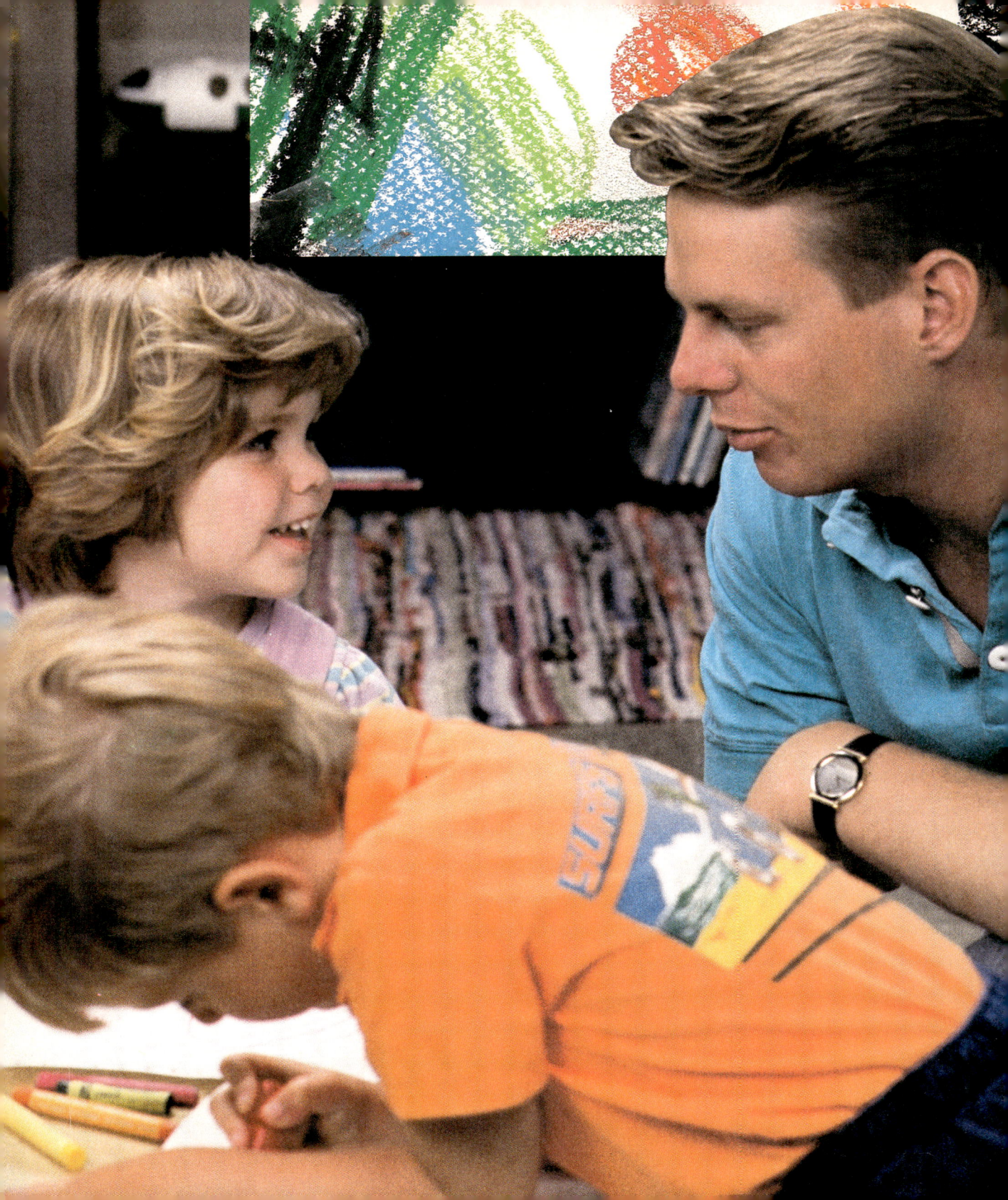

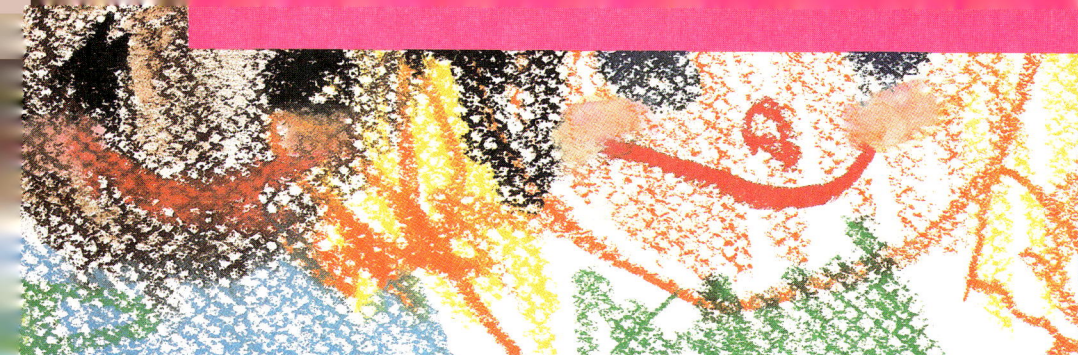

PART 2
Caring For Children

CHAPTER 6
Day Care Centers, Leadership, and Careers

OBJECTIVES

When you have finished this chapter, you will be able to

- Identify the purposes of centers for young children
- List and define the kinds of programs available for young children
- Describe the kinds of facilities that are appropriate for young children
- Discuss standards for indoor and outdoor spaces for children's groups
- Identify policies of child care centers
- Outline the legal concerns of centers
- Describe some career options in fields related to child care
- Prepare an application for employment and a resumé
- Demonstrate basic interview skills

Carol Louise Johnson held the car door open while her three-year-old son, Jonathan, took the long step to the asphalt. "Mommy, I want to stay home with you today," he said, and then grasped his mother's hand tighter than usual. Carol Louise had decided to return to work at the insurance office, so she had explained to Jonathan that he would soon be starting preschool.

"I'm not going to leave you here today," his mother replied. "You and I are just coming for a visit to see how we like La Casita. There are other children here and many things to do." Jonathan had been on the waiting list at La Casita Children's Center for two months. Then Mrs. Cisneros, the director, called to say that there was an opening and to invite them to visit.

Carol Louise pulled open the carved, wooden door of the old adobe building. Jonathan hesitated, then stepped onto the wooden floor. A small, pleasant-looking woman emerged from an office and extended her hand to Carol Louise. "I'm Mrs. Cisneros. You must be Mrs. Johnson," she said.

Carol Louise accepted the handshake and nodded. Looking down at her son, she said, "This is Jonathan."

Mrs. Cisneros bent her knees slowly, moving down so that her eyes were level with Jonathan's. She smiled warmly and said, "Jonathan, I'm so glad to meet you." Jonathan moved closer to his mother. Mrs. Cisneros waited a moment, then asked Jonathan, "Would you like to see where the boys and girls play?" He nodded and Mrs. Cisneros stood up slowly.

Jonathan now felt more comfortable with this pleasant lady. He liked her blue dress with the colored flowers embroidered down the front. She took his hand and together the three of them walked down a hall toward the three-year-olds' room. As they rounded a corner, Jonathan could hear children playing. When they arrived at the room, he looked inside and his eyes got big. Children were building roads with blocks and driving trucks and cars over them. Some were bathing dolls—with real water. One girl was painting with bright colors at an easel.

A young man wearing jeans and a bright blue sweatshirt came toward them and looked immediately at Jonathan. He bent his knees like Mrs. Cisneros had and spoke to him, "Welcome Jonathan! I'm the children's teacher, Mr. Marquez. Would you like to come in and look around?"

Jonathan wanted to play, but he still felt a bit nervous, so he shook his head no. Carol Louise said, "Jonathan, I am not going to leave. Let's sit over here and just watch the children play." He followed his mother, and they sat down in small chairs near the edge of the room. Mr. Marquez explained that the children chose where they would play and could move to another area after putting away the things they used in the first. Jonathan got more and more interested in all the things going on, and gradually stopped feeling nervous. He went over to a group playing with blocks and joined in their game.

CHILD CARE PROGRAMS AND FACILITIES

The purposes, programs, and facilities of child care centers vary. Based on what they believe, the directors of centers develop the curriculum and environment for the children. The number of children enrolled, along with several other factors, determines the classification of a child care center.

Purposes of a Child Care Center

Programs for children under six vary in purpose. Each center develops its philosophy and curriculum based on what the adults in charge believe is important for young children. Some common aims of child care programs are discussed in the following sections.

ASSISTING PARENTS WITH CHILD CARE

Parents who leave their children in any type of child care situation expect to have at least some help with child-rearing tasks. This help can go beyond basic physical care to include training in self-help skills, teaching of pre-math and language skills, and providing experiences that enrich children's lives.

FIGURE 6-1   Many parents today need assistance with child care during working hours, and they appreciate a high-quality preschool.

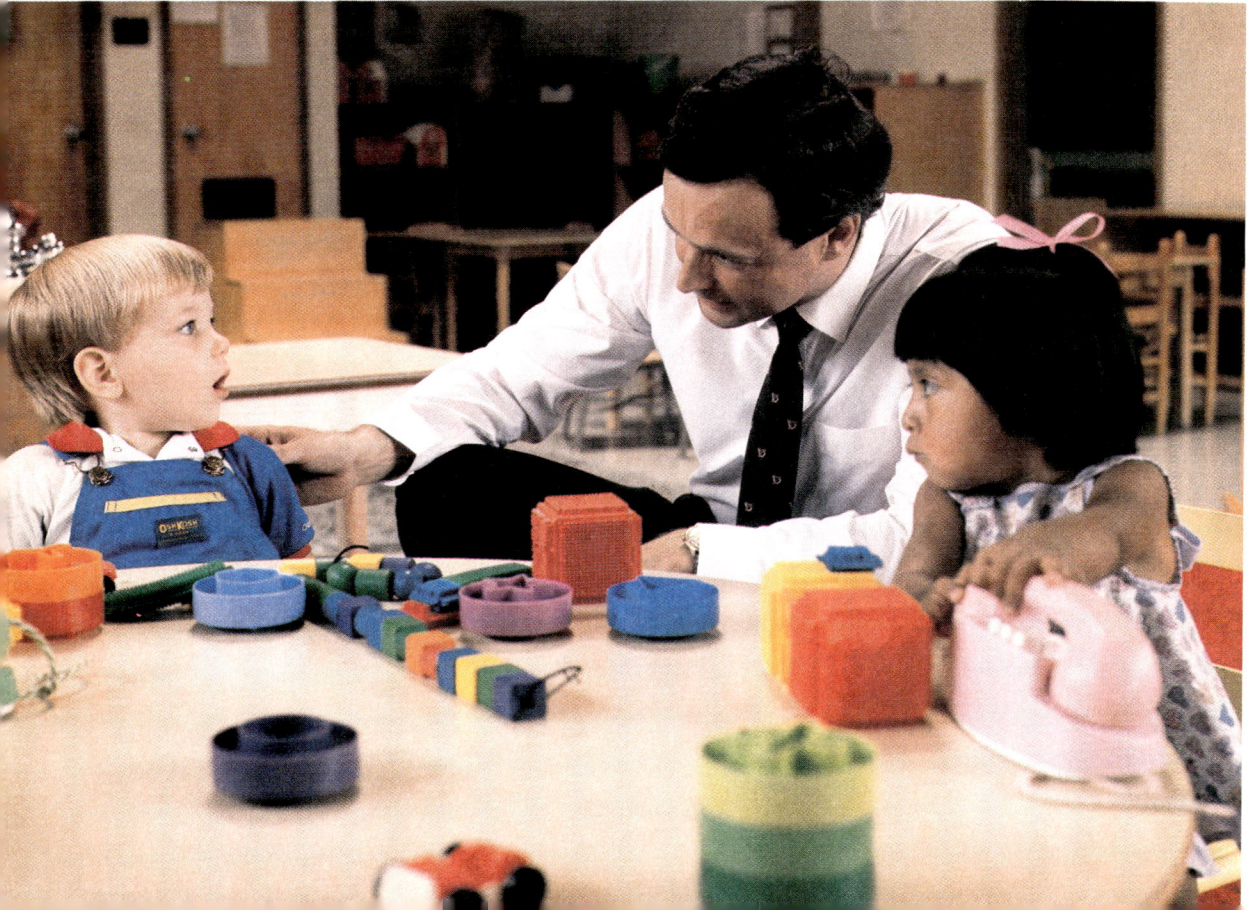

STRENGTHENING CHILDREN'S ABILITIES

Programs can be designed to strengthen children's natural abilities. Programs may also emphasize development of skills and special talents. Children with extraordinary abilities can benefit from programs that are designed to develop these strengths. Children whose abilities lag behind those of other children can benefit from programs whose teachers are trained to work with children having special needs.

IMPROVING CHILDREN'S SENSE OF SELF-WORTH AND SOCIAL SKILLS

Programs can help children learn to develop a good feeling about who they are and what they can do. Regular interaction with other children, as is provided by the supervised play in a well-run child care center, can help in developing social skills.

IMPROVING LANGUAGE SKILLS

Preschool children actively work at learning to speak and to understand others' speech. Preschools help children learn speaking skills as well as pre-writing and pre-reading skills.

DEVELOPING THINKING SKILLS

Children are natural investigators. Preschool programs can help children think about their discoveries and stimulate their natural curiosity.

DEVELOPING SELF-HELP SKILLS

Children want to gain control over their bodies and to be able to do things for themselves. Preschool programs can help children move toward this goal.

DEVELOPING IMAGINATION AND CREATIVITY

The early childhood years are a time of exploration and pretending. Preschool programs can stimulate children's imaginations and strengthen their creative abilities.

DEVELOPING MOTOR SKILLS

Children have a strong drive to use their muscles, especially the large muscles in the legs and arms. Motor abilities involving the large muscles are also called **gross motor skills.** Children also

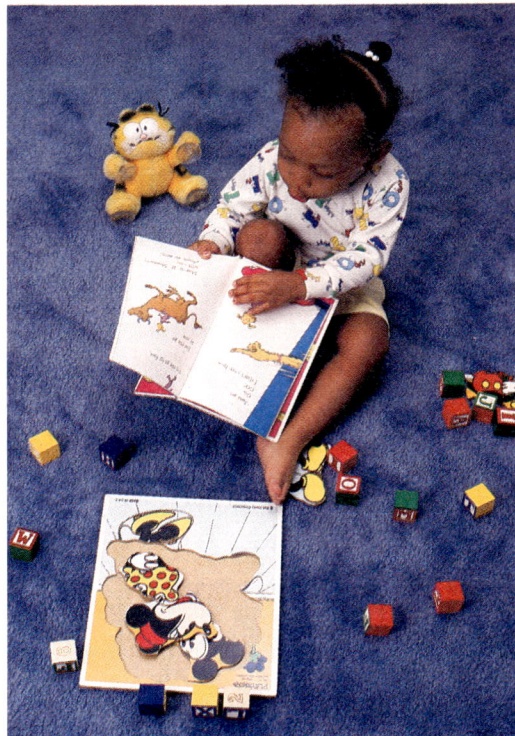

FIGURE 6-2
Turning the pages of a book involves fine motor skills, and so does playing with blocks and puzzles.

need to develop their **fine motor skills,** which involve the use of the muscles in the fingers and hands. Carefully planned activities can help children enjoy developing their motor skills.

IDENTIFYING AND REFERRING CHILDREN WITH SPECIAL NEEDS

Caregivers and teachers in preschool programs may be the first to discover that children need special help. They then work with parents and specialists to help these children overcome or deal with their handicaps or learning disabilities.

Kinds of Programs

The goals chosen by the leaders of a center will determine what kind of program is developed. Some programs are a blend of more than one kind of goal. The four basic kinds of programs are custodial care programs, developmental programs, structured educational programs, and special needs programs. The following sections discuss all of these, as well as special preschool programs run by schools and Head Start.

CUSTODIAL CARE PROGRAMS

Programs whose goal is custodial care are aimed at taking care of the physical needs of young children. **Custodial care programs** are designed to keep children safe and in a healthy environment. Caregivers see to it that children receive nutritious snacks and meals and that they have adequate rest.

DEVELOPMENTAL PROGRAMS

In addition to providing custodial care, **developmental programs** include activities that encourage children to develop mentally, creatively, physically, and socially and to develop language skills. In a developmental program planned activities are based on children's needs and on developmental tasks. **Developmental tasks** specify the mental and physical skills children need to master before they can move on to the next stage of development. Preschool children need to develop the following:

- A sense of self-worth
- Some ability to play well with other children and to get along in a group
- Some self-discipline
- Understanding of concepts basic to math, reading, and writing
- Basic language skills
- Self-care skills
- Physical skills, such as running, climbing, hopping, and manipulating small objects
- Personal values

A developmental program is designed to encourage children to participate in activities that will stimulate growth in the above areas. Teachers plan activities, ask questions, invite participation, and provide experiences that stimulate children's development. Developmental programs are child-centered but are planned and led by trained adults. Children in developmental programs can often be found building with blocks, climbing through tunnels, pretending to be firefighters or doctors, listening to or telling

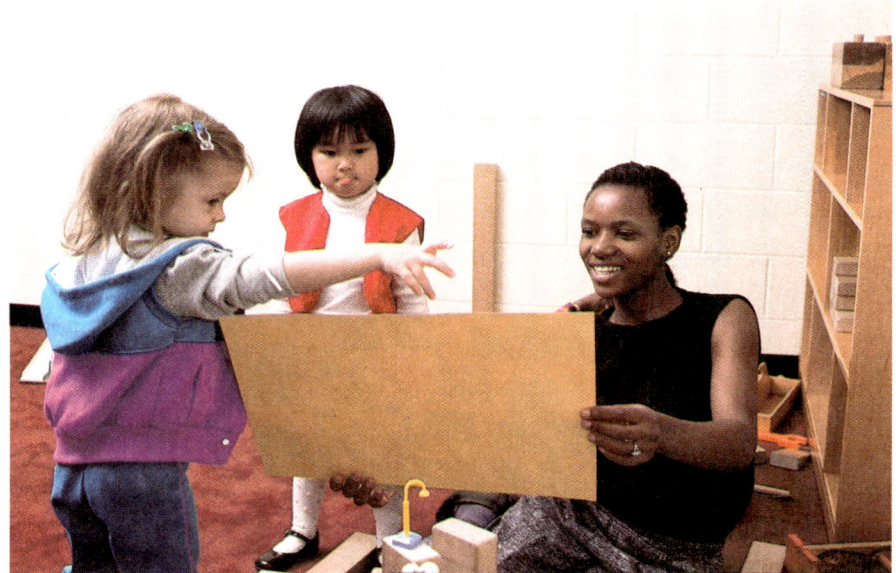

FIGURE 6-3 Developmental programs are based on children's needs and encourage them to learn by offering them a variety of planned activities.
Source: © 1985 by Blair Seitz/Photo Researchers, Inc.

stories, moving freely to music, or painting pictures of their own (not coloring in preprinted sheets).

STRUCTURED EDUCATIONAL PROGRAMS

The aim of **structured educational programs** is to teach children specific skills. Frequently these skills are ones children would usually learn in elementary school. The program may focus on early reading, writing, sports, dance, or music. Teachers usually lead or direct the children in their activities. Children in these programs may be found sitting at tables copying letters, coloring in drawings that are alphabet-related, playing soccer, practicing dance steps, or learning songs. Parents and teachers tend to emphasize performance and accomplishment in this type of program.

SPECIAL NEEDS PROGRAMS

The aim of **special needs programs** is to help children who are developmentally delayed or handicapped to function more effectively. Children in these programs can be found participating in a large variety of activities that are designed to help them strengthen their abilities and compensate for weak areas. Teachers are highly trained and design activities for children's individual needs.

SCHOOL-BASED PROGRAMS

Some school districts and private schools offer classes for preschool children. Frequently these **school-based programs** are directed toward handicapped or disadvantaged children. Poor children and children who do not speak English frequently have difficulty achieving in school. Early childhood programs help these children get equipped to function in elementary school. School-based programs are usually regulated by education agencies and therefore not subject to the regulations of day care licensing.

HEAD START

Since 1964 Head Start programs have been funded by the federal government. **Head Start** is designed to meet the developmental needs of three- to five-year-olds from poor families as well as prepare them to enter school. Program goals include improving language skills, helping children gain a positive self-image, and developing curiosity, healthy living habits, and self-discipline. Head Start programs are usually state-licensed unless they operate as part of a school-based program.

Professionals who specialize in early childhood education sometimes do not agree on which of these kinds of programs is best for young children. The type of program chosen for a center will be based on the beliefs and opinions of the adults in charge. This book will emphasize methods used in developmental programs.

Do preschool programs make a difference in children's development? The Something to Think About feature addresses this question.

Kinds of Facilities

A child care facility is characterized by the number of children attending, the building, equipment, and materials used, the way the facility is governed and operated, and the kind of program

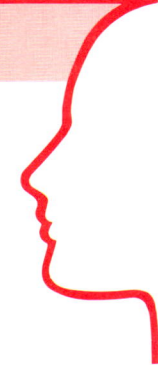

Something to Think About

Do Early Childhood Programs Make a Difference?

Dr. Burton White has said that there is nothing better for a child under three than a parent who is "absolutely nuts" about the child and can spend a majority of every day talking with and doing things with her or him.[1] Adults, especially those a child is most closely attached to, serve as consultants for the child—providing information about the world. The bond between young children and loving parents enables children to play freely and gain that information.

Not all parents can stay home with their children. An increasing number of parents must work. Do parents who stay home with children necessarily give them a good environment in which to grow? A parent's presence in the house does not guarantee that a child is receiving appropriate care and love. Some parents do not know how to be effective parents—how to help children develop and learn. Some are not even able to give basic physical care.

Children who benefit most from effective preschool programs are those whose parents cannot or do not offer them effective parenting. Good developmental programs can help disadvantaged children to have opportunities more nearly equal to those of children who have more advantages. Children who are handicapped also benefit from attending early childhood programs that are appropriately planned and have well-trained staff.

Should children whose parents can support them adequately and provide living experiences that encourage development be placed in child care centers? If so, at what age? How important do you think the parent-child relationship is in a child's development? What is best learned from parents or from being with groups of children? How important is the quality of the child care center and its staff? Is a child better off in a poor center or a disadvantaged home? Is a child who has a developmentally enriching home better off there or in a really good preschool program? What do you think?

[1]Dr. White is a leader in the field of child development who is profiled in the Leadership at a Glance feature in Chapter 11. The work referenced here is from conference notes: Center for Parent Education, Houston, Texas, February 1983.

offered. Facilities of the same general type will vary in some ways, however.

DAY CARE CENTERS

Day care centers serve children from birth through age five. They serve a minimum of ten children and are open on a full-time basis. Day care centers are licensed by most states.

FAMILY DAY HOMES

Family day homes serve fewer than ten children. Most are run by the owner in his or her home. A few owners employ a second person to assist with child care. These facilities are licensed in most states.

WORK-BASED CENTERS

Work-based centers usually operate like other day care centers but are set up by a business for its employees. Often the center is on the same property as the business. Child care may be offered by a company as part of a package of job benefits. Employers who supply child care often find that parents' absence from work is greatly reduced. Work-based centers are usually state-licensed.

COOPERATIVE CENTERS

Cooperative centers are similar to day care centers except that parents are expected to assist in the center a certain number of days each month, in exchange for lower fees. The advantages are that parents can spend more time with their own children and children have opportunities to play and interact with other children. Also, parents can improve their parenting skills by participating in a quality program. The disadvantage of these centers is that it can be difficult for working parents to participate unless they have flexible hours or are self-employed. Cooperative centers are usually state-licensed.

PARENT'S DAY OUT AND DROP-IN CENTERS

Parent's day out centers provide custodial care and sometimes developmental or educational activities. Most of these centers enroll children for only one or two days each week. Enrollment is usually on a monthly basis.

Some department stores and malls provide **drop-in centers**, which are essentially babysitting arrangements. Parents leave their children while they shop and pay according to the time the children are there.

Most states do not require parent's day out programs or drop-in centers to be licensed, so the quality of care in these facilities varies even more than in regulated centers.

CHILD CARE ENVIRONMENTS

The environment of a child care center is designed to care for children's physical needs and provide learning opportunities. What are the characteristics of a good environment for young children? The National Academy of Early Childhood Programs recommends that children's environments be safe, clean, attractive, and spacious. The environment of a child care center should allow children to progress developmentally.

Effective Environments for Children

Environments that provide for children's developmental and physical needs have specific characteristics. These are described in the following sections.

SAFETY

A safe environment has no sharp edges or dangerous surfaces, no splinters on wood furnishings, and nontoxic paint on walls and other surfaces. Electrical connections should be inaccessible to children. (Chapter 8 discusses safety in the child care environment more thoroughly.)

EASE OF SUPERVISION

Preschool children must have constant supervision, even in a relatively safe environment. The children's environment should be designed so that the adult or adults can easily supervise activities and view all the children.

CHILD-SIZED FURNISHINGS AND EQUIPMENT

Children spend much of their time in adult environments where they are too small to use the furnishings and equipment the way adults do. Child-sized furnishings and equipment make children more comfortable and give them the experience of having their world fit their size.

Chairs should be small enough that children can comfortably touch the ground with their feet. A child-sized stove and sink should be about waist-high for children, and the top of a refrigerator should be at about their eye level. Equipment in rooms for toddlers is, in general, smaller than that in rooms for three- and four-year-olds.

PERSONAL SPACE

Space for children's personal belongings is an important part of the preschool environment. Each child needs a place to put his or her personal things—a blanket for nap time, toys to cuddle, a change of clothes, wraps for cool weather, and perhaps lunch.

FIGURE 6-4   Small children feel comfortable with furnishings their size.
Source: © Erika Stone 1989

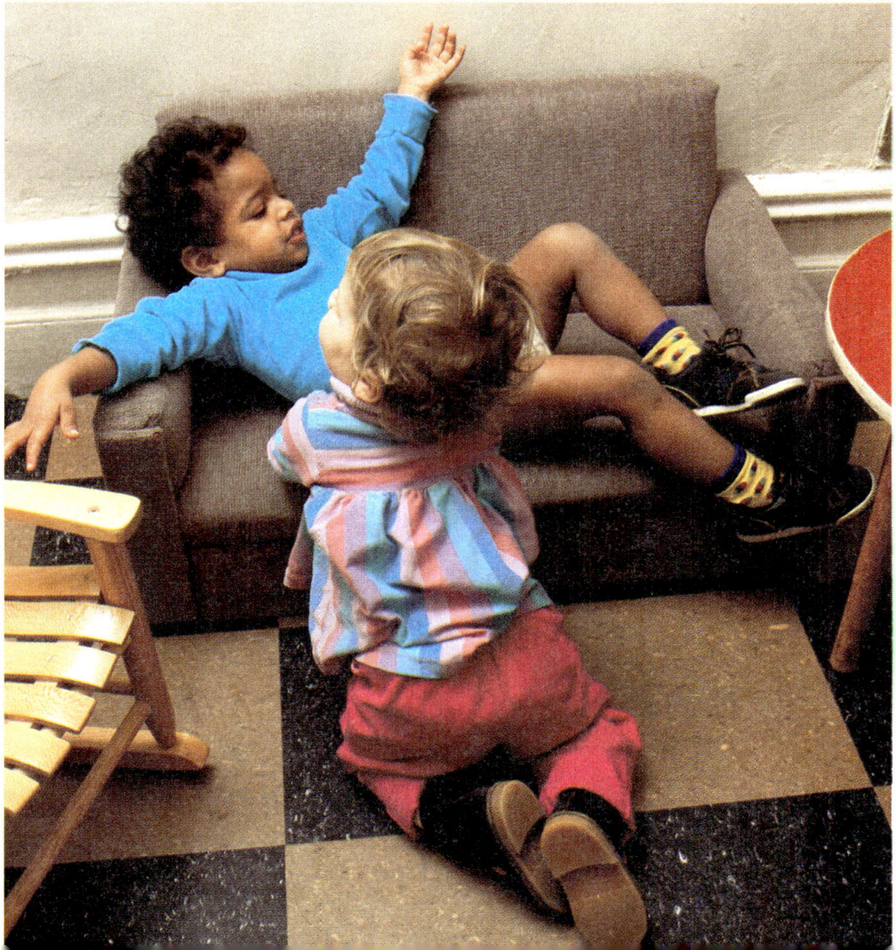

PRIVATE SPACE

Children need a place where they can sometimes get away from the group for a few moments—a place within the room that allows a child a bit of privacy. It can be a small space, such as a beanbag chair in the book center, a cozy space to crawl into, or an activity set up for just one child. This space, like all others in the children's environment, must be easily visible to the care-givers.

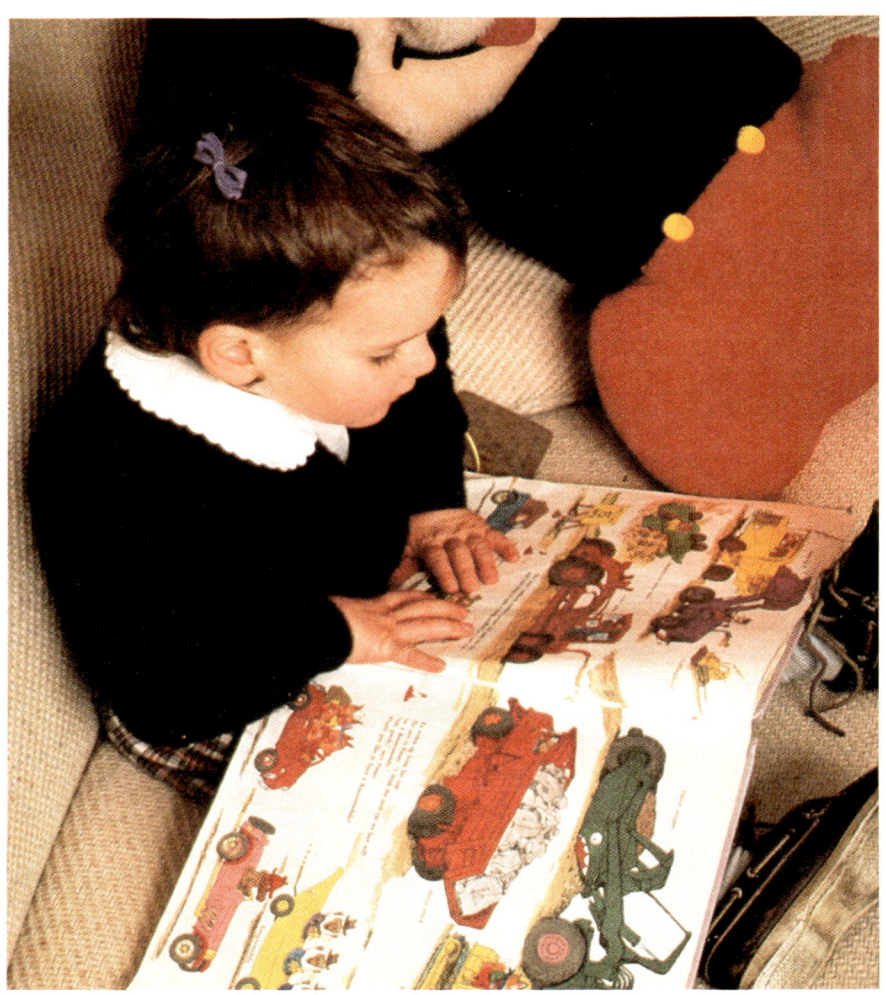

FIGURE 6-5 A private place in a child care center allows children to do quiet activities alone.
Source: © *Laura Dwight*

SOFTNESS

Children need softness in their environment. Softness can be provided by carpeting, wall coverings, furnishings, or equipment. A child-sized rocking chair can provide softness of movement; music can also soften the environment.

SOUND-ABSORBING PROPERTIES

Children, even in a supervised environment, tend to be noisy. When sound-absorbing materials are used in a room, the envi-

FIGURE 6-6   Arranging several large pillows on the floor in one area is a way to put softness into the child care environment. *Source: © Erika Stone*

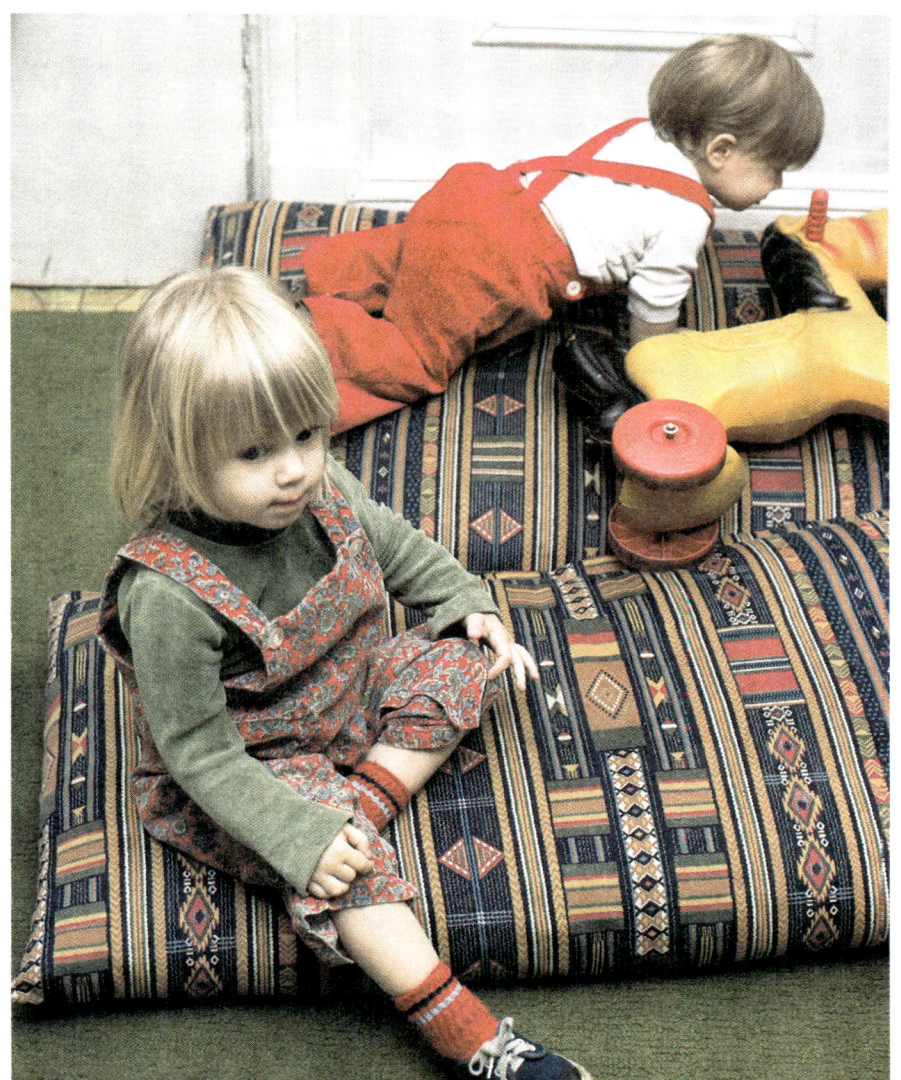

ronment is more pleasant for everyone. Sound-absorbing surfaces include carpeting, acoustical coverings for ceiling and walls, fabric coverings for walls and windows, and upholstered furniture.

Materials that reflect sound, and therefore increase noise, include masonry, glass, concrete, tile, wood, and metal. Some surfaces have to be sound-reflecting. For example, floors in art and eating areas must be easy to clean. These surfaces should be balanced with softer ones wherever possible.

POLICIES OF CHILD CARE CENTERS

When Carol Louise and Jonathan finished their visit in the three-year-olds' room, they stopped by the center's office. Carol Louise asked Mrs. Cisneros about the center's hours and dates of operation, fees, and how things would be handled if Jonathan became sick while he was at the center. Mrs. Cisneros gave her an enrollment packet for Jonathan and read through the policy handbook with her.

Policies of child care centers are sets of rules that outline how they do business. Policies concern children, parents, staff, and how the center is operated. Some policies may be determined by federal or state laws or by the center's governing board, if there is one. Directors of centers also have philosophies of teaching and caregiving that will determine policies. (A **philosophy** is a way of thinking and believing that often guides decision making.)

It is helpful to parents and staff if the center places its policies in a **policy handbook** and distributes it to each person concerned. Some centers, however, do not furnish a handbook. In such cases it is up to parents and staff to learn and adhere to word-of-mouth policies. Written policies are best because they provide consistency and prevent misunderstandings.

Policies Concerning Children

Policies about children explain the rules that affect children while they are at the center.

CHILDREN'S FILES

State agencies that regulate child care require that basic information for all children enrolled be on file in every center. This information usually includes the following:

- The child's complete name, home address, home telephone number, and birth date

- The parents' names, home and work addresses, and telephone numbers where they can be reached when the child is at the center

- Names (and possibly pictures) of people to whom the child may be released

- Name, address, and telephone number of the child's doctor

- Statement of child's health that includes past and present illnesses, injuries, recent hospital stays, allergies, and a list of medications the child takes regularly

- Current immunization record

- Statements giving members of the center's staff authorization to seek emergency medical care

- Permission (when applicable) for transportation to participate in gymnastics or water activities or to have pictures taken for publication

Children's files are considered confidential. **Confidentiality of files** means that only the staff, authorized licensing representatives, and the child's parents have access to what is in a file. People who see the files are not allowed to talk about what is in them to people outside the center. Parents have a right to see their child's file. It is not legal to keep any file on a child that parents cannot see.

FEES

Many centers charge an enrollment fee, which is usually used to pay for learning materials. The regular payment for attendance is called tuition. Some centers require payment weekly, others monthly. It is considered a good business practice to collect fees in advance of services. Therefore, some centers will require parents to pay the first month's charges before the child can attend.

Some centers add a late charge if the fee is not paid by a specified date. Others simply drop children from enrollment if payment is late. Some centers have strict rules about hours and charge extra when parents pick up children later than the scheduled time. Payment policies should be stated in the center's policy handbook.

ATTENDANCE

Days and hours of operation, as well as holidays, are given in the policy handbook. The center's policy for absences may also be stated.

ATTENDANCE DURING ILLNESS

Children who are ill are usually kept at home. A few centers, particularly those run by hospitals for their employees, have a special unit to care for sick children. Children who become sick during the day are cared for by a staff member, and parents are called to pick up the child. Parents are usually expected to come as soon as possible.

FIGURE 6-7 Child care centers must not practice racial discrimination.
Source: Gerber Products Company

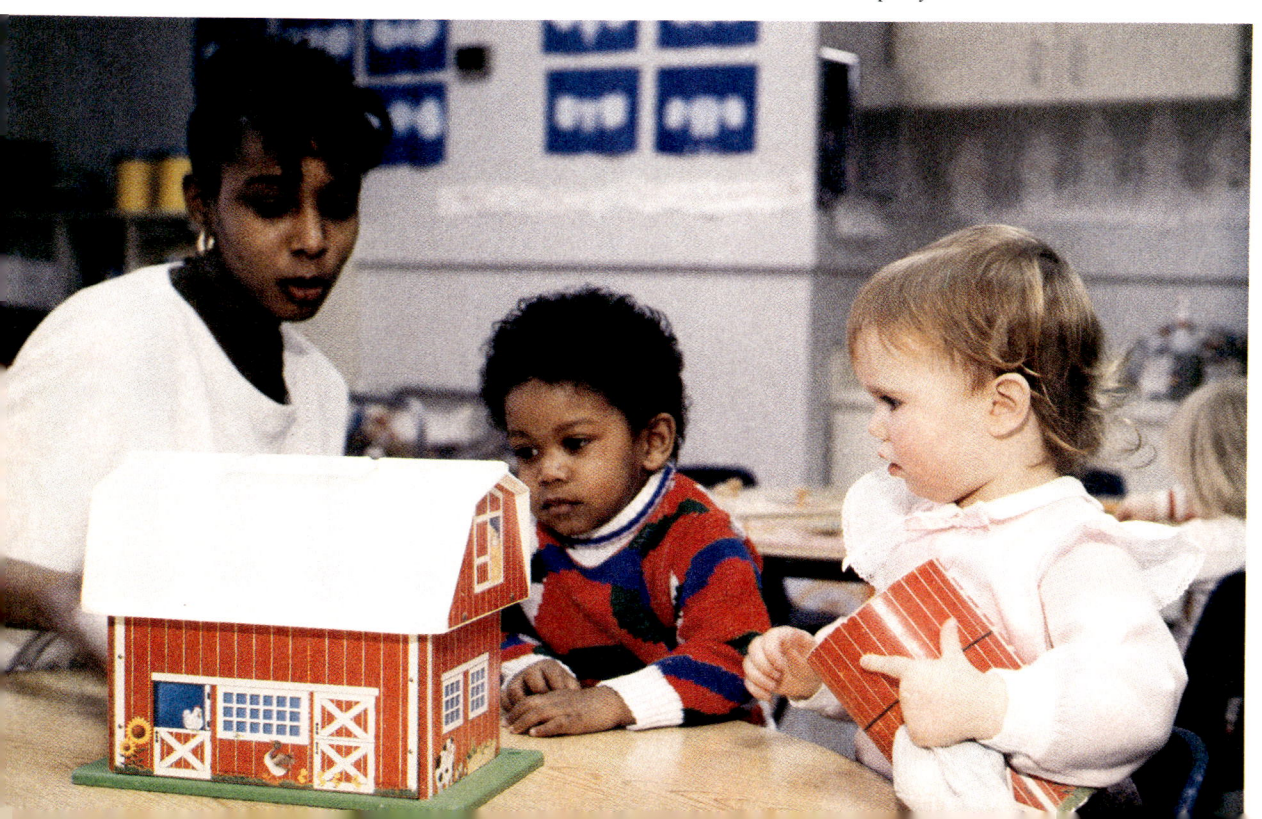

If a child develops a contagious illness, parents of all the children in the center are notified. A written notice is posted or given to parents and usually includes the name of the illness, the symptoms, and the period of incubation. The **period of incubation** is how long it takes for a child to come down with the illness after he or she came into contact with it.

MINORITY CHILDREN AND LANGUAGE DIFFERENCES

Centers are not allowed to discriminate against children for racial or cultural reasons. Children who do not speak the same language as the adults and other children should be included and helped as much as possible.

Bilingual teachers know two languages well enough to speak and teach in both of them. Having bilingual teachers or caregivers is an advantage to children who speak the second language at home. When a center employs bilingual staff, a statement of that fact is usually included in the policy handbook.

PERSONAL BELONGINGS IN SCHOOL

Most centers have policies stating what children may bring with them to the center. As a rule, teachers prefer that children leave toys and other belongings at home, except for a favorite toy or possession to be shared during circle time or to have close at nap time and a blanket and possibly a small pillow to use during nap time.

MEALS AND SNACKS

Most states regulate the kind of food that children can have at a center. Regulations usually specify that half of a child's nutritional needs must be met by the food given to the child at a center each day. Many centers establish a policy that children must not bring food or snacks from home, if these are provided.

PARTIES

Many centers provide, or allow parents to provide, parties for holidays and birthdays. Birthday parties should be similar for all children so each child will feel that his or her birthday is a special time.

Policies Concerning Parents

Policies concerning parents deal with information parents should receive from or give to the center, procedures for dropping off and picking up children, and visits by parents.

Members of the staff can use a variety of ways to communicate with parents, including monthly or weekly newsletters, regular parent meetings, bulletin boards, talks when children are dropped off and picked up, home visits, and telephone calls.

Parents need to take a moment in the morning and the afternoon to speak with their child's teacher. The teacher needs to know if the child has any special needs or concerns that may affect his or her day. At the end of the day parents can find out what interesting events or activities took place at the center. It will give them things to talk about with the child in the evening.

DROPPING OFF AND PICKING UP CHILDREN

Most centers have policies about how children should be dropped off and picked up. These are designed to protect children from danger and the center from liability and may include the following:

Dropping children off. Parents should bring children into the center, sign them in, and leave them with a teacher. Parents do not drop children at the front door of the center, even if a teacher is nearby.

Picking children up. Parents must come into the center to pick up children. Children may be picked up by parents or other persons they designate. Children will not be released to unauthorized persons.

PARENTS' VISITS

Centers that discourage parents' visits during any time of the day are not the best place for children to spend time. A center that is good for children allows parents to visit *at any time* whether or not the visit is scheduled. Parents should not be required to notify the center before they visit. They should be able to go directly to their child's room and to know what is going on at that time with the children. It is the responsibility of parents, however, not to be disruptive in their visits.

LEGAL CONCERNS OF CHILD CARE PROVIDERS

Child care is one of the most responsible and difficult professions. Young children are the responsibility of their parents because they are unable to care adequately for themselves. When parents purchase child care services, they are seeking adults who will also care responsibly for their children. Children are very vulnerable to disease, accidents, and emotional injury. Laws have been written and enacted to protect children while they are in child care facilities and away from their parents. These laws are enforced by agencies of the government, usually state agencies.

Minimum Standards

The government agency charged with the responsibility of enforcing child care laws develops a set of **minimum standards,** or rules that must be followed by anyone engaged in the business of child care. In most states somewhat different standards may be applied to family day homes, day care centers, and institutions that provide care around the clock. Standards address many of the following areas of concern:

- Organization of the center
- Hours of operation
- Enrollment procedures
- Types of records and methods for keeping records
- Transportation procedures
- Qualifications of directors and other staff members
- Training of staff members
- Discipline and guidance methods
- Number of children each adult is allowed to care for
- Amount of space needed indoors and outdoors for children's activities
- Furnishings and equipment for children
- Toilet and hand-washing facilities
- Fire, health, and safety precautions

- Health requirements for children
- Procedures for illness, injury, and medications
- Meals and nutrition
- Animals and pets at the center
- Procedures for emergencies
- Activities

Government agencies that regulate child care send representatives to visit centers to see that they meet the minimum standards. If a center does not, it must correct the problems or lose its license and be closed. Some situations may be so dangerous that the licensing representative will close the center down immediately, although this does not happen very often.

Liability

Child care providers are liable for the health, safety, and well-being of each child while the child is in their care. **Legal liability** means that a person must bear the consequences if something or someone he or she is responsible for is harmed. Adults who care for children are responsible for knowing what their needs are and how to meet them. These adults are also responsible for supervising the children carefully to be sure their needs are met and they are safe. If children are hurt or become ill, responsible adults can be held liable. Caregivers can be sued for damages or even criminally prosecuted if they do not care properly for children.

Child care centers and each adult employed in such a place should carry professional liability insurance. **Professional liability insurance** provides legal aid when a center or caregiver is sued. If the center or caregiver loses the lawsuit, the insuring company pays the amount awarded to those suing, up to the value of the policy. Professional caregivers carry liability insurance because even careful, caring providers may not be able to prevent an injury or harm to a child. Having good liability insurance coverage protects the caregivers from devastating losses.

PLANNING AND PREPARING FOR A CAREER

Selecting and beginning a rewarding career take careful preparation and planning. Chosen careers are more likely to be realized when education and experience are related to career goals.

Careers Related to Children

When planning a career, most people do not know exactly what job they intend to hold. Many aim for a type of job rather than a specific position. A **career cluster** is a group of jobs that are similar or related to one another. For example, there are a number of positions available in the child care field. There are also positions in other fields, such as medicine or law, allowing professionals to specialize in meeting needs of children.

CHILD CARE CAREERS

Child care careers include positions as caregivers, teachers, teacher's aides, cooks, program directors, administrative assistants, or center directors. The National Association for the Education of Young Children (NAEYC) has established four levels of qualifications for staff who teach young children. These are given in Table 6-1.

Note in Table 6-1 that the more qualified staff members have more responsibility and require less supervision. They also have more advanced education or training. As employees gain experience and training and accept greater responsibility, they become qualified to move to higher positions. Moving to a more responsible position is known as moving up the career ladder. A **career ladder** is the cluster of jobs in a field arranged according to level of responsibility and qualifications. Look again at Table 6-1 and decide which job is at the bottom of the career ladder and which is at the top.

Managers of child care centers are usually called **directors**. Managing a center involves many skills. Directors plan, organize, carry out plans, and evaluate results. Other necessary tasks include keeping financial records, purchasing, controlling costs, keeping records on children and staff, hiring and firing staff, and making sure that regulations are followed. Doing all of this involves a great deal of communication with people both inside and outside the center.

A director of a child care center may also be the owner of the business. **Entrepreneurship** means owning and operating a business. Being an entrepreneur means learning how to organize and manage a business. Entrepreneurs take the risks and enjoy the benefits of business ownership.

There are also jobs in the child care career cluster that are not in child care centers. One such job is being a nanny. **Nannies**

TABLE 6-1 Responsibilities and Qualifications of Early
Childhood Staff

Level of Professional Responsibility	Title	Training Requirements
Pre-professionals who implement program activities under direct supervision of the professional staff	Early Childhood Teacher Assistant	High school graduate or equivalent, participation in professional development programs
Professionals who independently implement program activities and who may be responsible for the care and education of a group of children	Early Childhood Associate Teacher	CDA credential or associate degree in Early Childhood Education/Child Development
Professionals who are responsible for the care and education of a group of children	Early Childhood Teacher	Baccalaureate degree in Early Childhood Education/Child Development
Professionals who supervise and train staff, design curriculum, and/or administer programs	Early Childhood Specialist	Baccalaureate degree in Early Childhood Education/Child Development and at least three years of full-time teaching experience with young children and/or a graduate degree in ECE/CD

Source: Accreditation Criteria and Procedures of the National Academy of Early Childhood Programs (*Washington, DC: NAEYC, 1984*), *19. Copyright by the National Association for the Education of Young Children.*

are trained professionals who are employed by families to care for children in their homes. Nannies are responsible for all the needs of a family's children during a forty-hour work week. Men who do this type of work are called **mannies.** Nannies or mannies

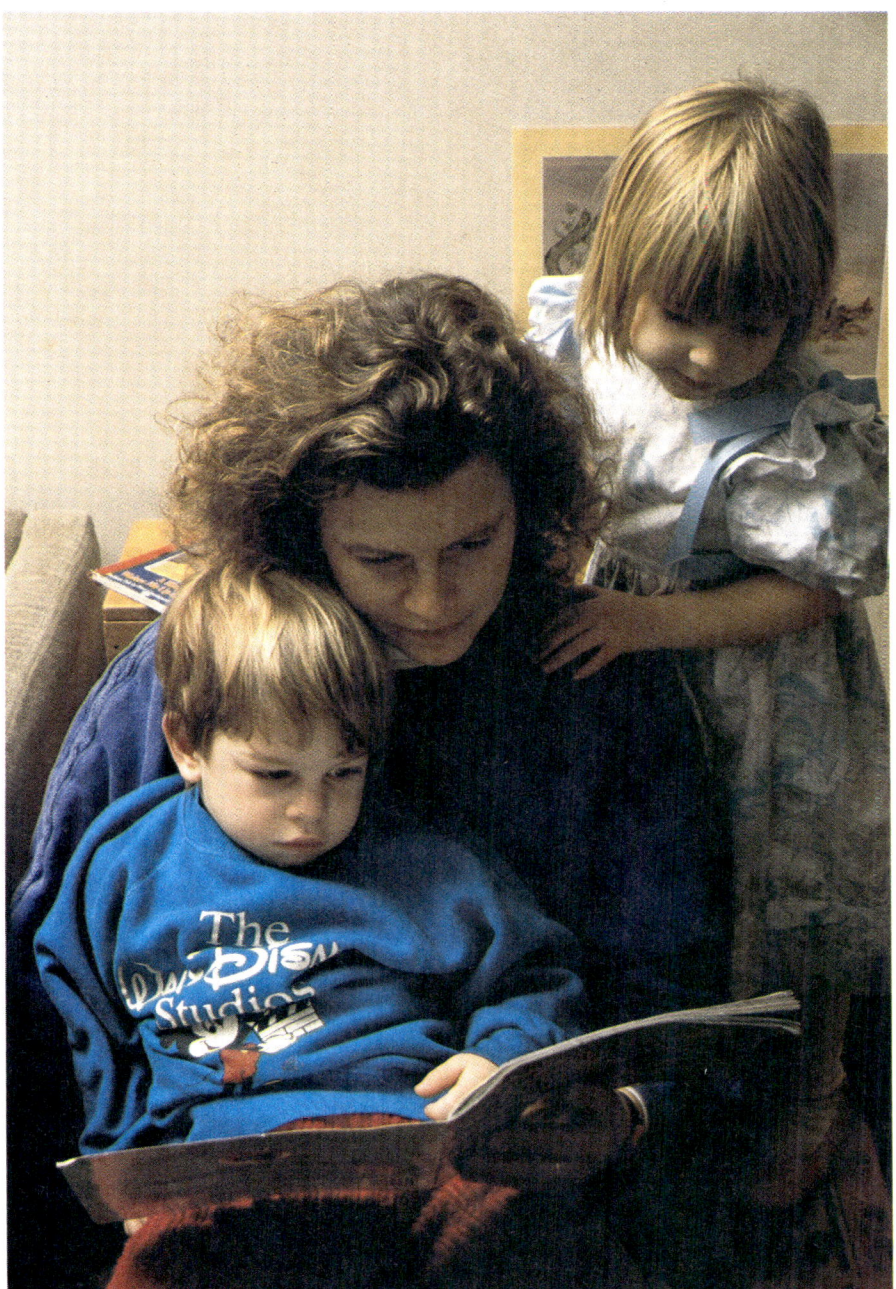

FIGURE 6-8   Being a teacher's aide, or assistant, is the bottom rung of one career ladder in the child care field.
Source: © Erika Stone 1989

may live in the family's home or they may work there and live in their own home. Nannies or mannies are primarily employed by wealthy families, usually ones with two professional parents but occasionally ones with a single parent. Special training for work as a nanny is available in large cities throughout the country.

House parents, as well as other types of professionals, work with children in institutions. These institutions include temporary shelters for abused or abandoned children, centers for children with health, emotional, or mental problems, and correctional institutions.

TEACHING AND RESEARCH

Preschool, kindergarten, special education, or elementary school teachers who have a bachelor's degree and a teaching certificate can be employed by either public or private schools. Another child-related career is that of home economics teachers who teach child development and family living courses.

Teachers who obtain advanced degrees may become counselors, administrators, college professors, or researchers. **Child development researchers** are professionals who scientifically study the development and behavior of children.

SOCIAL SERVICES

Professionals in **social services** work for public agencies that serve children and families. These workers usually have a degree from a two-year or four-year college program. Some social workers regulate child care centers. Others investigate reports of child abuse or work with foster parents. The growing number of homeless families with children presents special challenges for the future. Professionals who are trained to assist homeless and very poor families are needed in increasing numbers.

Private organizations also may offer services to children and families. These services may include help for homeless children, runaways, and children whose parents or other adults cannot help. Many religious groups employ education directors, counselors, and family life specialists.

MEDICINE

Nurses, doctors, and other specialists trained in pediatrics care for sick children. **Pediatrics** is the medical profession's term for children's health care. Highly specialized skills are necessary to give children the best medical care.

Professionals who work with children and families during hospitalization or extended periods of health care are called **child life specialists.** Their training focuses on child development with an emphasis on child life. This type of training is available in some colleges that offer degrees in home economics.

FAMILY COUNSELING AND CHILD PSYCHOLOGY

Family counselors and child psychologists have a master's or doctoral degree in family counseling or psychology. They are trained to help families think through problems and arrive at a solution. When there is a serious emotional problem, such as from abuse, a professional with these kinds of skills is often needed.

Sometimes tensions or problems are created in families because parents must try to satisfy both job demands and children's needs. The Something to Think About feature gives you an opportunity to consider the sources of such conflicts and how they might be resolved.

Something to Think About

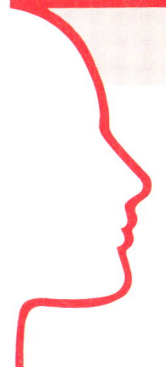

Work-Family Conflicts

More adults are employed outside the home today than ever before. Frequently both mothers and fathers of preschool children work. Children are cared for by child care centers or relatives or, in some cases, are left at home with little or no supervision.

Conflicts arise between parents and among family members in response to the pressures of jobs. Some possible sources of conflict include the following:

- *Work schedules.* Do parents work the same or different shifts? Do they work weekends or night shifts?

- *Child care.* Do fathers spend more time caring for and interacting with children when mothers work?

- *Household tasks.* Do fathers and other family members pitch in and give extra help with household tasks if the mother works, or does she have a work overload?

- *Traditional or nontraditional roles.* Do parents adhere to traditional roles of father as provider and mother as nurturer, or do they share both roles? Are they happy about their roles?

- *Lack of fairness.* Are work loads and leisure time balanced?

- *Job compatibility.* Do parents' jobs complement one another? Can both parents pursue chosen careers while maintaining a healthy family atmosphere? Can they enjoy talking with one another about work as well as about family and home?

- *Power.* Is personal power shared or does one parent dominate the other? How does each parent feel about the power structure? Does the fact that both parents are employed affect the balance of power?

- *Status.* How does the fact that both parents work affect the family's status within the extended family and within the social network?

- *Personal freedom.* How does being in a two-earner family affect the personal freedom of each parent and each child? Does being part of a two-earner family limit or enhance each parent's opportunities to progress in the workplace? Does having an employed spouse make one more or less free to change jobs or to get further education? Does having more money mean that family members do more of the things they enjoy together?

- *Time together.* How does having both parents employed affect the amount and quality of time they spend with one another and the children?

- *Effect on children.* When both parents work, do children do better or worse in school? How are children's attitudes about women and work changed when their mother works outside the home? How are children's values and sense of security affected?

As a child care professional, you will have many opportunities to assist families as they struggle with work-family issues. The way you think through these questions and work out their solution with the important people in your own life will have an effect on your competence in your career.

LAW

Lawyers who handle family problems such as divorce, child support, child abuse, and juvenile offenses are frequently in contact with children. Police and probation officers who handle cases involving juveniles also work with children, many of whom are troubled.

Applying for a Job

The first step in applying for a job is nearly always completing an application form. A resumé may be given to the potential employer with the application.

PREPARING AN APPLICATION

A completed application form is often an employer's first look at you. When you are hired, your application generally is kept in your employee file. It is part of your permanent work record. Applications make the best impression when they are carefully filled out. Basic rules for completing an application include the following:

- Type the information or print it in ink.

- Spell all words correctly and use correct grammar.

- Be as neat as possible.

- Answer all questions honestly and completely.

- Respond to every question. Put NA for "not applicable" if a question does not apply.

- If asked what salary you would accept, write "open" if you do not know what salary is offered or is appropriate.

- For references use only names you have received permission to use. Most applications ask for three.

- Write, rather than print, your signature at the end of the application.

Applications can be either mailed or delivered personally to a prospective employer. When mailing an application, be sure to include your correct name, address, and a telephone number where you can be reached. When delivering an application, you need to be prepared to be interviewed at that time.

PREPARING A RESUMÉ

A **resumé** is a document prepared by a person to show a potential employer his or her strengths. It advertises qualifications for a job to potential employers. Resumés usually include the following information:

- Complete name, address, phone number, and Social Security number

- **Career goals,** which are statements that spell out what kind of work a person intends to do, the type of position desired, and the contribution he or she wants to make

- **Employment history,** which is a summary of work experience that includes each company's name and address, the supervisor's name and phone number, dates of employment, the reason for leaving the job, and a brief summary of the duties (Experience that applies to the job being sought is given emphasis.)

- Education, including the name and address of each school, date of graduation, course of study, and diploma, degree, or certificate awarded

- Special training, certificates, and licenses, including the agency or group that issued each one and effective dates

- Special skills related to child care, which may include storytelling, puppetry, or musical skills

- Organizations and interests, including both school clubs and out-of-school organizations, offices held and responsibilities, and at least one interest that involves other people and perhaps one or two that are pursued alone

A resumé should be typed on good-quality white paper. All words should be spelled correctly. There should be no smudges or dirty spots on the finished resumé.

A resumé should be only one or, at most, two pages long. The most important thing to remember about creating a resumé is to be honest. Leave out any of the items listed above that do not apply to you.

Interviewing

Most employers schedule an interview only if they are favorably impressed by your application and have a position open for which you qualify. A **job interview** is a meeting between an employer and a job applicant for the purpose of exchanging information about the applicant's skills and other qualifications and the job's benefits and requirements. When you submit an application, find out about the procedures for obtaining an interview. If it is simply a matter of requesting one, schedule an interview as soon as possible.

Learning to interview successfully is a skill you will have a need for. Basic guidelines for interviewing include the following:

- Be clean and well-groomed, and wear clothes that look good, fit well, and are not flashy or revealing.

- Use colognes, perfume, or cosmetics moderately.

- Go to the interview alone.

- Bring your birth certificate, driver's license, diploma, Social Security card, completed application, and resumé.

- Arrive for the interview 10 to 15 minutes early.

- Remain calm.

- Shake hands warmly as you look the interviewer in the eye.

- Be polite, courteous, and tactful.

- Be enthusiastic but not overbearing.

- Be interested in the business or organization without being nosy.

- Give fairly short answers that are accurate and informative.

- Ask about the duties and responsibilities of the job.

- Express goals and be decisive.

- Save questions about salary, benefits, and working conditions until the end of the interview.

- Do not prolong the interview.

- Thank the interviewer for talking with you.

- Leave promptly.

The Chain of Command

In any well-run business there is an organizational structure called the **chain of command.** This specifies whom each person supervises and to whom each person reports. The organizational

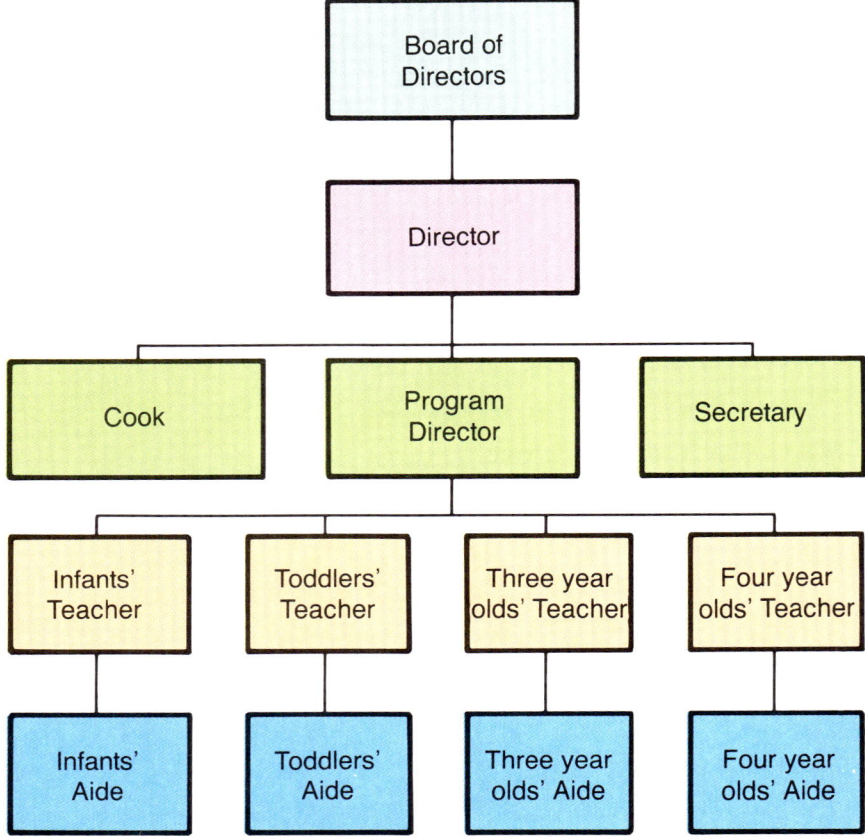

ILLUSTRATION 6-1 An organizational chart for a child care center shows the chain of command and the lines of authority.

chart in Illustration 6-1 shows the chain of command for a child care center. Each rectangle represents a position. The positions toward the top of the chart supervise the positions below them. The lines show the relationships between various positions and who reports to which supervisor and are called the **lines of authority.**

Where there are no lines of authority, there is no direct responsibility and usually no reason to report. For example, there are no lines of authority in Illustration 6-1 between the aide in the infants' room and the toddlers' teacher. Therefore, the toddlers' teacher does not supervise the infants' aide, and the infants' aide does not report to the toddlers' teacher.

Each job has responsibilities. When a caregiver accepts a responsibility, he or she should also be given the authority needed to fulfill it. If an aide is responsible for supervising a group of six toddlers, the aide needs to have the authority to discipline them appropriately and to carry out activities with them. Problems arise when responsibility and authority do not match.

PROFESSIONAL RESPONSIBILITIES

Being a professional involves more than holding a job that is designated as a professional position. It includes a person's attitude and approach to his or her work, as well as his or her commitment to doing the best job possible.

Participating in Professional Organizations

Groups of professionals form organizations in order to strengthen their profession and form a network of support for themselves. Being a member of one or more of these organizations is one part of being a responsible professional. Organizations for professionals who work with young children include the National Association for the Education of Young Children (see the Leadership at a Glance feature); the Southern Association on Children Under Six (SACUS, P.O. Box 5403, Brady Station, Little Rock, AR 72215); and the Association for Childhood Education International (ACEI, 11141 Georgia Avenue, Suite 200, Wheaton, MD 20902).

Upholding Professional Ethics

Ethics describe standards of conduct. Professional ethics are based on the values and knowledge commonly held by those in a given profession. The written statement that outlines such standards of conduct is called a **code of ethics.**

A committee of the National Association for the Education of Young Children has recently developed a set of standards for early childhood professionals in that organization. The code is based on commonly held values, including the following:

■ Appreciation of childhood as a unique and valuable stage of the human life cycle

Leadership at a Glance

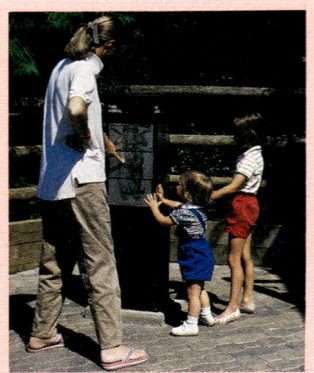

Source: Courtesy of the Cincinnati Zoo and Botanical Garden.

National Association for the Education of Young Children

The National Association for the Education of Young Children (NAEYC) is a professional organization whose purpose is to improve the quality of care given to young children. The NAEYC publishes a journal entitled *Young Children* as well as many books and other educational materials designed to help teachers, directors of child care centers, and parents do a better job.

Members of NAEYC include students, teachers, and people from all walks of life who are concerned with children. They recognize and support the very important role of parents in the lives of young children.

Each year NAEYC and its affiliates hold conferences where the democratic process is used to make decisions concerning how the members will promote the needs of young children and lend support to parents and families. These conferences also provide members with current information about working with young children and their families.

You can obtain more information about NAEYC publications and membership by writing to this address:

National Association for the Education of Young Children
1834 Connecticut Avenue, N.W.
Washington, DC 20009

- Recognition that knowledge of child development is the foundation for sound programs
- Acknowledgment of the interconnection between child and family
- Recognition that children are best understood in the context of family, culture, and society

- Respect for the dignity, worth, and uniqueness of each individual (child, family member, or colleague)

- Commitment to helping children and adults achieve their full potential in the context of relationships that are based on trust, respect, and positive regard

The code addresses the responsibilities of professionals who deal with young children and the behavior of those professionals toward children, families, colleagues, community, and society. The first principle addressing professional conduct toward children is as follows: "Above all, we shall not harm children. We shall not participate in practices that are disrespectful, degrading, dangerous, exploitative, intimidating, psychologically damaging or physically harmful to children. *This rule has precedence over all others in these standards.*"[1]

DEVELOPING LEADERSHIP SKILLS

Your community and our nation need strong leaders. Participating in organizations is one way to develop leadership skills and provide service to others.

The Future Homemakers of America, Inc., is a youth leadership organization for students enrolled in home economics or related courses. The organization is featured in a Leadership at a Glance feature.

Being a leader in a group may or may not mean being an officer of it. Leaders are those who think responsibly, act with care, and have the strength to do what they believe is right—regardless of pressures or circumstances. They carry out responsibilities with consideration for others and the organization's purposes.

If you want to become a leader, it is important to develop **leadership skills**—qualities and abilities that help make a person effective as a leader. A good leader is confident and cooperative and has good communication skills. Illustration 6-2 lists the traits of an effective leader.

Carol Louise was impressed with the variety of things children were doing at La Casita and with the pleasant and competent

---

[1]S. Feeney and K. Kipnis (1989). "Code of Ethical Conduct and Statement of Commitment," *Young Children*, 45 (1).

Leadership at a Glance

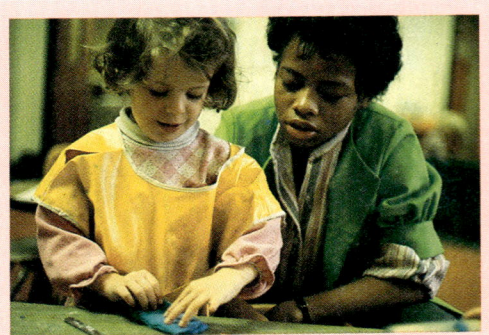

Source: *Future Homemakers of America, Inc.*

Future Homemakers of America, Inc.

Chapters of Future Homemakers of America exist in many junior and senior high schools in connection with home economics classes. There are three kinds of chapters: FHA chapters for consumer and homemaking classes, HERO chapters for occupational classes, and FHA/HERO chapters that have both types of members.

You may have an opportunity to participate in an FHA or HERO chapter in connection with this course. Membership opens up the following opportunities:

To grow individually through the "Power of One" achievement program

To strengthen occupational skills through competition in "STAR Events"

To develop leadership skills

To attend state and national leadership meetings

You can find out more about participating in FHA or HERO from your teacher or by writing to the national headquarters at this address:

Future Homemakers of America, Inc.
1910 Association Drive
Reston, VA 22091

adults who worked there. She was also impressed with how much the children seemed to enjoy what they were doing and the way the adults paid attention to and encouraged the children. Jonathan said he liked La Casita so Carol Louise decided to enroll him. Carol Louise felt more comfortable returning to work because she knew Jonathan would be learning and enjoying his days as well.

ILLUSTRATION 6-2 An effective leader of a group has certain traits related to working with others, working for the group, and management.

Working with others
- Works well with both students and adults
- Helps develop leadership qualities in others
- Communicates well with chapter members and leaders and is a good listener
- Involves everyone, considering individual abilities and interests in delegating responsibilities
- Shows appreciation and gives recognition as earned

Working for the group
- Works to instill confidence and pride in the group
- Shows genuine interest and involvement in the chapter's activities
- Places group interests above self-interests
- Takes pride in the goals of the organization

Management
- Encourages other students to participate and work toward group goals
- Demonstrates efficiency and competence
- Accepts responsibilities and follows tasks through to completion
- Makes decisions and stands by them, yet is flexible when change will benefit the group
- Manages time, energy, and resources well

Source: Future Homemakers of America, Inc., Handbook for Youth Centered Leadership, *1982, p. 43.*

Summary

Purposes of a child care center include assisting parents with child care, strengthening children's developing abilities and skills, and identifying and helping children with special needs. Child care programs may be custodial care, developmental, structured educational, special needs, school-based, or Head Start. Types of facilities include day care centers, family day homes, work-based centers, cooperative centers, and parent's day out or drop-in centers. Child care environments include enough space, private and personal areas, softness, and sound-absorbing surfaces.

Children's centers have policies concerning children and parents. These are frequently printed in a policy handbook and discussed with parents when they enroll children. Centers also have legal concerns. Most states set and enforce minimum standards for child care facilities. Adults who provide child care are liable for children's safety and well-being.

Planning and preparing for a career is important for high school students. Career clusters are groups of related jobs. A career ladder shows how you move from entry-level jobs to jobs with more responsibilities. In child care you can work as a nanny or manny, caregiver, teacher, assistant teacher or aide, program director, or director. Related careers include teaching at higher levels, research, social services, and medical or legal careers that specialize in children and families.

To get a job, you not only need to find an available one you are qualified for, you also need to develop skills in writing resumés, filling out applications, and interviewing. Succeeding in a job includes understanding and respecting the chain of command.

Child care professionals follow ethical practices. These include maintaining confidentiality, showing respect, giving assistance, providing opportunity, and gaining knowledge.

Membership in professional organizations is another professional responsibility. Members have opportunities to develop leadership skills.

Terms and Concepts

Gross motor skills

Fine motor skills

Custodial care programs

Developmental programs

Developmental tasks

Structured educational programs

Special needs programs

School-based programs

Head Start

Day care centers

Family day homes

Work-based centers

Cooperative centers

Parent's day out centers

Drop-in centers

Policies of child care centers

Philosophy

Policy handbook

Confidentiality of files

Period of incubation

Bilingual teachers

Minimum standards

Legal liability

Professional liability
insurance

Career cluster

Child care careers

Career ladder

Directors

Entrepreneurship

Nannies

Mannies

Child development
researchers

Social services

Pediatrics

Child life specialists

Resumé

Career goals

Employment history

Job interview

Chain of command

Lines of authority

Code of ethics

Leadership skills

Checking Your Understanding

1. Explain the role a child care program may play in the lives of families.

2. List and briefly describe each type of child care program. Select the one you think is preferable and explain briefly why you think it is best.

3. Name the kinds of child care facilities. Discuss circumstances in which each kind might be selected by parents.

4. Describe how you might create private spaces and softness in a preschool room.

5. List the contents of children's files. Explain why it is important to have each of the items on file.

6. Why do you think information in a child's file must be kept confidential? How can staff members keep children's files confidential?

7. What problems might arise if children were allowed to bring personal belongings to the center?

8. Why is it important to keep parents informed about what is happening at the center?

9. How does a policy allowing parents to visit at any time help ensure that children are treated properly in a child care center?

10. What is legal liability? Describe what being liable means to a child care worker. Why is it important for each center and each adult employed there to carry professional liability insurance?

11. Name the career options in the child care career cluster and write a very short job description for each.

12. List eight guidelines for filling out an application for employment.

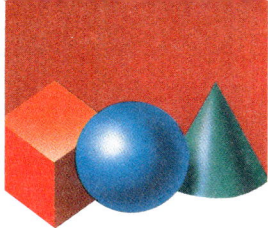

6 HANDS ON WITH CHILDREN

TEACHING CHILDREN ABOUT WORK

Children learn about work from adults. By the time they are eighteen months old, children are highly interested in participating in work. What are some ways to help young children develop healthy attitudes about work and begin to prepare them for careers?

- *Teach children order.* Have materials children use placed where they can be easily reached and put away.

- *Teach children self-care skills.* Help children learn to wash their hands, toilet, dress, and feed themselves.

- *Provide opportunities to observe adults doing their jobs.* Point out people at work. Talk about the things they do. Take children where they can safely see different kinds of work being done.

- *Provide opportunities to imitate adults.* Dress-up clothes and dramatic play areas offer children opportunities to "try on" adult roles and see how it might feel to be a teacher, truck driver, or engineer.

- *Tell stories and provide experiences related to jobs.*

- *Find value in children's contributions and express your appreciation.* Give children manageable tasks to do and allow them to experience the good feelings from making a contribution. Give them a sense of real achievement.

- *Encourage a hopeful attitude.* Help children see their own possibilities.

Learning about work is closely related to developing a sense of self-worth. Children's development of a sense of self-worth depends on two seemingly opposing conditions. First, when children experience achievement, they conclude that they are of worth. Second, when they sense that they are loved and that nothing will change that love—even if they do not achieve—their sense of worth is confirmed.

CHAPTER 7
Health Care and Illness

When you have finished this chapter, you will be able to

- Classify foods into four basic food groups
- Help children prepare and serve food
- Check children's health and immunization records
- Discuss ways to prevent the spread of diseases through sanitation and hygiene
- Notify parents of children's illnesses
- Evaluate a child care center for basic health standards
- Check children for signs of illness
- Identify symptoms of communicable diseases
- Care for a sick child in the child care center
- Teach children self-care routines

Geoffrey had been enrolled in La Casita for a week when one of the children in the group became ill. When Geoffrey's parents, Jerome and Donna, picked him up on Thursday, they were handed a note informing them that a child at the center had been diagnosed as having chicken pox.

Geoffrey's parents were not happy to find out that he had been exposed to this illness. However, the outbreak of chicken pox was the first such occurrence at La Casita that year. Also, they knew that being with other children—even in a good center like La Casita—would increase the chances that he would be exposed to illnesses.

Mrs. Cisneros followed the center's established policy when notifying parents that children had been exposed. The note gave the symptoms that needed to be observed, the incubation period, and the recommended action. Knowing that Mrs. Cisneros and her staff handled an outbreak of illness in the center according to accepted procedures was reassuring to Geoffrey's parents. They were impressed with the efforts of the staff to prevent illness, to help children learn about caring for their health, and to create a sense of good health.

HEALTH CARE BEGINS WITH GOOD NUTRITION

Children's nutritional needs are similar to those of adults. Knowing what foods children need and in what amounts is necessary for parents and child care professionals.

The Four Food Groups

Foods are grouped by nutritionists according to their main contributions to the body. Usually foods are categorized in four

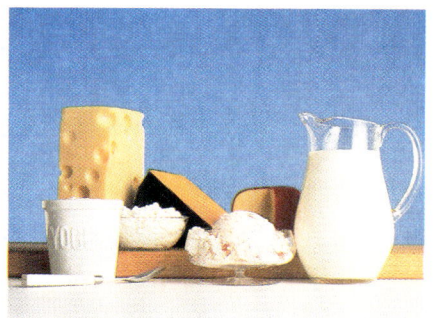
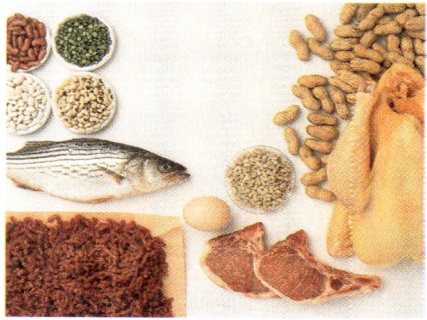
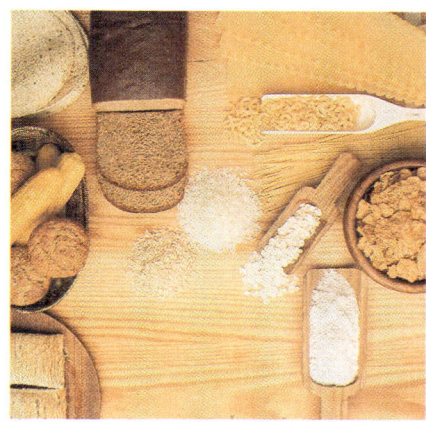
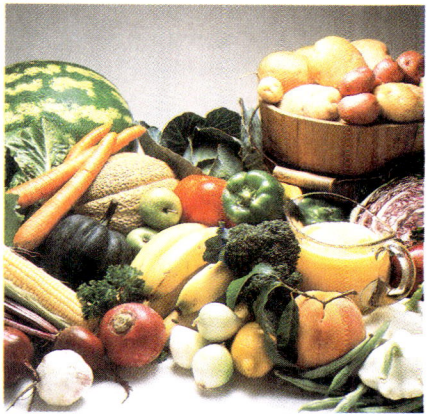

FIGURE 7-1   The four food groups are (clockwise from upper left) the milk group, the meat group, the fruit and vegetable group, and the bread and cereal group.
Source: USDA photos

groups: the milk group, the meat group, the fruit and vegetable group, and the bread and cereal group.

THE MILK GROUP

Foods from the **milk group** provide calcium, phosphorus, protein, vitamins A and D, and some B vitamins. Low-fat milk, skim milk, whole milk, yogurt, cottage cheese and buttermilk are recommended sources of these nutrients. Other dairy products, including cheese, ice cream, custards, and flavored milks, have varying amounts of these nutrients and should be served only once each day.

Serving fruit-flavored milk may encourage children to drink milk. However, chocolate in milk can interfere with the body's ability to absorb the important bone-building calcium. Chocolate milk should not be served more than once or twice each week.

Children need two to three servings from the milk group each day. A serving is 8 ounces of milk (1 cup) or 1 ounce of cheese.

THE MEAT GROUP

Foods from the **meat group** provide protein, iron and B vitamins. The foods in the meat group include fish, chicken, beef, turkey, and pork. Other protein foods can be substituted for meat. These include eggs, cheese, and cottage cheese. Vegetable sources of protein such as peanut butter and dried beans can be substituted for meat if they are served with a whole-grain bread such as cornbread or whole wheat crackers.

Children should have two to three servings from the meat group each day. Toddlers get about 2 tablespoons for each serving, and preschool children get 4 tablespoons (about $\frac{1}{4}$ cup). Serving sizes increase as children grow.

Children should be given tender meats that are not highly seasoned. Meat should be cut into bite-sized pieces. Skin, bones, and extra fat are removed from the meat. Children need a variety of meats that are cooked until well-done but are still moist.

THE FRUIT AND VEGETABLE GROUP

Foods from the **fruit and vegetable group** provide a rich variety of vitamins, minerals, natural fiber, and water. Some fruits and vegetables are particularly rich in vitamin A, and others are particularly rich in vitamin C.

Fruits and vegetables rich in vitamin A are usually bright yellow or green. Carotene, the plant form of vitamin A, is yellow in color. Good sources of vitamin A include pumpkin, carrots, spinach and other leafy green vegetables, winter squash, sweet potatoes, cantaloupe, broccoli, dried apricots, peaches, and tomatoes.

Foods providing large amounts of vitamin C include brussels sprouts, strawberries, oranges, broccoli, grapefruit, leafy green vegetables, cauliflower, cantaloupe, tangerines, cabbage, tomatoes, asparagus, raspberries, blackberries, and potatoes. Nearly all fruits and vegetables have some ascorbic acid.

Children need to eat one serving of a bright yellow or green fruit or vegetable every other day and at least one food rich in ascorbic acid every day. Serving sizes for fruits and vegetables are one small piece. Servings of cooked, chopped, or mashed fruits are one tablespoon per year of age up to eight. That is, two-year-olds' servings are 2 tablespoons, and five-year-olds' servings are 5 tablespoons.

Fruits and vegetables are most enjoyable and nutritious if they are fresh or very lightly cooked. Overcooked vegetables lose their flavor and texture so children do not like them as well. Fruits and vegetables rich in vitamin C are often well liked by children. This vitamin is easily destroyed so these foods should be prepared just before eating. Leaving them in open air, soaking them in water, or overcooking can destroy much of their nutritional value.

THE BREAD AND CEREAL GROUP

Foods from the **bread and cereal group** provide generous amounts of iron and the B vitamins. Whole-grain foods also provide fiber. Foods included in the bread and cereal group come from the grain, or seed, part of grasslike plants. The most common grains are wheat, oats, rye, rice, barley, and corn. Many interesting and good-tasting products have been developed from these grains.

Whole-grain bread and cereal products should be labeled "100% whole grain." If a product is labeled simply "whole grain," this gives no indication whether there is a great deal of fiber or just a little fiber. If bread and cereal products are not whole-grain, they should be enriched. Enriching restores many of the vitamins and minerals lost during the milling process.

Children need four servings from the bread and cereal group each day. A serving for toddlers is a half slice of bread, $\frac{1}{4}$ cup of cooked cereal, or ½ cup of prepared (cold) cereal. Servings for five-year-olds may be twice those amounts.

Poorly Nourished Children

Children who do not receive the right kind of food over a period of time begin to show signs of being poorly nourished, or undernourished. Generally their health is poor. They are often overweight or underweight. They seldom sleep well but are not alert when awake. They may be irritable and hard to get along with. Other signs of being poorly nourished include the following:

- Skin may be pale, loose, rough, or delicate.
- Posture may be poor, with shoulders rounded.
- Eyes may be red, itching, and sensitive to light.
- The child may be a picky eater and have a poor appetite.
- The child may have irregular bowel movements, be constipated, or have diarrhea.
- Teeth may be irregular and decayed, and gums may bleed or be spongy.
- Hair may be dull or even coarse.
- Muscles are underdeveloped.
- If overweight, the child is flabby.
- A severely undernourished child may have a protruding abdomen (lower belly).

Children with Food Allergies

One part of the enrollment form for a child care center concerns the child's health. This part should include a question asking about allergies. Teachers and caregivers need to be informed about children's food allergies. The center will keep written records on allergies children have. Many centers post a list somewhere near the eating area where caregivers can check it regularly.

Helping Children Prepare and Serve Food

Preschool children can begin to help prepare food and to assist with mealtime routines. Recipes can be written so children can read them. Children can prepare simple foods as long as they use equipment that is safe for them and are well supervised. They can also help set the table and clean up after meals and snacks.

Preschool children enjoy the opportunity to see food being made. They enjoy tasting things and watching them cook, for example, through a glass door on an oven with a light inside. They like the smells and enjoy the feeling of accomplishment when they eat what they have prepared.

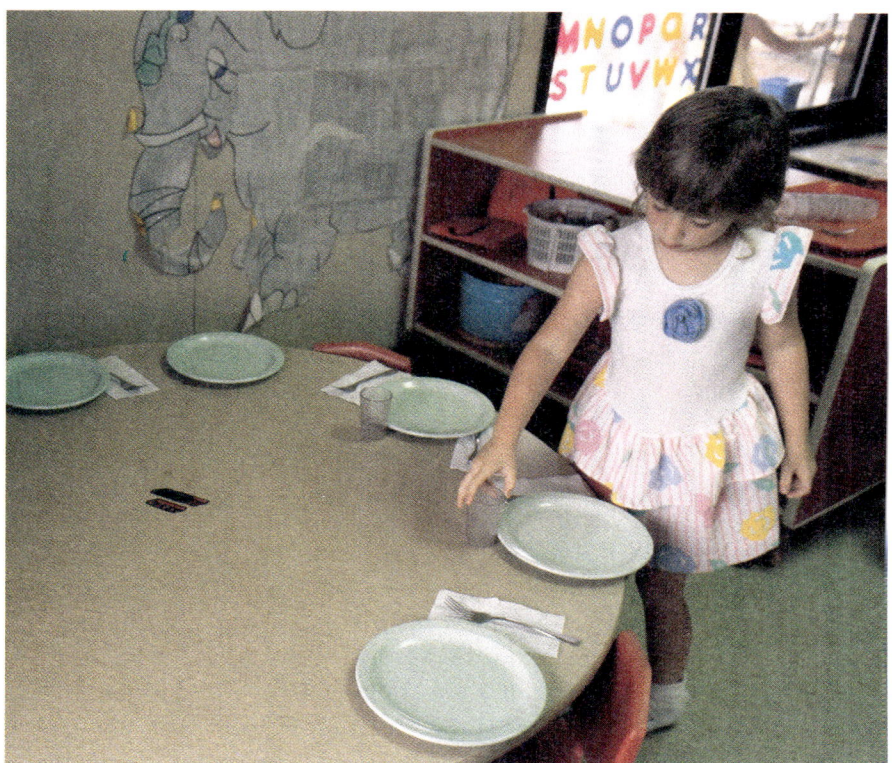

FIGURE 7-2 Preschoolers can help at mealtimes by setting the table.

What can a preschool child do to help prepare and serve meals?

▪ Get out equipment that he or she can reach and carry safely

▪ Get out ingredients

▪ Spoon ingredients into a measuring cup

- Pour ingredients into a bowl
- Stir with a wooden spoon in a plastic or metal bowl
- Place biscuits or cookies on a pan
- Watch while food cooks—from a safe place
- Carry some foods to the table
- Serve food onto his or her own plate
- Carry dishes to the sink or dishwasher
- Assist in washing nonbreakable dishes and utensils that are not sharp
- Help put dishes away

Preschoolers need help with some tasks related to meal preparation. Older preschoolers should be carefully supervised if they are allowed to use knives or electrical appliances. All preschoolers should be supervised very closely when they are around a hot stove or oven. Preschoolers need to be helped when ingredients, equipment, or dishes are too high for them to reach or too heavy for them. They also need to be helped with carrying, passing, washing, and putting away dishes that are hot, heavy, or breakable.

Children need praise and appreciation for the help they give. They are not able to do things as carefully and correctly as adults, so adults need to be accepting about the way things turn out. The process of helping is more important than a perfect product. It is very important not to redo something a child has done, even if redoing it makes the product better. Help the child make the change or let it go as it is. Careful supervision and guidance during the cooking process will keep errors to a minimum.

PREVENTING ILLNESS

What does it mean to be healthy? Some people would say it means not being sick. Child care workers can help prevent illness in centers by following practices that promote good health and by monitoring children's health.

Promoting Good Health in Child Care Centers

Children under three are more likely to experience certain illnesses if they are in child care. Children over three do not seem to be as affected by attendance at preschool.

Everything an effective staff does in a well-run developmental child care center aims to promote each child's well-being, or health. In addition, certain specific tasks need to be done to foster good physical health. These include maintaining adequate immunization and health records and using appropriate sanitation and hygiene procedures.

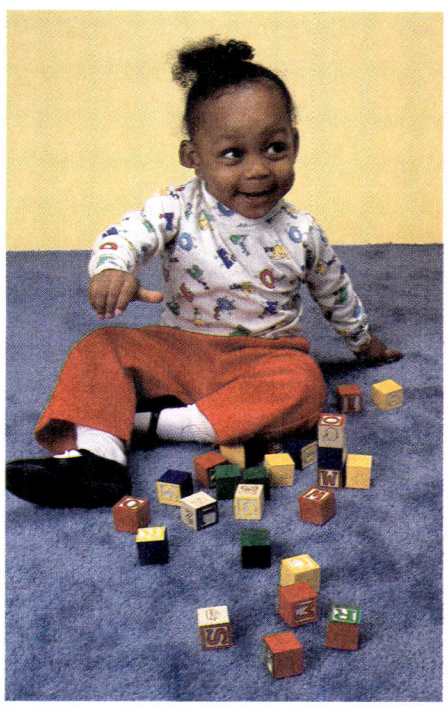

FIGURE 7-3
The promotion of a child's well-being, or health, concerns parents and caregivers.

IMMUNIZATION AND HEALTH RECORDS

Immunizations are doses of vaccines. **Vaccines** are low-level doses of active or inactive viruses that are given to children to help them establish their own immunity to diseases. **Immunity**

is the greatly increased ability of the body to resist infection by a specific disease.

Diseases for which vaccines are given are usually highly contagious, or easily passed from one person to another. Diseases

Leadership at a Glance

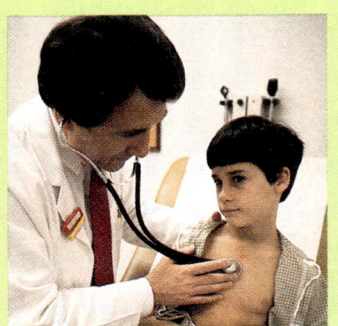

Source: *Children's Hospital Medical Center*

American Academy of Pediatrics

The American Academy of Pediatrics is an organization of doctors who provide health care for children and adolescents. Their main purpose is to help their young patients be as healthy as possible, both mentally and physically.

In addition to being medical specialists, pediatricians are advocates for children and youth. They work to ensure that children's health needs are considered in legislation and public policy. They promote laws designed to protect children, such as those related to the use of car safety seats and seat belts, child abuse, and immunization programs.

Family crises sometimes cause problems for children. Pediatricians are often aware of these and may serve as a family counselor. They can give advice about coping with problems and may become a child's friend.

Pediatricians also teach children and their parents about proper nutrition, accident and disease prevention, and athletic conditioning.

The American Academy of Pediatrics publishes information about careers in pediatrics. If you would like to know more about such careers, about this organization, or about the materials it publishes, you can write to this address:

American Academy of Pediatrics
P.O. Box 927
Elk Grove Village, IL 60007

common to children for which vaccines are regularly given include the following:

- Diphtheria
- Tetanus
- Pertussis (whooping cough)
- Polio
- Measles

- Meningitis
- Mumps
- Rubella (German measles)
- Hepatitis B

The American Academy of Pediatrics has established a recommended schedule for administering vaccines, shown in Table 7-1. Vaccinations are recorded on forms called **immunization records.** Most states require that children entering child care receive certain vaccines and that their immunization records be kept on file in the center.

SANITATION

Keeping surfaces free from bacteria and viruses that might make people sick is called **sanitation.** Faucets and table surfaces are often contaminated with germs. To stay sanitary, these and other surfaces must be regularly treated in a way that kills the bacteria and viruses. Heat or chemicals may be used to sanitize surfaces. Effective sanitizing reduces the number of cases of diarrhea and strep among children in a center.

How is sanitary different from clean? Clean means no dirt can be seen and things are put away; however, clean does not mean germ-free. Sanitary means clean and germ-free.

Sanitizing by heat. Clothing and linens can be made germ-free by being dried in a clothes drier. Dishes can be processed through dishwashers with sufficiently hot water or a heated drying cycle to make them germ-free.

Sanitizing by chemicals. Bacteria and viruses may also be killed by using solutions of water and certain chemicals for cleaning. Sanitizing chemicals are available commercially. These chemicals must be selected with care—some may be harmful if misused or used too frequently. Chemicals must be stored where children cannot get at them and in a place away from food so they are not mistaken for food.

TABLE 7-1 Recommended Schedule for Immunizations

Age	DTP (Diphtheria, Tetanus, Pertusis)	Polio	TB Test	Measles	Mumps	Rubella	Hib-Conjugate	Tetanus-Diphtheria
2 months	✓	✓						
4 months	✓	✓						
6 months	✓							
1 year			✓					
15 months				✓	✓	✓		
18 months	✓	✓					✓	
4–6 years	✓	✓		✓	✓	✓		
5–21 years								
14–16 years								✓

Source: "Protecting Your Child Against DTP," American Academy of Pediatrics, revised 1989. Reprinted with permission.

A common sanitizing chemical is chlorine bleach. Chlorine bleach sanitizes when used with water in the following amounts:

- Dishwater: $\frac{1}{4}$ cup per gallon of water
- Laundry: 1 cup per load (18-pound capacity washer)
- Surfaces: $\frac{1}{2}$ cup per gallon of water

Surfaces to be sanitized. All surfaces children come in contact with have to be sanitized often, according to a regular schedule. Since children under three are more susceptible to diseases, surfaces in the infant and toddler rooms need to be sanitized daily. Feeding and diaper-changing areas should be sanitized after each use.

Surfaces in areas used by children over three have to be sanitized at least once each week. Toileting and hand-washing areas should be sanitized daily. Feeding areas need to be sanitized after each use. If there is an outbreak of a contagious illness in the center, all rooms should be sanitized more frequently to minimize the spread of disease.

HYGIENE

Keeping caregivers and children free of bacteria and viruses that cause communicable diseases is more successful where practices of good hygiene are followed. **Hygiene** means conditions or practices that promote good health. Such practices include the following:

- Washing hands frequently
- Bathing daily
- Wearing clean clothes to work
- Keeping nose free from mucus
- Avoiding sneezing or coughing on children or children's food

Hand washing. The dirtiest surfaces in a child care center are nearly always the hands of caregivers. Hand washing must be frequent and routine among caregivers in order to avoid spreading germs that cause diseases. Frequent hand washing along with other good hygiene practices protects the health of children and caregivers alike.

Hands should be scrubbed with soap for a full minute under running water. Caregivers' hands are washed at the following times:

- Before the day's work begins
- Before and after handling children's food
- Before and after wiping a child's nose or giving any kind of bodily care
- Before and after changing a diaper
- Before and after giving medication
- At the end of the day

Cleaning up blood. Since many viruses that cause serious illnesses thrive in blood, it is important that blood be cleaned up immediately and carefully. All blood spills must be cleaned up immediately with a solution that is made by mixing 10 parts of water and 1 part of chlorine bleach (for example, 10 cups of water and 1 cup of bleach). Use paper towels and disposable plastic gloves. Avoid allowing blood to come in contact with mucus membranes or openings on the skin of caregivers or children.

Monitoring Children's Health

An important part of maintaining a healthy environment in a child care center is observing children for signs of illnesses. When a sickness is identified early, the affected child can receive proper care sooner. Also, the spreading of the illness among the other children is more likely to be prevented. Centers can also provide for tests for particular problems and notify children's families of the results.

HEALTH CHECKS

One way children's health can be protected in a center is by frequently making sure that everyone is healthy. A **health check** is a quick daily procedure by which caregivers determine whether any of the children are ill. As children are brought into the center each day by parents, caregivers are responsible for checking for these symptoms:

- Itching or rash
- Bad skin color

- Face flushed or pale
- Red eyelids, circles under eyes, watery or glassy eyes, yellowed or bloodshot whites of eyes, or swollen eyes
- Runny nose
- Throat red or swollen
- Spots in mouth or throat
- Wounds, injuries, or bruises
- Bluish tinge to fingernails

In addition, caregivers can touch children to check for these symptoms:

- Fever (skin should be normal temperature)
- Lumps under jaw (swollen lymph glands)

Finally, caregivers can listen for

- Barky cough
- Cough that sounds wet, or as though mucus is being coughed up
- Wheezing
- Rattled breathing
- Breathing through the mouth
- Shallow, rapid breathing
- Comments about symptoms

During the day caregivers can be alert for general signs that a child is not feeling well. For example, a child may not seem to be acting like his or her normal self. Or a child may show a lack of appetite at snack or meal times.

HEALTH SCREENINGS

Many health problems of children can be identified by health screenings. **Health screenings** consist of tests that reveal particular problems in young children, such as vision problems, hearing problems, or speech problems. These tests are often provided free of charge or at a very low cost by organizations interested in the

ILLUSTRATION 7-1 Following these steps will ensure that an accurate thermometer reading is obtained.

Step 1   Hold the thermometer at eye level with the ridge toward you and the white surface away from you.

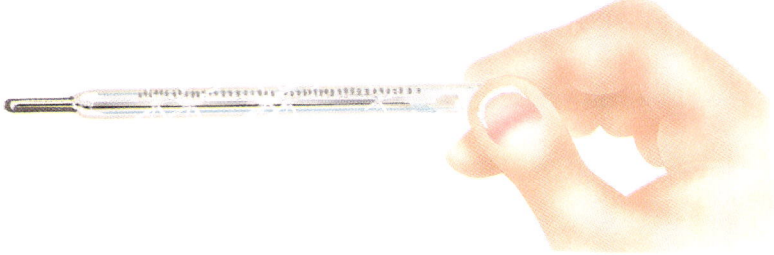

Step 2   Gently twist the thermometer until you see a flash of silver. The temperature is the exact point at which the silver ends.

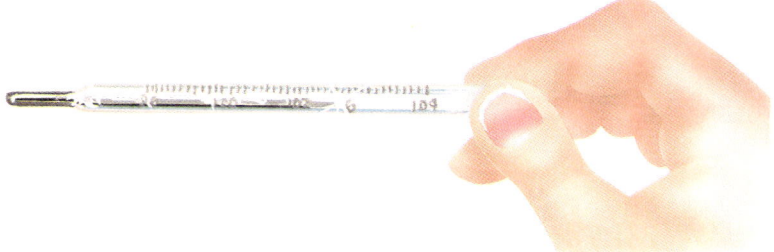

Step 3   Read the temperature. Thermometers are marked in tenths of degrees. An arrow points to normal body temperature, which is 98.6°F. The degrees are marked with longer lines. A number is usually written by every other degree. For example, the thermometer shown is marked at 98, 100, 102, 104 and 106. Each short line between degree markers indicates two-tenths of a degree. To read a thermometer, find the last long line the flash of silver goes past. That is the number of degrees. Count the number of short lines after the long line that the silver goes past. Multiply this number by 2. Add that number of tenths to the degree. For example, on the thermometer shown, the silver flash goes 3 marks past 102. Since 3 × 2 = 6, six-tenths of a degree is added to 102. This temperature is written 102.6° and said aloud as "one hundred two and six-tenths."

health needs of young children. Some screening tests can be conducted by members of a center's staff who have completed special training.

TAKING A CHILD'S TEMPERATURE

Thermometers are devices for measuring temperatures. Children's temperatures may be taken rectally, orally, or axillary (in the armpit). With children who are very small or very ill, temperatures are taken rectally. Older children's temperatures are taken orally. Axillary temperatures are taken when children strongly object to the use of a rectal thermometer but are too young or too sick to use an oral thermometer safely.

When a child is sick, the doctor needs to know exactly what his or her temperature is. It is important that a caregiver be able to read, write, and say the correct thermometer reading. Illustration 7-1 shows how to read a thermometer.

Caregivers can also take a child's pulse (heart rate) and respiration rate (breathing rate), record them, and report to the

ILLUSTRATION 7-2   These are accepted methods for taking a child's pulse and respiration rates.

Pulse Rate

To take a child's pulse rate, place the tips of your fingers about one finger's width below the child's left nipple. Count the number of beats for 15 seconds. Multiply that number by 4. The normal pulse rate in children ranges from 70 to 170 beats per minute. Infants average about 120 beats per minute; five-year-olds average about 100 beats per minute.

Pulse rate = number of beats in 15 seconds × 4

Respiration Rate

To take a child's respiration rate, count the number of times he or she breathes in and out in 15 seconds. Multiply that number by four. The child should not be aware that you are watching because this could cause the breathing rate to change. The normal respiration rate for an infant is 30 per minute.

Respiration rate = number of breaths in 15 seconds × 4

parents or doctor. Illustration 7-2 presents the accepted methods of taking a child's pulse and respiration rate.

COMMUNICABLE DISEASES AND CHILD CARE

At a child care center, it is important to keep as many children healthy as possible. Young children in child care are especially susceptible to illnesses that can be easily passed from one to another. Although many of these illnesses are no longer as common as they were because of immunizations, many still affect children. Children are particularly vulnerable to illnesses because they have not yet built up immunity to many of them and because the number of people they come in contact with increases as they get older.

Children with immunity disorders, those with leukemia or other forms of cancer that are present throughout the body, and those who are taking medications that affect the immune system are especially likely to catch contagious diseases. Parents whose children are vulnerable to illness for these reasons need to make teachers and caregivers aware of that fact.

Communicable Diseases in Child Care Centers

Communicable diseases are those that are passed from one person to another. They are caused by bacteria or viruses. Common childhood diseases are listed and described in Table 7-2.

Communicable diseases are passed in various ways in a child care center, including the following:

- Through mucus membranes, by handling tissues with mucus or kissing the mouth of an infected child

- Through contact with feces, by handling dirty diapers or failing to wash hands thoroughly after changing an infected child's diaper

- By breathing the air in which an infected child has sneezed or coughed

- By eating food that has been handled by a person who is sick

- Via unsanitized surfaces (some bacteria can live on unsanitized surfaces and will be transferred through contact)

TABLE 7-2 Common Communicable Diseases Affecting Children

Disease	Symptoms	How passed
Chicken pox	Slight fever, loss of appetite for 24 hours, red rash that becomes blisters	Contact with mucus from an infected person or with skin blisters
Diphtheria*	May resemble a common cold or may involve sore throat and fever, hoarseness, cough, and difficulty breathing (children sometimes die in 6 to 10 days when diphtheria is severe)	Direct contact with an infected person, someone who carries the disease but does not have it, or contaminated objects
Fifth disease	1. Rash on cheeks may look like child was slapped 2. Red spots appear on arms and legs and eventually whole body 3. Rash disappears, but may come back if exposed to sun, heat, or cold or if irritated	Contact with blood, urine, or mucus from an infected person
German measles*	Low fever, headache, looking and feeling sick, sore throat, and cough, followed by rash that begins on face and spreads down the body and is usually gone in three days	Contact with mucus of an infected person, or sometimes blood, urine, or feces of an infected person
Measles*	Fever, feeling and looking sick, cough followed by rash that lasts 3 to 4 days	Contact with mucus, blood, or urine of an infected person
Mumps*	Fever, feeling and looking sick, pain in ears, especially during chewing, lack of appetite for about 24 hours, swelling and tenderness in cheeks and neck	Contact with mucus or saliva of an infected person

(cont.)

TABLE 7-2 (cont.)

Disease	Symptoms	How passed
Roseola	High fever for 3 to 4 days, followed by pink rash that appears on trunk and spreads to arms and legs and lasts 1 or 2 days (usually found in babies and toddlers up to age two)	Unknown
Polio*	Fever, sore throat, headache, vomiting, stomach pain, and stiffness in back, neck, and legs (can cause children to be paralyzed)	Contact with feces or mucus of an infected person
Scarlet fever	High fever, fast pulse, vomiting, headache, and stomach pain	Contact with mucus from an infected person or with contaminated articles (such as tissue), or from contaminated milk or other food
Tuberculosis	May be no apparent symptoms, or may be fever, weakness, cough, and weight loss	Direct contact with mucus of actively infected person
Whooping cough*	Sneezing, cough, and low fever, followed in about a week by dry, hacking cough ending in a high-pitched sound; eyes may bulge and tongue protrude	Mucus from infected person

*Children can be immunized against these illnesses.

Symptoms of Communicable Disease

Jerome and Donna learned the symptoms of chicken pox and watched Geoffrey daily for signs of the illness, until the incubation period had passed. Fortunately he did not come down with it.

What are the most common signs that a child has a communicable disease? Fever and sore throat are often symptoms of communicable disease. A rash is sometimes a symptom. Children having these symptoms should not be admitted to a room with the other children. The parents should be called if the symptoms appear during the day.

Symptoms that require immediate medical attention include the following:

- Fever over 101°F with pain, vomiting, or diarrhea
- Breathing difficulties
- Bleeding that does not stop or is fast
- Sleep that cannot be interrupted
- Projectile vomiting (throwing up in a shooting stream)
- Stomach pain with a slight fever
- Dry mouth and skin and no wet diaper for 6 hours
- Something in the eye that tears will not remove

Most states do not allow children to come to a child care facility if they have symptoms of illness. Although most parents will keep children at home when they are ill, some will not, in spite of this regulation. It is up to caregivers to send children home when they are ill.

Caring for Sick Children

Some states provide special licensing for centers who accept sick children. Work-based child care facilities may seek this type of license. Special isolated areas and trained staff must be present when centers allow ill children to stay. Medical and child care professionals are working together to develop safe and effective methods for caring for mildly sick children in child care facilities.

Children often have concerns about illness, particularly their own illness. They need help coping with pain and with feeling badly. Children who are expecting to go to the hospital may be particularly fearful. The Hands On with Children feature for this chapter deals with helping children prepare for a hospital stay.

Sometimes children begin to show symptoms of illness while they are at their regular child care center. What measures do caregivers take when a child becomes ill? They isolate the child, call one of the child's parents, and stay with the child. They need to get help from a doctor if the symptoms listed above are observed.

ISOLATING THE CHILD

When a child develops symptoms of an illness, he or she should immediately be separated from the other children and observed carefully by a trained staff member. The child's temperature should be taken.

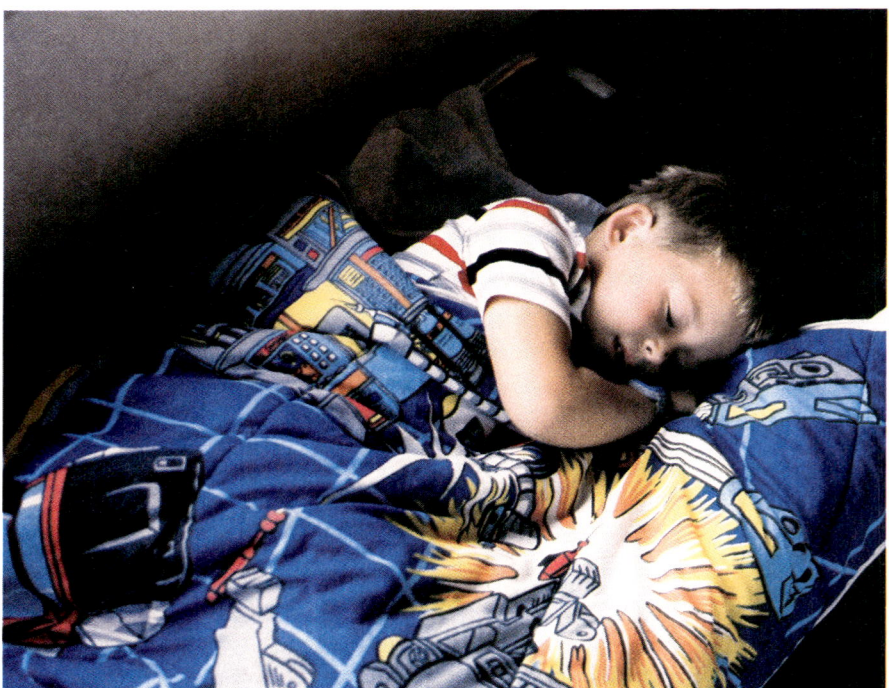

FIGURE 7-4   A sick child may need to rest in an isolated area until a parent can pick him or her up.

CALLING A PARENT

Let a parent know as soon as possible what the child's symptoms are and when they were recorded. Tell the parent to come and get the child.

GETTING MEDICAL HELP

If a child's symptoms indicate that he or she needs immediate medical attention, call an ambulance if one is reasonably close or take the child to a doctor or emergency room.

STAYING WITH THE CHILD

All children need to be watched constantly, but particularly a child who is ill. When a child is ill, a staff member stays with the child in the isolated area until a parent or medical help arrives. The caregiver can comfort the child and make him or her comfortable. *Aspirin or other medication is never given without first consulting the child's doctor and informing him or her of the child's symptoms.* Aspirin given to children who have some communicable diseases may cause the development of a potentially serious condition called Reyes syndrome.

Caregivers who must care for an isolated sick child for more than a few minutes can help the child in several ways. A caregiver in this situation can do the following:

- Follow any doctor's orders exactly.
- Prevent the spread of the disease by washing hands frequently and properly disposing of tissues or other articles containing mucus or other body fluids.
- Provide a quiet activity for the child to help take his or her mind off being sick.
- Keep the child comfortable.
- Monitor and record the child's temperature, heart rate, and respiration rate.
- Provide emotional support.

Recording Incidents of Illness

It is important for caregivers to write down a child's symptoms and any action taken when caring for a sick child. If a doctor

LA CASITA CHILDREN'S CENTER
Record of Illness

Child's name   _David Fuentes_   Date _Jan. 12, 1992_
Time parent contacted _9:42 am_ Parent's directions _Call doctor._
Mother will pick David up about 10:00 am.
Symptoms _102°F fever, pain in stomach_

Child's doctor contacted? _yes_   Time _9:55 am_
Doctor's orders _Bring David into office right away._

Record of Action Taken

Time	Pulse	Respirations	Temperature	Medications/Treatment
9:30 am	85 /min	22 /min	102°F	Sponged with cool water
	/min	/min		
	/min	/min		
	/min	/min		

Other action taken _David rested in isolation area while waiting for his mother._

Kim Liu
Signature of Staff Member

Yolanda Cisneros
Signature of Director

ILLUSTRATION 7-3   This type of record should be kept on any illness that occurs in a center.

gives orders over the phone, write them down. Give the parent a copy of the record and keep a copy in the child's file. A copy of a form that might be used for recording illness is shown in Illustration 7-3.

Notifying Parents of Children's Illnesses

When a child becomes ill in a center, one of his or her parents must be called immediately. Parents often become upset when their children are ill, so it is important that caregivers who call parents to notify them remain calm and speak reassuringly. However, it is equally important to give parents the facts. Be specific about what has happened. If it is important for parents to come immediately, tell them so. Then reassure them that you will be with the child and that appropriate action has been taken.

If one of the children in a center has been diagnosed by a doctor as having a communicable disease, parents of all the children have to be notified. The notice should contain at least the following information:

- Name of the disease
- Date on which the first child was diagnosed as having it
- Number of days in the incubation period (the number of days until symptoms may appear)
- Symptoms
- Action that needs to be taken

Minimum standards established by a state government often dictate how such a notice has to be given. If no specific guidelines exist, the notice should be posted in several very visible places around the center at parents' eye level. In addition, it is a good idea to send a copy of the notice home with each child.

Infections in Child Care Centers

Infections are conditions caused by bacteria, viruses, fungi, or parasites and usually affecting a limited area of the body, such as the intestinal tract, skin, or hair. Children in child care facilities are at risk for picking up infections from contact with other children. Infections commonly passed among children are described in Table 7-3.

TABLE 7-3 Common Infections

Infection	Description	Symptoms	Treatment
Head lice	Parasites found in hair or on scalp; passed by sharing combs or sleeping where an infected person has slept	Itching scalp	Apply lice treatment available at a drugstore or by prescription from a doctor.
Impetigo	A highly contagious skin infection that itches and oozes; caused by streptococcus or staphylococcus bacteria	Itching, oozing skin lesions	A doctor should be consulted.
Pinworm	A parasite that lives in the lower intestine	Itching around the rectum during sleep, possibly mild stomachache, appearance of threadlike worms around rectum or on bedding or under-clothes	A doctor should be consulted.
Ringworm	A fungus infection that usually appears in the scalp area; caught by sharing combs or direct contact	Small red spots that expand into an increasingly larger ring	A doctor should be consulted.
Scabies	An itchy condition of the skin caused by a tiny parasite; passed by skin-to-skin contact	Itching skin	A doctor should be consulted.

Giving Medication to Children

Parents who bring medication to the center to be given to their children need to sign an authorization each day. This form gives the staff permission to give the medication and states the times it is to be given. Only medication prescribed by a doctor and ordered by parents should be given to children. Under no circumstances should any member of a center's staff give a child medication that has not been authorized in this way.

The *right* medicine must be given to the *right* child in the *right* amount at the *right* time. Any mistake could be deadly to a child.

Medications must be stored out of children's reach, preferably in a locked cabinet. Medications that need refrigeration should be stored in a refrigerator located outside the children's room. If they have to be kept in a refrigerator in a children's area, they should be placed where they are hard for children to reach. In this case caregivers also need to be sure that children do not open the refrigerator without adult supervision.

FIGURE 7-5 A special kind of spoon for giving medicine to children enables caregivers to measure doses correctly.

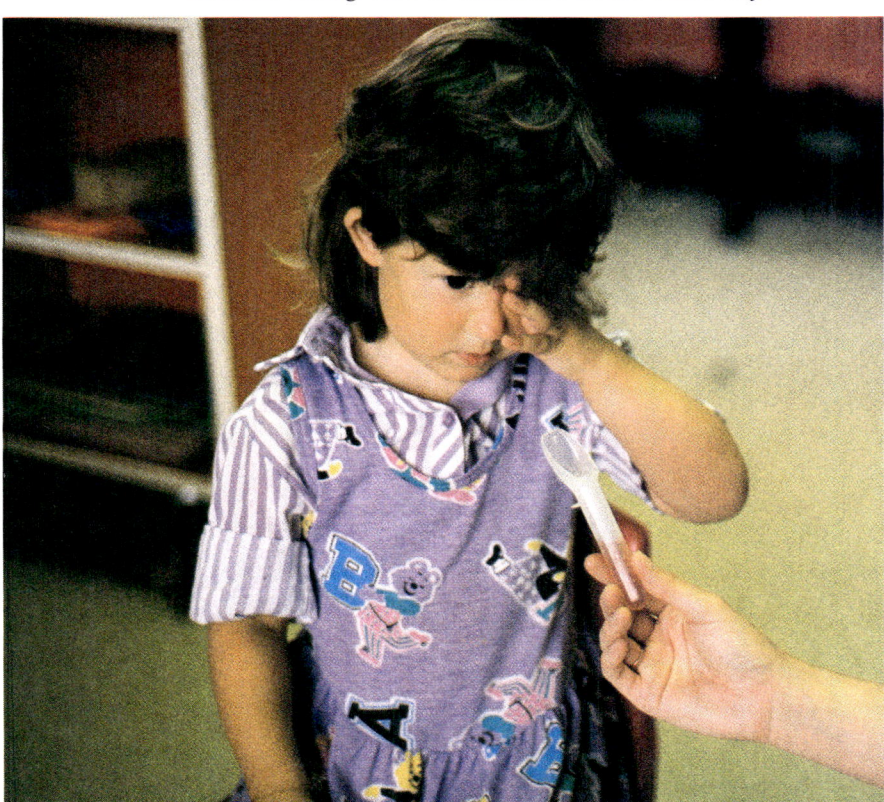

When giving medication to children, carefully measure the dose before going to the child or picking her or him up. A toddler or preschooler needs to sit in a comfortable position to take medication. Babies need to be held in an upright position. Use a spoon designed for giving children medicine or a dropper. Each child who receives medication must have his or her own spoon or dropper. Place the end of the spoon into the child's mouth and use a pouring motion to help the child swallow the medication. Praise the child for accepting the medication.

HELPING CHILDREN WITH SERIOUS ILLNESSES

Sometimes children have to deal with serious illnesses. Occasionally children remain in child care during these times. Their teachers and caregivers can help them deal with their serious problems.

Chronic Illnesses

A long illness, particularly one that is serious, is called a **chronic illness.** Chronic illnesses that may affect young children include those acquired after birth and those caused by birth defects or handicaps. Chronic illnesses may be lifelong and may result in early death. Examples of chronic illnesses include the following:

- Diabetes
- Asthma
- Cystic fibrosis
- AIDS
- Leukemia and other forms of cancer
- Heart, lung, and kidney disorders
- Cerebral palsy

Families of children with chronic illnesses experience shock when they first learn of the illness. Family members are often disappointed that the child is no longer perfect. Sometimes they feel guilt or resentment because of the child's condition. They may feel helpless. With time, most families adjust. Some eventually accept the illness and the child, becoming realistic in their expectations. Unfortunately, some do not ever again really accept the child. Chronically ill children in child care centers may have families or family members who have different reactions to the child's illness.

Chronic illness makes development more difficult. The key to helping children with a chronic illness is enabling them to carry out the main developmental tasks for their age level.

Children with AIDS

AIDS (acquired immune deficiency syndrome) is a serious disease that has no known cure. A report from the U. S. Health Service Centers for Disease Control states that "it is a disease caused by a virus that can damage the brain and destroy the body's ability to fight off illness."[1]

AIDS is thought to be transferred through the following body fluids, especially if fresh:

- Blood
- Feces
- Semen
- Saliva
- Urine
- Vaginal secretions

The four most common ways in which the AIDS virus is passed from one person to another are

- Sexual intercourse (any type)
- Sharing needles (usually among illegal drug users)
- Blood transfusion (if donor was infected)
- Birth to an infected mother

For approximately 2.5% of AIDS cases, the sources have not been confirmed or clearly identified.

AIDS is not thought to be transferred through casual contact. Hugging, holding, rocking, or playing with an infected person are not considered to be ways of spreading the virus.

Very few children have AIDS. Most who do were born to an infected mother. Some have received blood transfusions; many of these have hemophilia, an inherited disorder that causes blood not to clot properly. It is possible for children who have been sexually abused to develop AIDS.

---

[1] *What You Should Know About AIDS*. Atlanta, GA: U. S. Public Health Service Centers for Disease Control, n.d.

Children who have AIDS have the same needs as other children. In addition, they have a devastating illness that frequently causes them to feel sick. They need the same compassion as children who have leukemia, diabetes, or any other chronic illness. The Something to Think About feature discusses caregivers' responsibilities concerning children with AIDS.

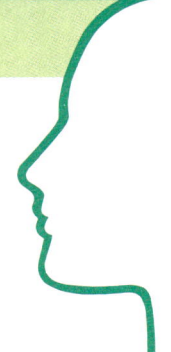

Something to Think About

What Are Caregivers' Responsibilities Concerning Children with AIDS?

Children who have AIDS can certainly be considered to be innocent victims of the disease. Informed caregivers know that AIDS is not spread by the kind of touching that is appropriate for them to give to children at a child care center. Children with AIDS need plenty of tender loving care and to be treated as much as possible like other children. Caregivers can safely give them what they need.

Any adult caring for children has a responsibility to stay healthy. A caregiver should not take the risk of exposing himself or herself to AIDS in any possible way. Caregivers need to follow a special procedure for handling body fluids of AIDS-infected children (see the text). Any center accepting an AIDS-infected child should contact local medical authorities for assistance in establishing safe caregiving procedures.

There is a real need for child care centers that will accept chronically ill children, particularly those with AIDS. Is caring for an innocent child worth the risk? How much risk do you think is involved? Would you accept an assignment to care for an infant with AIDS as his or her primary caregiver? In today's world these issues are clearly something to think about. What do you think?

When handling body fluids of AIDS-infected babies and children, caregivers need to exercise extra care to ensure that fluids do not come in contact with other children or themselves. When handling these body fluids, a caregiver uses the following steps:

Step 1 Before changing a diaper, dressing a wound, or handling body fluids in any way, put on a sterile (never used) pair of surgical gloves.

Step 2 Dispose of any body fluids collected in a sealed, covered container.

Step 3 Disinfect diaper area (or wound area) with a medically approved disinfectant.

Step 4 Dispose of surgical gloves.

Step 5 Disinfect hands with a medically approved hand disinfectant.

Step 6 Clean all blood spills immediately with chlorine bleach solution (a mixture of 10 parts water to 1 part bleach). Use paper towels and disposable plastic gloves.

LEARNING ACTIVITIES ABOUT HEALTH

An important part of taking care of children's health is helping them to learn about health and health care. Activities can be planned to support this learning during the children's day.

Self-Care Routines

Self-care routines are ways children learn to care for their own health. Child care centers are well-suited to helping children learn self-care skills.

Learning to care for oneself begins with receiving appropriate care from adults. When infants are changed regularly and their faces and noses are kept clean, caregivers are teaching them the feeling of being clean—a feeling most children like. Wiping infants' hands with a damp cloth before feeding time prepares them for later hand-washing routines.

What self-care skills should be taught to young children and when? Child care centers can help toddlers start to learn how to wash their own hands, use the toilet, get enough rest, and brush their own teeth.

WASHING HANDS

As soon as children can walk well, they can be helped to hold their hands under warm, not hot, running water. Soap can be applied by caregivers, who will also need to help the children rinse and dry their hands. Hand washing needs to be practiced before and after meals and before and after toileting.

TOILETING

A major task of toddlers is learning to use the toilet rather than soiling diapers. As children approach two, most of them begin to become annoyed with having dirty diapers. Some tell caregivers as soon as they soil a diaper, or even just before. Many become fascinated with the functions of the bathroom and various forms of water play. All of these behaviors suggest that children may be ready to learn toileting habits.

Toilet training also goes on at home; therefore, it is most important that caregivers work in a friendly way with parents to make sure that what is being done in the center is the same as what is being done at home.

A chart that can be useful for gathering information on a child's elimination habits is shown in Illustration 7-4. Caregivers check a child's diapers every 15 minutes for a week and record the times when they are wet or soiled. This record lets caregivers know what times of day the child is most likely to wet or soil diapers. If the child is wetting or soiling at fairly consistent times and if the between wettings is about two hours, most children are ready to toilet train.

The chart in Illustration 7-4 can be used effectively to toilet-train a child. Once a chart is completed for a child, caregivers follow the steps given in Illustration 7-5.

RESTING

Children need to rest during the day. Some sleep; others just rest. Caregivers help children learn to rest by establishing a set time for daily naps and by creating a restful environment. Most child care centers schedule a few minutes of sitting quietly in the morning and time for napping after lunch. Environments that help children to rest have the following features:

■ Lowered levels of light (not total darkness)

■ Comfortable, clean mats or cots

LA CASITA CHILDREN'S CENTER

Weekly Record of Wetting and Soiling

Child's Name _Sarah_   Week Beginning _Sept. 18_

TIME	MONDAY	TUESDAY	WEDNESDAY	THURSDAY	FRIDAY	SATURDAY	SUNDAY
7:30		WET	WET				
7:45	WET				WET	WET	
8:00				WET			
8:15					BM		BM
8:30	BM					BM	
8:45			BM	BM			
9:00		BM					
9:15							
9:30			WET			WET	
9:45	WET	WET		WET	WET		
10:00							WET
10:15							
10:30							
10:45							
11:00							
11:15							
11:30			WET		WET	WET	WET
11:45	WET	WET		WET			
12:00							
12:15							
12:30							
12:45							
1:00							
1:15							
1:30							
1:45			WET				WET
2:00	WET	WET		WET		WET	
2:15					WET		
2:30							
2:45							
3:00							
3:15							
3:30							
3:45							
4:00			WET				
4:15		WET		WET	WET	WET	
4:30	WET						WET
4:45							
5:00							
5:15							
5:30							

ILLUSTRATION 7-4   By keeping records of children's wetting and soiling patterns on a form like this, caregivers can help them develop successful toileting habits.

ILLUSTRATION 7-5 Caregivers can follow these steps to help children with toilet training.

Step 1 Place the child on a child-sized toilet for a short time at the time of day when he or she usually wets, or just a few minutes earlier. If the child resists, do not insist.

Step 2 Allow the child to stay for about 15–30 seconds, or 1 minute at most.

Step 3 If the child does not produce urine or feces in the toilet, do not make any comment. Just help him or her with clothes and allow to resume play. Most will wet or soil diapers shortly.

Step 4 Repeat the procedure the next time as indicated on the chart. The child should soon be ready.

Step 5 If a child succeeds, compliment him or her gently. Help the child clean himself or herself.

Step 6 If a child tells you he or she wants to use the toilet, allow this, even if the chart does not indicate that he or she is probably ready. Children need to know they can get the adult help they need when they use the toilet.

Step 7 Encourage parents to replace diapers with underwear once the child is successful at toileting.

- Blankets, usually the child's own, for warmth and comfort
- Good ventilation (fresh air)
- Comfortable temperature
- Soft, soothing music

Children who have difficulty settling down to rest or going to sleep may need to have a caregiver gently rub or pat their backs for a time. A caregiver may lie down beside a child who is having difficulty. Children who resist resting regularly may need to have nap time in an area separate from the other children and supervised individually. All children need to be supervised by an alert adult during rest and sleep periods.

BRUSHING TEETH

Children need to learn to brush their teeth after snacks and meals. Dental assistants may come to the center to show children how to brush teeth.

Toothbrushes need to be carefully marked with children's names and hung where they can air-dry. Toothbrushes should not be close enough to touch one another. Children need to be supervised during toothbrushing routines to ensure that they are brushing adequately and using only their own toothbrushes.

FIGURE 7-6   Learning to brush teeth correctly and regularly is a basic self-care skill.

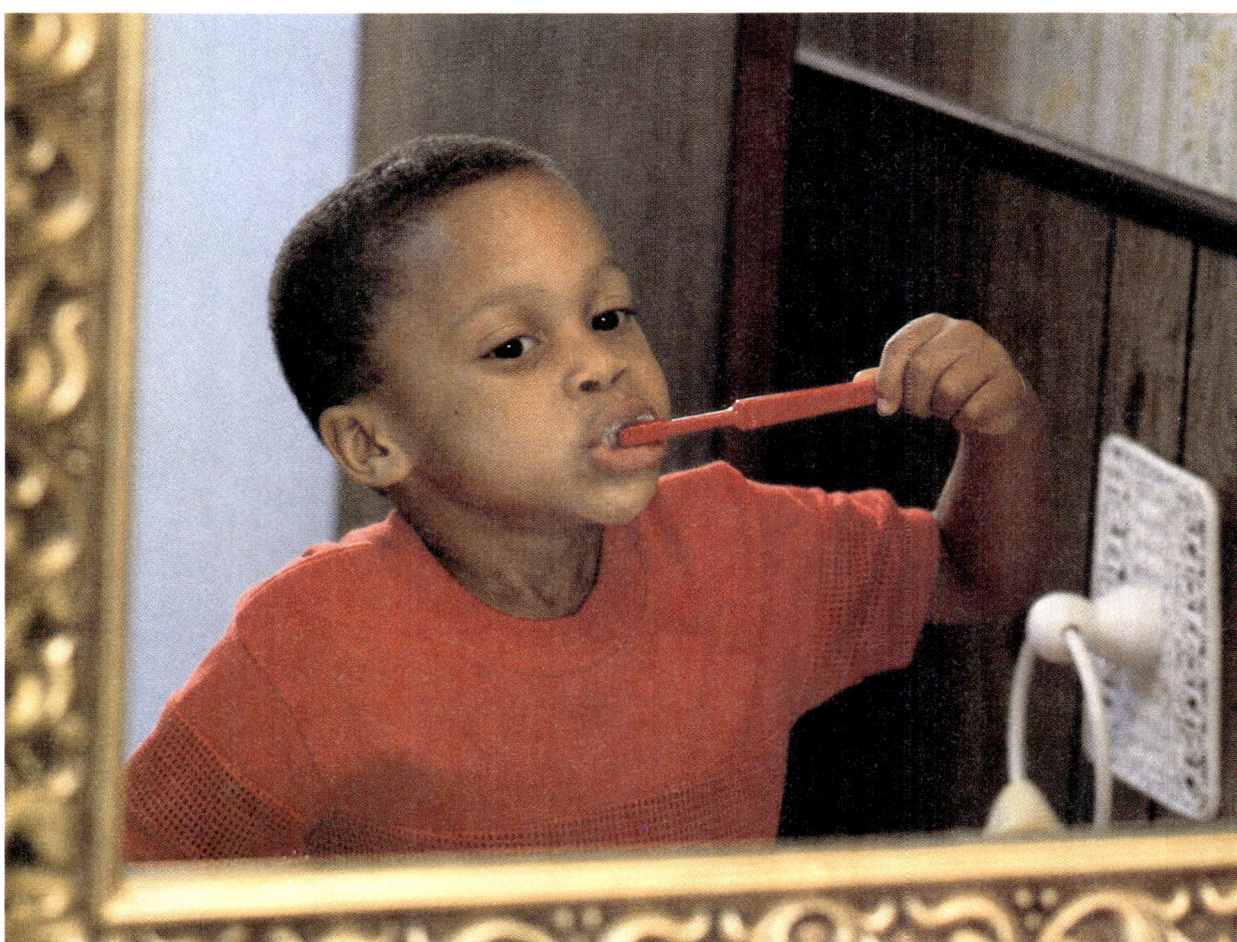

Learning About Health Care

In addition to learning self-care skills, children can learn to take care of their own health through activities at the center. Activities that lend themselves well to learning about health care include stories and puzzles about health care, dramatic play with health care props, and music and art activities with a health-related theme.

Jerome and Donna were impressed with the concern shown at La Casita for Geoffrey's health. They had no idea that caring for children's health in groups required so much effort. They

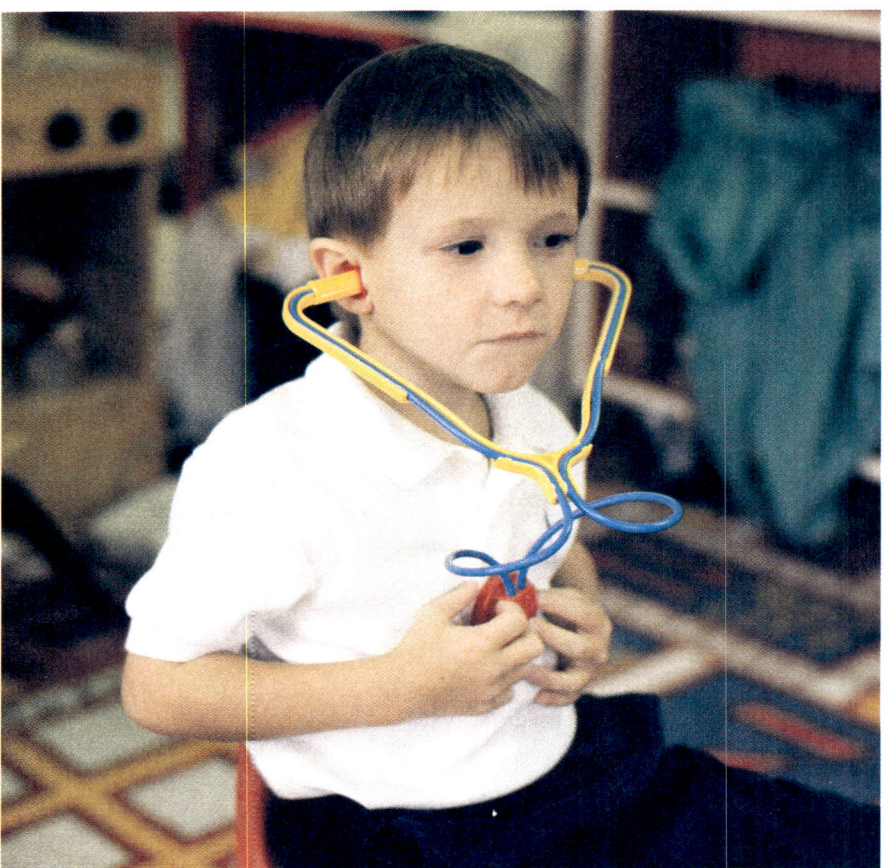

FIGURE 7-7   Dramatic play with health care props such as a toy stethoscope improves children's awareness of health and health care.

expressed appreciation to Mrs. Cisneros for the care she took to make La Casita a healthy, as well as an educational, experience for Geoffrey.

Summary

Foods can be divided into four food groups: the milk group, the meat group, the fruit and vegetable group, and the bread and cereal group. Poorly nourished children show signs that can be easily seen. Some children are affected by food allergies, which must be known to caregivers. An important part of teaching pre-school children about food is helping them assist with preparing food and with mealtime routines.

Staff members are responsible for getting health records of children and keeping immunization records current. Staff members prevent illness by following correct measures for sanitation and hygiene. They also check children daily for signs of illness.

Communicable diseases are common among children. When children spend time together in child care facilities, they are readily exposed to many illnesses. Symptoms of communicable diseases can be identified by trained caregivers. Caregivers may have the responsibility of caring for a sick child while waiting for parents or medical help to arrive. They need to isolate the child, call the parents, and get medical help if needed.

Infections may also occur in child care centers. Because infections can spread readily among children, care needs to be taken to notify parents and to treat the infection effectively.

Chronic or serious illnesses are among the health problems of young children. Children and their families can be helped to cope with the problems arising from such illnesses.

Child care centers also assist in maintaining children's health by teaching self-care routines. The activities offered at a center include opportunities for learning about health.

Terms and Concepts

Milk group	Immunizations
Meat group	Vaccines
Fruit and vegetable group	Immunity
Bread and cereal group	Immunization records

Sanitation   Communicable diseases

Hygiene   Infections

Health check   Chronic illness

Health screenings   Self-care routines

Thermometers

Checking Your Understanding

1. Name the four basic food groups and list two foods for each group.

2. Give five symptoms that can be seen in poorly nourished children.

3. Give six examples of things a child can do to help with food preparation and meal routines.

4. What is the difference between a clean surface and a sanitary surface?

5. Name two methods of sanitizing surfaces.

6. What is hygiene?

7. What is the dirtiest surface in a child care center?

8. Describe the technique used to wash hands properly. List six times when caregivers need to wash their hands.

9. Use the lists of symptoms given in the chapter to make a simple chart that could be used for a morning health check in a child care center.

10. Why is it important to know how to take and record a child's temperature, pulse rate, and respiration rate?

11. List the main ways in which communicable diseases are passed on in child care centers.

12. List eight symptoms that may indicate the presence of a communicable disease.

13. List four things a caregiver needs to do when a child becomes ill at a center.

14. List five infections that may occur in a child care center.

15. What information is included on a notice to parents about a contagious illness in the center?

16. Select one of the chronic diseases that affect children and report on it to your class.

17. Describe how you would help a child learn to wash his or her hands.

18. Discuss why it is important for caregivers and parents to work together on toilet training.

19. Make a list of props that might encourage children to role-play their fears concerning illness or hospitalization. (See the Hands On with Children feature on following pages.)

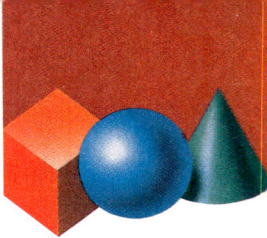

7 HANDS ON WITH CHILDREN

PREPARING CHILDREN FOR HOSPITALIZATION

Hospitals are unfamiliar places for children. Having to go to the hospital may cause a child to feel fear—of the unknown, of abandonment, of strangers, or of pain. Children can work through these fears with the help of parents and caregivers.

Caregivers can help children develop coping skills for handling pain, illness, and hospitalization. When a child expresses a concern, adults need to respond by listening carefully, then responding to the child's statement. It is important to encourage the child to express feelings and fears without causing more fear or worry.

Dramatic play provides opportunities to act out fears and other emotions concerning medical care. The family or block center can be set up as a hospital room or doctor's office. Children can role play being doctors, nurses, and patients. Role play is adult-stimulated dramatic play. Props that encourage role play include the following:

- Admission kit
- Stethoscope
- Bandages (can be torn from an old sheet)
- Band-aids
- Gloves
- Tape
- Thermometer
- Alcohol pads
- Syringes (without needles!)

- Oxygen mask
- IV tubing (less than 12 inches long)
- Doll
- Child-sized bed (crib mattress is sufficient)
- Surgical mask and gown
- Doctor's cap and coat
- Nurse's cap
- Uniform

This kind of role play requires the supervision and interaction of attentive adults.

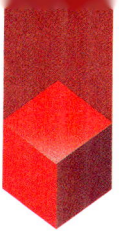

Puppets provide an excellent opportunity for children to work through their fears. Puppets can say things to children that adults may not be able to get away with. Children will tell puppets things they will not tell adults.

Pediatrics units in many hospitals invite parents to bring children in for a visit a day or so before admission to meet the people and see the place they will be going. A talk with a friendly, understanding nurse or hospital staff member can do a great deal to calm a child's fears.

CHAPTER 8
Safety and Emergencies

OBJECTIVES

When you have finished this chapter, you will be able to

- Identify causes of injuries to children
- Assist in child-proofing the child care environment
- Explain how child care centers can promote safety and prepare for emergencies
- Assist with evacuation drills
- Describe appropriate first aid for minor injuries and medical problems
- List important safety rules for a child care center
- Help children learn about community helpers

When Jerome and Donna rounded the corner to pick up Geoffrey at La Casita one afternoon, a fire truck was sitting in front of the building. Firefighters in full gear were pulling hoses from the truck. Children were standing in line outside the building. Jerome quickly parked the car, and they jumped out, looking for Geoffrey. Mrs. Cisneros came to them quickly, smiling. "Geoffrey's fine. The fire company brought the truck over to show the children the equipment, and we had a fire drill. Everything is fine."

Jerome clasped Donna's hand, and they both sighed with relief. Fire drills and learning about community helpers were part of La Casita's ongoing safety education program. La Casita had a good safety record. The staff members put a lot of effort into preventing injuries.

CHILDHOOD INJURIES

Children under six are injured more often than people of any other age group. Many childhood injuries may be prevented by removing hazards from the environment. **Hazards** are any situations, objects, or substances that might cause injury or create an emergency.

A very effective way of preventing injuries to children is supervising them closely. Alert supervision involves not only watching closely what children are doing but also developing the ability to assess what they are developmentally able to do. Infants have no idea of danger. Toddlers are so full of curiosity that they seldom see hazards. Preschool children are somewhat aware of risks and have better judgment than toddlers, but they still need careful supervision.

Something to Think About

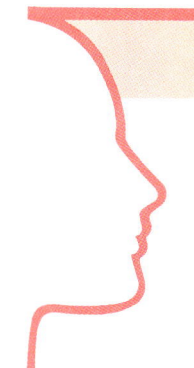

Preventing Injury Versus Taking Risks

How careful should caregivers be? Is it possible to keep children too safe? If children are never allowed to take chances, how will they learn to manage risk?

People who work with children strive to help them grow to be competent adults. Learning means meeting new challenges, and challenge involves risk. If children are never presented with new and challenging situations, how can they grow, learn, and develop?

One question caregivers must consider is this: When does risk become danger? The answer is not always clear and may change as children grow. Part of being a professional is developing the ability to make this type of judgment on a daily basis.

There is another question caregivers must consider: Do caregivers have the right to expose children to risk in the name of learning? What if a caregiver makes a mistake? What if a child is hurt while trying something new?

Lawsuits are very common in our society. Although professional liability insurance can help protect caregivers from lawsuits, sometimes the coverage is inadequate. Does a caregiver want to jeopardize his or her family's future income by taking the chance of being sued?

Where does a professional child care worker draw the line between preventing injury and allowing children to take measured risk? What do you think?

The following are important aspects of preventing childhood injuries:

■ Child-proofing the environment
■ Careful and consistent supervision of children
■ An understanding of children's developmental stages
■ Teaching children basic safety habits
■ Teaching children how to get adult help

Causes of Childhood Injuries

Falls are the most frequent cause of children's injuries in child care settings. The second most common cause of children's injuries is an accident involving some mechanism or object. The most common injuries are bruises, scrapes, and open wounds. Children are more likely to be injured on the head, face, and forehead than on other parts of the body. Children are most frequently injured in the outdoor play (climbing and running) areas of a child care facility. Boys are more likely to be injured than girls.

Injury can be caused by any situation or substance a child does not know how to manage. Most accidents are preventable. Some injuries, however, will occur no matter what precautions are taken by adults.

The following sections describe the most common types of injuries received by children.

INJURIES FROM AUTOMOBILE ACCIDENTS

The major cause of accidental injury and death in children under four is automobile accidents. Children are frequently injured or killed when they are in a car that is involved in an accident. They are much more likely to be harmed if they are not properly restrained in a car seat or by a seat belt. Many children are hit by cars as pedestrians or while playing in the street.

BITES

Children are often bitten by insects, snakes, pets, or other animals. Most bites occur because young children are not adequately aware of the danger or because they inadvertently provoke the animal.

Children sometimes bite each other. This most commonly occurs among toddlers. When a child bites someone, it is often due

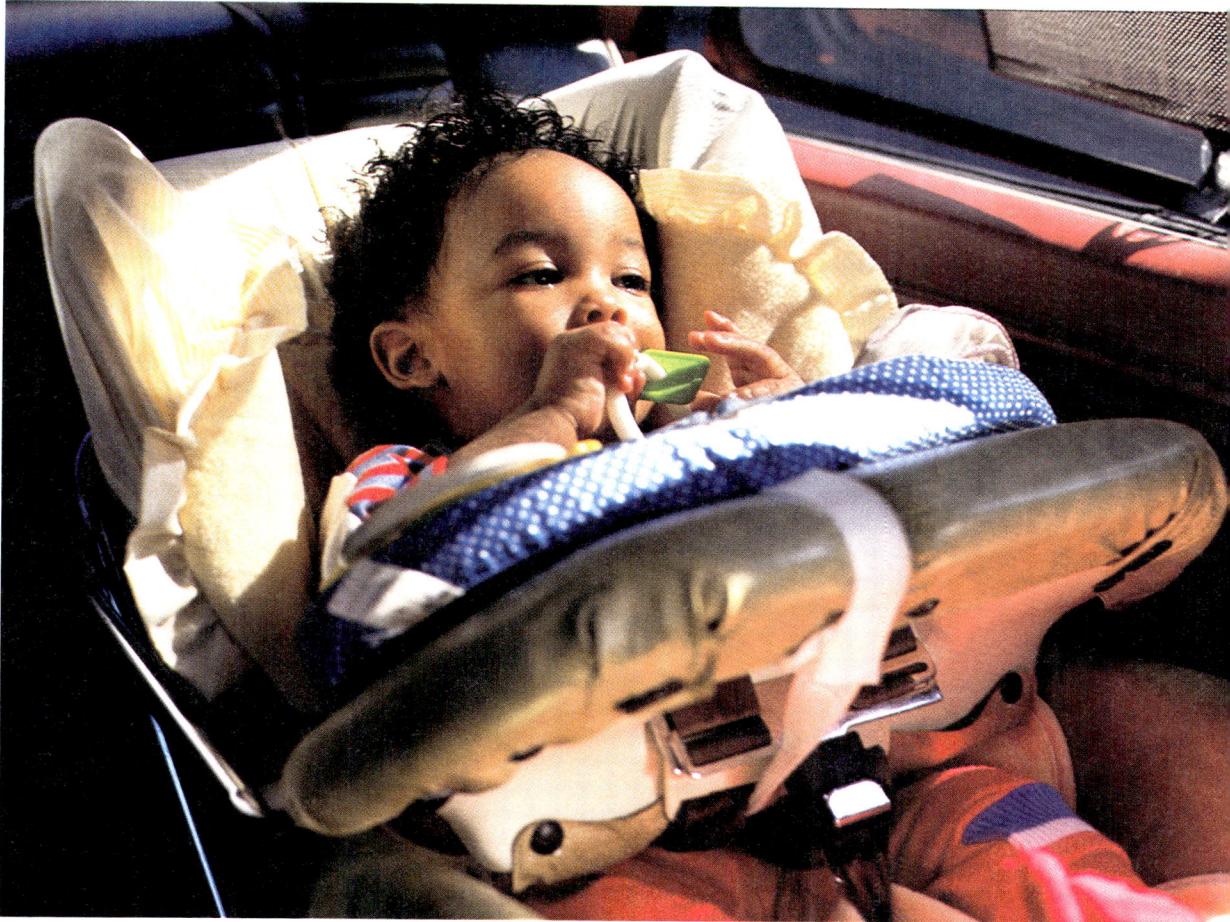

FIGURE 8-1   If young children are always correctly buckled into safety seats when they ride in a car, they are much less likely to be injured in automobile accidents.

to frustration. Frustration occurs in young children when they cannot say what they want to say or make their bodies do the things they want to do.

BURNS

Children are most frequently burned by hot appliances, heaters, radiators, furnaces, pots whose handles stick over the edge of the stove, hot foods, hot water from a faucet or other source, matches or cigarette lighters, cinders from fireplaces, or open flames. Sometimes they are burned by adults or older children with irons or other hot appliances, cigarettes, hot water, or hot grease or food. When children are accidentally burned by other people, it is often the result of carelessness. When a child is intentionally burned, that is physical child abuse. Chapter 9 discusses child abuse in more detail.

Children may also be burned electrically. Electrical burns may be accompanied by shock or cause death. Electrical burns most often occur when children place fingers or objects into electrical outlets, when they use electrical appliances without adequate supervision, or when they use appliances in the presence of water. All of these situations are *very hazardous* for children.

CHOKING

Children can choke on anything they can get into their mouths. Babies and toddlers often choke on items they find on the floor because they naturally explore and learn by tasting and feeling with their mouths. They do not know the difference between safe and unsafe objects. Objects that are unsafe in this sense include toys, buttons, pins, pen caps, balloons, and marbles. Young children may also choke on foods such as dried beans, carrots, popcorn, chunks of meat, hard candy, grapes, raisins, chunks of peanut butter, hot dogs, and peanuts.

DROWNING

Children can drown in as little as 2 inches of water in as short a time as 20 seconds. They can drown in swimming pools, wading pools, bathtubs, and even sinks. Children are fascinated by water and love to play in it. Children, especially toddlers, should *never* be left alone near water. Knowing how to swim does not make a young child safe around water.

FALLS

Babies can fall from any surface on which they are placed. Babies wriggle, move, push, roll over, and creep. If left unprotected, babies are likely to fall from changing tables, high chairs, beds, chairs, or sofas.

Babies between 7 and 12 months old begin to climb. Toddlers climb onto and into everything in sight. Since they cannot climb down, however, they often fall. For example, they can climb up stairs before they can climb down them, so they often fall down stairs. They may also climb into refrigerators, out of windows, and into wells.

Preschool children do not fall as often as toddlers. They usually fall from play equipment or structures onto which they have climbed.

POISONING

Babies between 7 and 12 months old put everything in sight into their mouths for the purpose of exploring. Saying no is not enough. All substances that might poison children must be kept where children cannot find them or get to them. Toddlers love to climb, and some can climb to the top of a refrigerator once they get a start from a chair left near a cabinet. Caregivers must assume that there is no place a toddler cannot reach. Any poison or medication kept in an unlocked cabinet or one with a lock that children can open is a hazard.

Children can be poisoned by a wide variety of substances, including household chemicals, prescription and nonprescription drugs, parts of some plants, garden and automotive products, cosmetics and lotions, fumes, and lead (usually from old paint). It is the responsibility of caregivers to see that children do not have access to poisonous substances. Caregivers should know which local plants are poisonous. A brochure containing this information may be available from the state health department or a local poison control center.

SUFFOCATION AND STRANGULATION

Children can suffocate in a plastic bag or in an airtight space such as an old refrigerator. They can strangle if they get their heads caught between rigid bars. Some older cribs have slats that are placed far enough apart to be hazardous for a small child. Cords, ropes, belts, or any objects that are long and flexible can get wrapped around a child's neck and strangle him or her.

Age of Child and Type of Injury Likely to Occur

Developmental characteristics affect the kind of risks children take and the type of injuries they tend to receive. Children are more susceptible to injuries and accidents at certain ages. Children under two are especially susceptible to injuries. A summary of developmental characteristics of children that may contribute to accidents is found in Table 8-1.

TABLE 8-1 Developmental Characteristics and Likely Accidents

Age Range	Developmental Characteristics	Likely Accidents	Comments
0–6 months	Rolls over Creeps Sits with support	Falls Suffocation	Infant develops rapidly and may gain skills adults are not aware of, resulting in dangers.
7–12 months	Sits alone Crawls Stands Climbs up Walks	Falls Choking Poisoning	Mobility means child can get into new places and get hurt in an unlimited number of ways; curiosity increases, and child does not perceive danger.
1–2 years	Climbs down Runs Investigates everything Learns by trial and error Crawls into small spaces	Falls Burns Cuts Scrapes Poisoning Choking	Safety and learning due to curiosity must be balanced. Child responds to verbal commands, but must be watched constantly.
2–4 years	Strength and coordination increase Pedaling and jumping skills develop Experiments Uses imagination to think of more things to try	Falls Burns Cuts Scrapes Poisoning Drowning Choking	Although child has more self-control, he or she must be constantly supervised. Child responds to reward and punishment. Active mind requires challenges, which adults must provide with a reasonable amount of safety. Child needs to learn to handle risk without harm.
4–6 years	Interest in people outside family increases Starts to be interested in accomplishing new feats Plays increasingly with other children Influence by older children and other adults increases	All of the above plus accidents involving balls and wheels and injuries from fighting	Teaching of safety rules should increase. Adults begin to give the child some opportunity to handle risk and challenge with supervision. Careful monitoring of other adults associated with the child is increasingly important.

SAFETY IN CHILD CARE ENVIRONMENTS

Not all family day homes and child care centers have been made safe for children. Common unsafe conditions in some facilities include the following:

- There are no impact absorbing surfaces under playground equipment.
- Unprotected space heaters are accessible to children.
- Playground equipment is unsafe.
- There is no fence around the playground.
- The center does not have a bottle of syrup of ipecac (given for some cases of poisoning) or has an expired bottle.
- The tap water is too hot.
- Stairways are unprotected (have no safety gates).
- Cabinets containing toxic materials are accessible to children.
- There is no fire extinguisher or smoke detector.

Child-Proofing the Environment

Child-proofing simply means developing an awareness of potential hazards and removing those hazards from the child's surroundings. Hazards that cannot be removed can be shielded so children cannot get to them.

One technique that can be helpful in child-proofing is crawling on hands and knees all around the home or the child care center. Getting down on their hands and knees helps adults to see the environment from the eyes of a child.

Caregivers or parents who are child-proofing the places where children live and play need to look for and deal with many potential hazards. These include the following:

Hazards Causing Choking or Suffocation

- Overstuffed cushions among which children could become wedged and suffocate
- Plastic bags or other forms of lightweight plastic that could cause suffocation

- Drapery cords or electrical cords children may wrap around their necks
- Hard or sticky chunks of food

Hazards Causing Burns

- Hot tap water (Water heaters in child care centers should be set at 120°F or lower.)
- Fireplaces and fireplace tools
- Matches and cigarette lighters
- Pan handles sticking over edge of stove where children can reach
- Furnace grates in floors
- Unprotected space heaters
- Heated liquids and hot foods

Hazards Causing Cuts, Bruises, or Puncture Wounds

- Sharp corners or edges on furniture
- Straight pins
- Knives and other dangerous objects in drawers
- Dishes or decorative items made of glass that might break and cut children
- Breakable bottles
- Broken toys
- Wood with splinters
- Places where small fingers could become pinched
- Lawn and garden or carpentry tools
- Glass tops on tables

Hazards Causing Electrical Shock or Burns

- Uncovered electrical outlets into which children may poke fingers or other objects
- Power tools
- Irons on ironing boards

- Wet floors near appliances
- Appliances near bathtubs, sinks, or showers
- Small appliances (such as hair dryers) left plugged in so children can turn them on
- Electrical cords children might bite

Hazards Causing Falls

- Windows that children might crawl through
- High chairs placed where children can reach things that might hurt them
- Furniture that is unstable or that slides easily
- Any object allowing children to climb onto something they could fall from
- Unsafe climbing equipment

Hazards Causing Poisoning

- Ashtrays containing cigarette butts
- Bathroom cleansers
- Cosmetics
- Detergents and bleaches
- Peeling paint (Old layers of paint may contain lead.)
- Pesticides and mothballs
- Fertilizers and plant foods
- Kerosene
- Poisonous plants
- Paint and paint remover
- Unlocked medicine cabinets
- Medicines left within children's reach

Other Hazards

- Any unsupervised activity
- Garbage cans with broken glass, cigarette butts, tin can lids, and decaying food

■ Insecticides sprayed where children play

■ Items in purses

No environment is completely safe. The better the child-proofing however, the more likely it is that children will not be injured when adults are briefly distracted.

Safety Indoors

At a child care center, the children's rooms should be spacious enough for the number of children who will be there. The National Academy of Early Childhood Programs recommends a minimum of 35 square feet of usable floor space per child. Good ventilation is necessary to provide a free flow of fresh air that is a comfortable temperature (usually 68–74°F). Materials on the walls are sound-absorbing to reduce noise. The paint or wall covering is one that reduces glare and does not contain lead or other poisons. Electrical outlets are covered with dummy plugs.

Furniture must be sturdy, stable, and child-sized. Storage areas should be easy for children to reach. Safe climbing equipment is broad-based and stable and has mats underneath to cushion falls. Carpeting is not sufficient.

Children are easily hurt in a cluttered environment. Hallways and exits need to be clear. Narrow hallways or blocked exits may prevent escape in an emergency.

There should be cleaning and sanitizing routines that are followed regularly and enforced. Carpeting collects dirt and germs and has to be well-vacuumed daily and cleaned frequently. Infants laying on carpeted floors need to be placed on a washable mat, blanket, or sheet.

Children need to be taught basic rules of safety to follow indoors. These rules include the following:

■ Walk rather than run when indoors.

■ Close doors (some adult help may be needed).

■ Keep cupboard doors closed.

■ Only teachers plug in or turn on anything electrical.

Safety Outdoors

Outdoor play areas must be securely fenced. Children need to be able to see through or over part of the fence, but its protective ability should not be diminished to provide this. Part of the play area should be shaded so children will be less likely to get sunburned. A sunny area gives children a place to warm up when they are playing outside on chilly days. There should be some kind of windbreak to block gusts of wind. Strong winds can cause children to fall or blow objects into their faces. Surfaces should drain quickly after rain.

Climbing equipment must have an impact-absorbing surface placed underneath it. **Impact-absorbing surfaces** are those made

FIGURE 8-2 A climbing structure and slide made of metal and plastic is sturdy and free of splinters.
Source: Gerber Products Company

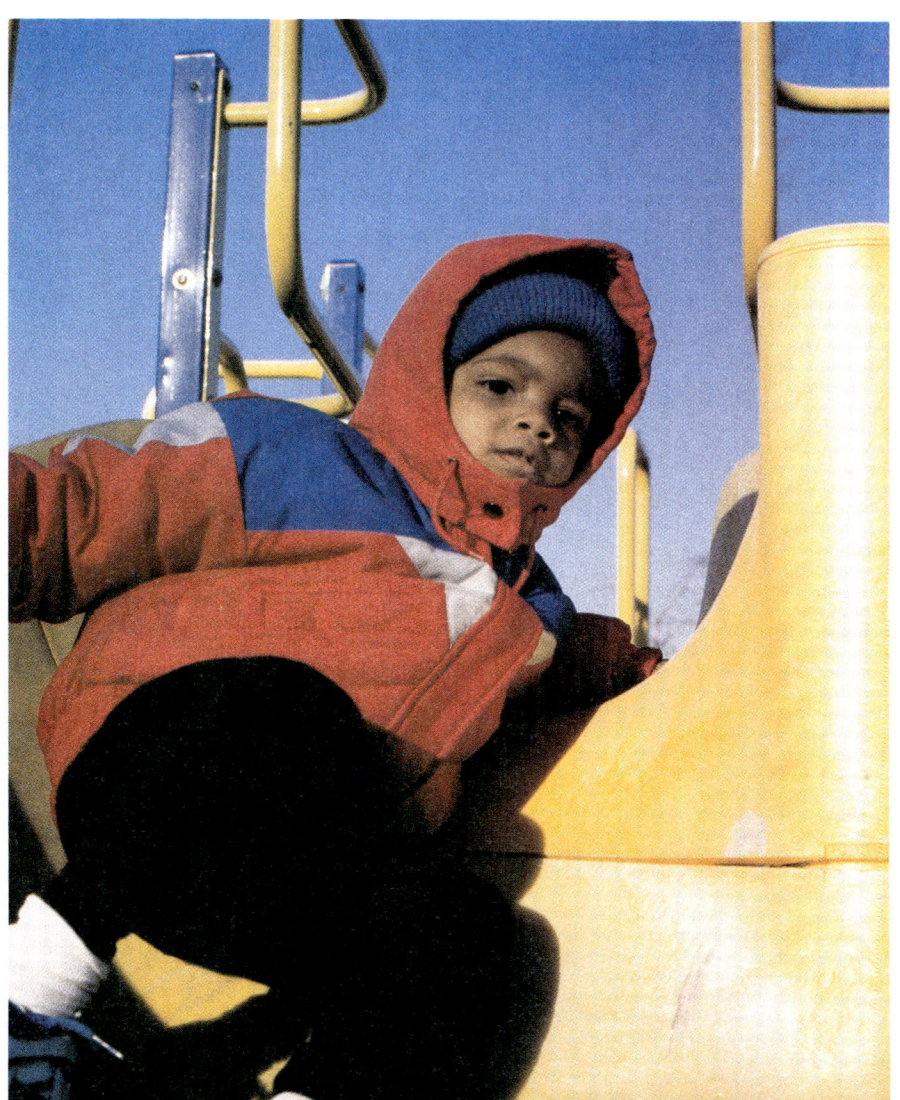

of some material that breaks a fall without injuring the child. Some common impact-absorbing surfaces are sand, pea-gravel, and shredded tires.

Play equipment should be sturdy enough to support adults and installed securely so that it does not tip or shift while children play. The equipment should be free of splinters and have no places where small heads or fingers might get caught. Play equipment should be arranged so that one piece does not get in the way of children playing on another piece. All equipment has to be easy to supervise visually at all times.

Some traditional forms of play equipment are now considered unsafe for children. These include see-saws, merry-go-rounds, and most swings. Swings can injure children by knocking them down. Swings with wooden or metal seats are particularly dangerous. Those made from tires or ones with canvas seats are less hazardous. Swings used by children under three should support them completely and not go very high. Swings must always be placed over an impact-absorbing surface. Children need to be closely supervised whenever they play on or near swings.

Sand can be excellent for creative play and is a favorite play material for many children. It is inexpensive and is found on nearly all playgrounds. Sand can be hazardous to children, however. When they play in sand, they should not be allowed to throw or eat it. Cats sometimes use unprotected sand as a litter box. Insects sometimes make their home in sandpiles. Dangerous objects such as nails and pieces of glass can become embedded in sand and injure children during play. Potentially harmful fibers are sometimes found in sand.

In parts of the country where the sun is very hot, children need protection when playing in sand outdoors. Fair-skinned children can burn within 10–15 minutes. Exposure to the sun without skin protection is a cause of skin cancer.

Sandboxes can be made safe by taking certain precautions:

- Keep cats and other animals out of sandboxes or sandpiles by covering them when not in use. Check daily for signs of animal contamination.

- Do not allow food on the playground—it might draw ants and other insects.

- Keep sandbox shaded so children will not get sunburned.

■ Set up and enforce basic guidelines for playing safely with sand, including a rule about not throwing sand.

Other Safety Precautions

There are several other general types of safety precautions that are necessary to make child care safe for children. These precautions concern fire safety, safe use of appliances and utilities, automobile safety, and water safety.

FIRE SAFETY

Homes and child care centers can take certain precautions to reduce the risks of fires and injuries from fires.

FIGURE 8-3 Children love to play in sand, but it can be hazardous.
Source: © 1981 Dario Perla/International Stock Photography

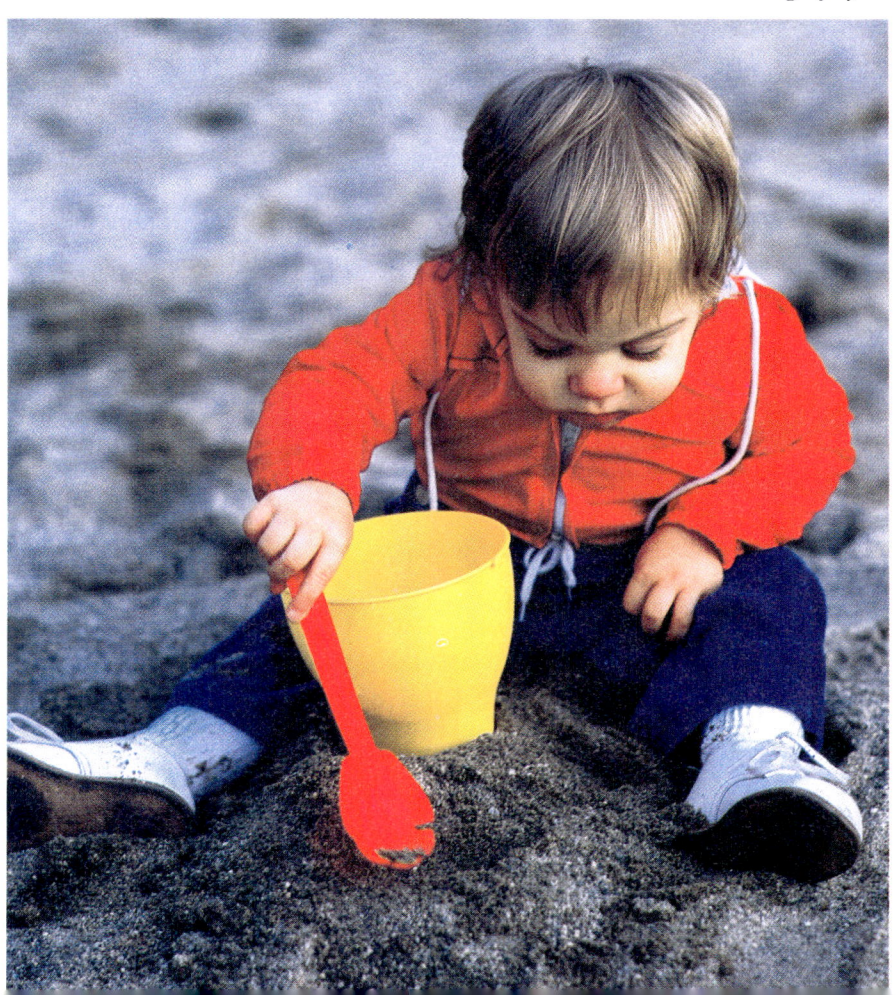

- Install smoke alarms in all areas of the center and see to it they stay in working condition
- Establish fire evacuation plans and practice them
- Use screens around space heaters and fire places
- Do not overload circuits
- Allow circulation of air around television sets
- Place matches and lighters where children cannot get to them
- Store gasolines and other flammable substances in tight metal containers
- Use flame-retardant materials in the building
- Dispose of rubbish and garbage regularly. Do not let old newspapers pile up.

SAFE USE OF APPLIANCES AND UTILITIES

Appliances, whether gas or electric, must be used properly and given regular maintenance to be safe. There are some additional precautions that will help ensure safety. For example, appliances should have a certification seal from a national testing organization.

All heating and cooling systems should be inspected annually by qualified professionals. Gas systems must be checked by a qualified gas plumber at least once each year. Gas burners have to be properly adjusted. Space heaters should have semi-rigid connections and protective guards. Gas appliances and heating equipment should be properly vented. Gas burners should light as soon as the gas is turned on.

If you smell a small amount of gas, follow this procedure.

1. Open a window.
2. Check pilot lights and burners.
3. Try to locate the source of the gas by brushing a solution of equal amounts of soap and water on gas pipes and connections and looking for bubbles. *Do **not** use a match or cigarette lighter to locate a gas leak.*
4. If you cannot find the source, call the gas company.

If you smell a great deal of gas, *get everyone out of the center immediately.* Then send a staff member to another location to call the gas company. *Do* **not** *light a cigarette, strike a match, use an electrical appliance, turn on lights, use the telephone, or turn on a flashlight.* Any spark could cause an explosion.

AUTOMOBILE SAFETY

Child care centers sometimes plan field trips for children. Some centers provide transportation to and from children's homes. Each child must be in a seat belt or car safety seat while being transported in a car or van. **Car safety seats** are safety restraints designed to reduce or prevent injuries to young children in case of an automobile accident. Only approved crash-tested seats that are used in the back seat are considered safe. To be approved, car safety seats must be padded and free of sharp or hard edges. They must fit in the car's seats and be usable with seat belts. If car seats are not used correctly, they are not safe or legal. Some car safety seats have a five-point harness that reduces seat belt injury in case of a crash. Children under four riding in a vehicle always need to be in a correctly placed and secured car safety seat. Children over four can usually be placed safely in a seat belt.

WATER SAFETY

Water play activities are part of many quality child care programs. Preferred activities involving water include bathing dolls, washing clothing and other items, painting with water, and playing at the water table.

Sometimes wading pools and even swimming pools are used by child care centers. However, children are not safe in water. They must be constantly supervised by an adult who is close enough to pull them out of the water if they get in trouble. An adult must remain within arm's reach of an infant or toddler. Preschoolers should not be more than a few feet from a supervising adult. A **supervising adult** is a full-grown person who is familiar with the abilities of children, recognizes hazards, watches carefully, and can act appropriately in case of immediate danger.

Even children who can swim cannot be allowed to play in water unsupervised. Children who say they can swim should be checked by a supervising adult. Swimming as an activity at child care is usually reserved for older children. Pools are hazardous and having one will increase a center's insurance rates.

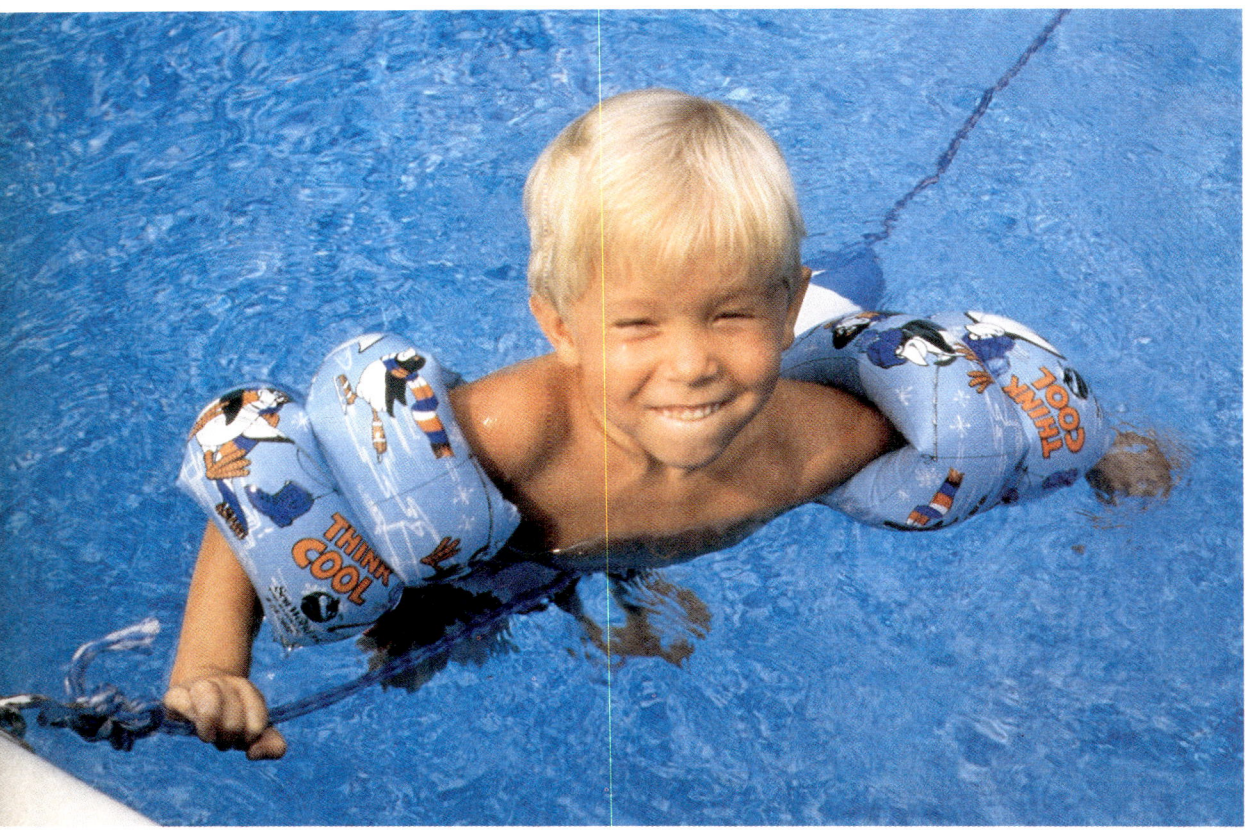

FIGURE 8-4   When children are in or near a pool—even if they are wearing flotation devices or know how to swim—they must be constantly supervised at close range.
Source: March of Dimes Birth Defects Foundation

Portable wading pools and other water containers should be put away when not in use. Wading pools have to be cleaned daily with disinfectant.

Permanent swimming pools must be surrounded by a fence at least 6 feet high with a locked gate to prevent children from getting into the pool. Pools with drains should have securely placed traps, and an attendant should be available to turn off a pump immediately in case a child is sucked into a drain. Pool chemicals must be securely locked away from children. Sharp objects should not be used in the pool area. A pool should be cleaned regularly. Swimming lessons should be given only by someone who has a lifesaving certificate.

Preparing for Emergencies in Child Care Centers

Being prepared for emergencies is the responsibility of every caregiver. An important consideration in planning for emergencies is ensuring that at least two qualified adults are present in a child care center at all times when children are present. While one adult handles an emergency, the other adult can supervise the children. In family day homes there is often only one adult caregiver; in these situations it is important that that person can call on another adult close by as a back-up to assist with emergencies.

When an emergency occurs, the teacher must remain in control of the situation and the people involved. The following steps are very important:

Step 1   Stay calm. Think.

Step 2   Get help. If other adults are present, have one of them call an ambulance. Ask others to help you control the children.

Step 3   Use correct CPR and first aid techniques as required.

Step 4   Stay with the child or children and continue to give aid until qualified help arrives.

If you are in a rural area far from hospitals and ambulances, arrange for other caregivers to stay with remaining children. Have another person drive you and the injured child to the closest doctor or hospital. On the way continue to give CPR and first aid if necessary.

Being prepared for emergencies includes having a trained staff, keeping first aid kits supplied, and establishing plans and procedures for evacuations.

TRAINING OF STAFF

Laws in most states require that every center have at least one caregiver who is fully qualified in first aid and CPR (cardiopulmonary resuscitation) on duty at all times. All caregivers need to take classes in first aid and CPR. In addition, charts showing basic first aid techniques and poison antidotes should be posted in every room where there are children.

FIRST AID KITS

A first aid kit is supplied with a minimum set of essential supplies to take care of minor injuries and other medical problems. A list of required and optional items for a first aid kit is found in Illustration 8-1.

Medicines in first aid kits should be replaced before their expiration date. Other items, such as sterile gauze bandages, need to be replaced when half has been used. There must be at least one first aid kit in the center and one in each van or automobile used to transport children.

EVACUATION AND HAZARDOUS WEATHER DRILLS

Plans for evacuating a child care center in case of a fire or other dangerous situation inside the center should be posted where staff will see it. Practice in carrying out the planned procedures is called an **evacuation drill.**

Procedure for fire drills. Fire extinguishers that have been regularly inspected must be located in every area of the building. Each room should have two clearly marked exits. If one is a window, it should be clearly marked and easy to open. A plan for exiting in case of a fire should be made and posted in every room. It should be clearly marked "Fire Evacuation Plan." Local fire officials can help set up safe evacuation plans for any building. Parents need to be informed about the plan.

Practice drills for fire evacuation should be conducted at least every three months. The following is the basic procedure for such drills:

Step 1   *Sound a prearranged signal.* Establish a signal that is used only for practice drills or an actual fire. One person is assigned to sound the signal. A bell or whistle is commonly used.

Step 2   *Get the children out of the building.* The teacher should lead the children out of the building to a prearranged, marked spot. It should be about 200 feet from the building. If a second adult is in the room, he or she should be the last one out and should make sure that no children have remained inside. When a second adult is not in the room, teachers can group as they leave the building, sharing the responsibility to see that all children are with them. Infants should be put into cribs in groups

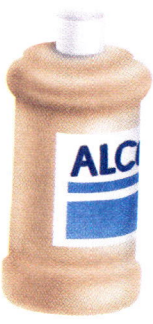
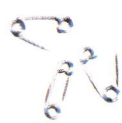

Required items

- Adhesive bandages (various sizes and shapes)
- Adhesive tape
- Alcohol
- Antiseptic soap
- Blanket
- Cotton balls
- Cotton swabs
- Gauze bandages (1-inch and 2-inch rolls)
- Medicine dropper
- Mineral oil (a poison antidote)
- Ointment for burns
- Safety pins
- Scissors
- Splints
- Sterile gauze pads (various sizes)
- Syrup of ipecac (a poison antidote)
- Thermometer and disposable shields
- Tongue depressors
- Triangular bandages
- Tweezers

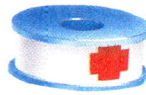
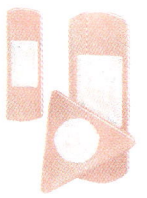
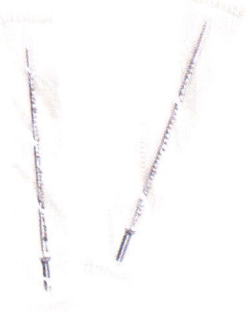
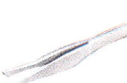
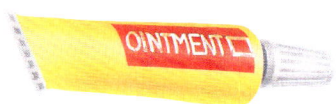

Optional items

- Basins for vomiting or bathing wounds
- Disposable cups
- Disposable tissues
- Hot water bag
- Ice bag
- Paper towels

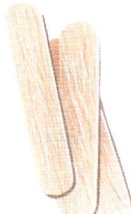
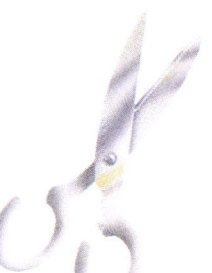

ILLUSTRATION 8-1   A first aid kit for a child care center contains certain supplies.

of four or five and rolled out of the building by adults. Toddlers need the most assistance. Some will have to be carried out or taken by the hand.

Step 3   *Be sure everyone is out.* Check to be sure that each child you are responsible for is at the prearranged, marked spot. Call each child's name and identify each by voice and by appearance. If the children are infants or toddlers, check and double check that each one is with you.

Step 4   *Return only on prearranged signal.* The assigned person sounds the signal to return from the practice drill.

Step 5   *Return by the same route.* Go back into the building following the same route taken when leaving the building.

This procedure is appropriate for evacuating the center when any hazardous condition has made it unsafe to remain inside.

Procedure for hazardous weather drills. A plan for protecting children inside the center during hazardous weather should be posted in every room. It should be clearly marked "Severe Weather Plan." Hazardous weather includes lightning, high winds, and sometimes flooding. In the case of high winds or tornados, children are safer in small rooms on lower floors with shock-absorbing cushions over them. If flooding occurs, it may be necessary to take children to a second floor. Recommended procedures for the severe weather likely to occur in the area of the country in which the child care center operates need to be learned and followed. For example, some areas are more likely than others to experience tornados.

It is important to remember that utilities may not function properly in hazardous weather. Gas lines can be uprooted leaving buildings without heat. If gas escapes, it might cause a fire or explosion. Electricity may be cut off. Loose, live electric wires can cause electrical shocks, burns, or death. The water supply can become contaminated.

Unlike fire drills, drills for hazardous weather situations bring the children to a safe area inside the building. The procedure for hazardous weather drills is as follows:

Step 1   Sound the prearranged signal.

Step 2   Get the children to the designated shelter.

Step 3   Have them put their heads down, and, if possible, cover them with shock-absorbing objects (such as pillows or mattresses).

Step 4   Check to be sure everyone is in the shelter.

Step 5   Return only on prearranged signal.

Step 6   Return by the same route.

Emergency Numbers

Emergency telephone numbers should be posted by every telephone and in every room of a child care center. These numbers should be posted even if all staff members have memorized them. It is very easy to forget or confuse numbers in an emergency.

Emergency numbers include the following:

- Emergency services number, usually 911
- Number for poison control center or hot line
- Number for fire department
- Number for closest hospital emergency room
- Emergency number for each child enrolled

Notifying Employees of Hazardous Substances

Employers are required by law to inform their employees of possible exposure to hazardous chemicals on the job. Employees must be given sheets that explain in detail the hazards of each chemical present in the work area. Employees must be trained about the nature of such hazards and how they can protect themselves. Names and telephone numbers of representatives of the companies that make the chemicals must be available to the local fire department on request.

Generally few hazardous chemicals will be found in child care centers. Some cleaning materials may contain such chemicals, but these would be locked up when not in use.

HANDLING INJURIES

Most injuries to children can be handled by a caregiver in the child care center. Some, however, will have to be treated by a doctor. Some injuries will require emergency help and perhaps hospitalization.

Basic First Aid

Every caregiver needs to be qualified to administer basic first aid. A handbook that describes procedures must be on hand in the center at all times. The following procedures are recommended by the American Academy of Pediatrics.

FIRST AID FOR SKIN WOUNDS

Skin wounds that children are likely to receive include bruises, scrapes, cuts, puncture wounds, and splinters.

Bruises. Rest the injured part of the body. Apply cold compresses, making sure that there is no ice next to the skin, for about a half-hour. If the bruise comes from a wringer or bicycle spokes, call the child's doctor immediately.

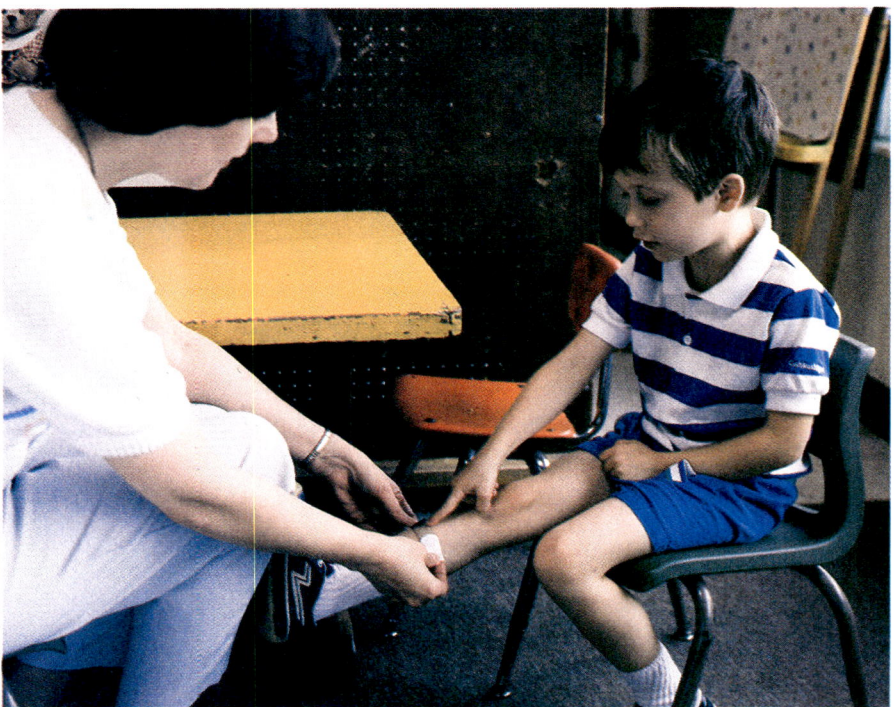

FIGURE 8-5   A simple scrape or cut is cleaned and covered with a sterile dressing.

Scrapes. Use gauze or cotton wet with clean water and soap to gently clean the wound. Apply a sterile dressing, preferably the kind that will not stick.

Cuts. If the cut is small, simply wash with clean water and soap, using gauze or cotton. Hold the wound under running water. Apply a sterile gauze dressing. If the cut is large, apply a dressing, pressing firmly to stop the bleeding. *Do not use iodine or other antiseptics.* Get medical help.

Puncture wounds. Get medical help.

Splinters. Wash area with clean water and soap. Remove splinter with tweezers. Wash again. If wound is deep, get medical help.

FIRST AID FOR BITES

Children may be bitten by insects (including being stung by bees) or by animals.

Insect bites. Remove the stinger, if present, with a scraping motion of the fingernail. Do not pull it out. Apply cold compresses. Get medical help if any of the following occur: rash, weakness, nausea, vomiting, "tightness" in the chest, nose, or throat, change in skin color, or unconsciousness.

Animal bites. Wash the area immediately with clean water and soap. Hold under running water for 2–3 minutes if the wound is not bleeding profusely. Apply a sterile dressing and get medical help. It is important to catch and keep the animal so it can be observed for rabies. Notify the police or animal control officer immediately.

Snake bites. Bites from nonpoisonous snakes are treated in the way cuts are. If the bite is from a poisonous snake, *stay calm and work fast.* Calm the child, getting him or her to rest as quietly as possible. Apply a constricting band (not too tight) above the wound and get medical help immediately.

If a caregiver does not know whether the snake is poisonous or nonpoisonous, he or she should treat the bite as a poisonous one. It is the responsibility of caregivers to learn to identify poisonous snakes in their area.

FIRST AID FOR BURNS

The treatment for a burn depends on its severity.

Burns of limited extent. If caused by heat, minor burns on arms and legs may be immersed in cold water. Wet packs can be applied to areas on the trunk or face. Cooling must be constant until pain disappears. Cover the burn with a nonadhesive dressing. Do *not* break the blisters. Get medical help.

If a burn is caused by chemicals, wash the burned area thoroughly with water. Get medical help.

Extensive burns. Keep the child in a flat position. Remove clothing from the burned area unless it is sticking to the skin. If clothing sticks, leave it alone. Cover the burned area with a clean cloth. Keep the child warm. *Get medical help immediately. Do not use ointments, greases, powder, etc.*

Electrical burns may be accompanied by shock, and the child may require CPR. If the child is touching the electrical source, pull him or her away using a nonconductive material, such as a folded cotton towel, between your hands and the child. *Do not use your bare hands.* The child's body can conduct the electrical burn and shock to the rescuer through bare hands.

FIRST AID FOR FRACTURES AND SPRAINS

Fractures or sprains are suffered in limbs and sometimes the back. The child will probably not be able to use the affected part until it has been treated.

Fractures. If a limb or other body part is deformed in any way, there is probably a fracture. *Do not move the child if a fracture of leg, neck, or back is suspected.* Get medical help *immediately.* If you must immobilize a fracture to transport a child to medical help, use a splint.

Sprains. Elevate the injured part. Apply cold compresses for a half-hour. If there is a great deal of swelling, do not allow child to use the injured part. Get medical help.

FIRST AID FOR INJURIES TO FACE OR HEAD

Injuries to the face or head require care that is specific to the injury.

Objects in Eyes. To remove an object from an eye, use a moist cotton swab. Work very gently. If the object cannot be easily removed, get medical help. If there is pain in the eye because of an object, a scrape, a scratch, or a cut, tape the eyelid shut until you can get medical help. If chemicals get into the eyes, flush with plenty of plain water. Do *not* use drops or ointment.

Nosebleeds. Have the child sit. Get him or her to blow out all clot and blood from the nose. Insert a wedge of cotton moistened with any common nose drops into the bleeding nostril. (Cold

Leadership at a Glance

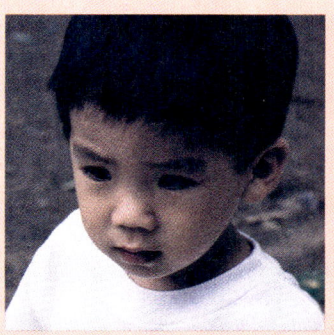

The National Committee for Prevention of Child Abuse

The National Committee for Prevention of Child Abuse is an organization whose purpose is to involve everyone concerned about child abuse in helping to prevent it. The organization's goals include educating the public and making people more aware of child abuse, developing prevention programs and programs that strengthen families to help prevent abuse, and researching and evaluating new ways of preventing abuse.

Since preventing child abuse is most effective at the local community level, the National Committee for Prevention of Child Abuse works through local chapters in all fifty states, as well as the District of Columbia, to develop programs locally. The people involved include volunteers from concerned groups and individuals in the community. The organization has an office in Chicago that provides support to local programs.

If you would like to know more about the National Committee for Prevention of Child Abuse, you can write to this address:

The National Committee for Prevention of Child Abuse
P.O. Box 94283
Chicago, IL 60690

water or peroxide solution may be used to moisten the cotton if no nose drops are available.)

Head injuries. Have the child rest as quietly as possible. Get medical help immediately. Tell the doctor if any of the following conditions occur:

- There is loss of consciousness.
- The child falls asleep and cannot be awakened.
- The child vomits and keeps vomiting.

- The child cannot move one or more of his or her arms or legs.

- Blood or watery fluid oozes from the ears or nose.

- The child has a headache that lasts over one hour.

- The child is dizzy for an hour or more after the injury.

- The pupils of the eyes are different sizes; one is larger than the other.

- The child is pale and weak and does not return to normal within a short time.

FIRST AID FOR POISONING

The first priority for cases of poisoning is to get the poison out of the child or off the skin or to dilute it. *Always* call the poison control center, doctor, hospital, or rescue unit immediately.

Swallowed poison. If a child has swallowed any poisonous substance, the following steps should be taken:

Step 1   Call for medical help.

Step 2   Dilute the poison by giving the child one glassful of water.

Step 3   *Do not make child vomit if he or she is unconscious or is having convulsions.* Do not make the child vomit if the poison swallowed is a strong corrosive (lye, strong acid, or drain cleaner) or if it contains kerosene, gasoline, or other petroleum products. If you do not know what the child swallowed, smell his or her breath. If there is any hint of gas, oil, or kerosene smell, do not cause the child to vomit. Vomiting can increase the damage in these instances.

Step 4   To make the child vomit, give 1 tablespoonful of syrup of ipecac plus 4 to 6 ounces of water if the child is between one and five years old. Children over five should be given 2 tablespoonfuls of syrup of ipecac with 6 to 8 ounces water. If the child does not vomit within 20 minutes, repeat the dosage *once only*. Do *not* give salt water.

Step 5   If instructed to do so, take the child to a medical facility, taking the package or container with the label and a pan with the child's vomitus.

Poison on skin. The procedure for cases where a child has spilled poison on his or her skin is as follows:

Step 1   Wash skin off immediately with a large amount of water, using soap if available.

Step 2   Remove any contaminated clothing.

Step 3   Call the poison control center or child's doctor for further help.

FIRST AID FOR OTHER PROBLEMS

Fainting, convulsions, and choking are treated in specific ways.

Fainting. Keep the child in a flat position. Loosen clothing from around his or her neck. Get medical help. Keep the child warm and his or her mouth clear. Do not give the child anything to swallow, and do not splash water on the child's face.

Convulsions. Get medical help. Lay the child on his or her side with the head lower than the hips. Apply cold cloths to the head, and sponge with cool water. Given nothing by mouth.

Choking. The Hands On with Children feature at the end of this chapter outlines the first aid procedures recommended by the American Academy of Pediatrics for infants and children who are choking.

Other Medical Emergencies

Children sometimes need emergency medical help at times when they have not been injured. Allergic reactions, insulin reactions, and attacks of appendicitis are occasional emergencies in child care centers.

ALLERGIC REACTIONS

Allergic reactions can be caused by medications, insect bites, foods, and so on. They range from mild to severe. Mild allergic reactions often involve a rash or itchiness. If a reaction becomes severe, there is **respiratory distress,** or difficulty in breathing. *This is an emergency. Get medical help immediately.*

INSULIN REACTION

Children who have diabetes sometimes have rapid changes in the amount of sugar and insulin (a hormone necessary for the body to convert sugar to energy) present in their blood. An **insulin reaction** is a condition that occurs when there is too much insulin in the blood. The following are symptoms of an insulin reaction:[1]

- Dullness, headache, irritability, crying
- Shaking, sweating, lightheadedness
- Hunger, change in mood or behavior
- Numbness of lips or tongue, pale skin, weakness, moist skin

If untreated, a child having an insulin reaction may lose co-ordination. The child's speech may become slurred, and he or she may become confused or even unconscious. Caregivers may help by giving the child a small glass of orange juice or milk. The insulin reaction should be reported immediately to the child's parents, and an incident report should be written. Parents should be encouraged to notify their doctor of the reaction.

If a child shows the above symptoms or excessive thirst or appetite for sugar-loaded foods, he or she may be an undiagnosed diabetic. The parents should be encouraged to seek medical help.

APPENDICITIS

A child who has a low fever (about 100°F), nausea, and pain in the lower abdominal area should be checked for appendicitis. **Appendicitis** is an inflammation of a small part of the lower intestine. If the child expresses discomfort when you press the lower abdomen and release it, or if the child seems to be getting sick rapidly, get medical help. Notify the parents.

Writing Incident Reports and Notifying Parents

Any time there is an injury at a child care center, a staff member should write an incident report. Copies of the report are provided to parents and the child's doctor and placed in the child's file. A sample form for incident reports is shown in Illustration 8-2.

---

[1]J. Ranch and M. McWeeney, "Managing Your Diabetes" (Indianapolis, IN: Eli Lilly and Co., 1986).

LA CASITA CHILDREN'S CENTER
Incident Report

Child injured _Bryan Hamilton_

Date _October 22_   Time _10:45_

Location where accident occurred _Playground by tire swing_

Description of accident _Bryan walked into swing area as swing came toward him. David's shoe struck him in the chin._

Description of injury _cut, about 1 inch long, with bleeding_

Description of action taken _Wound was cleaned. Bryan's parents were called. They took him to the doctor, who placed 3 stitches on the wound._

Yolanda Cisneros
Signature of Staff Member

ILLUSTRATION 8-2   A form like this can be used by staff members in preparing reports on children's injuries.

LEARNING ACTIVITIES ABOUT SAFETY

An important part of children's learning concerns how to stay safe. Children need to learn safety rules and to learn about community helpers.

Safety Rules

The children are not responsible for safety in a child care center; the caregivers are. However, toddlers and preschoolers need to be taught basic safety. Infants must have all safety provided for them.

Toddlers are dangerous to themselves and others because they are not able to judge situations accurately and decide how to act in a safe way. They do understand "no!" Caregivers need to be consistent about saying no, and they need to back it up. Toddlers should not be allowed to crawl to places where they might fall, to touch electrical outlets or switches, to play in an unfenced area, or to have any involvement with water without direct supervision.

Preschool children can learn to walk rather than run when they are indoors, to wipe up spills, to read traffic signs, to cross the street with adult supervision, and to latch gates. They still need constant supervision, however.

Activities for teaching children about safety rules might include putting traffic signals and signs in the block center and outdoor play area. Children can learn that objects marked with a red circle with a slash are not to be touched. Puppets, stories, songs, and finger plays can be used to teach concepts of safety. Children can be helped to play in safe ways. They will have to be reminded of safety rules regularly before they will remember to follow them.

Community Helpers

Community helpers include doctors and nurses, police officers, firefighters, ambulance drivers, paramedics and rescue drivers, ministers, priests, rabbis, and teachers. Children can learn about these helpers and what their jobs involve. Since community helpers are sometimes present during situations that are painful or fearful for children, helping children to have positive feelings about these people is important.

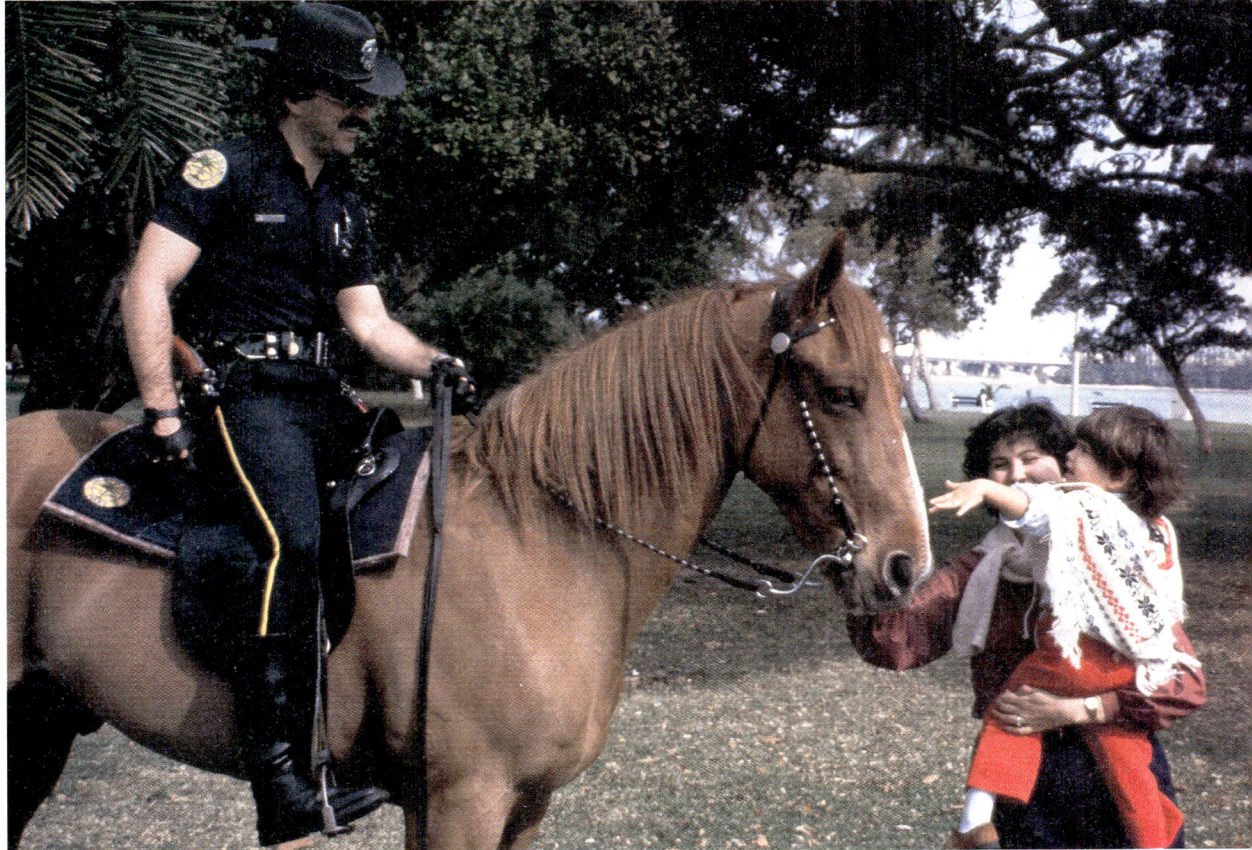

FIGURE 8-6   It is helpful for young children to learn about and meet
community helpers, such as police officers.
Source: Florida Department of Tourism

Children can learn about community helpers through stories,
puppets, songs, and dramatic play. Simple kits for learning about
these people can be assembled and kept from year to year in a
well-marked storage area.

Jerome and Donna were particularly pleased with the extra
measures taken by Mrs. Cisneros and her staff to ensure a safe
environment at La Casita. The staff worked at preventing accidents and were prepared for any emergency. Jerome and Donna
were also thankful that Geoffrey was learning to be responsible

for his own safety. An understanding of safe habits and an appreciation of community helpers would stay with him long after he left La Casita. This learning was part of the kind of child care they felt parents should provide for their children.

Summary

Common childhood injuries include those received from automobile accidents and falls, bites, burns, choking, drowning, poisoning, suffocation, and strangulation. To child-proof the environment, adults need to look closely at the surroundings as children see them. They need to pay careful attention to any hazard that could cause an injury to a child. Both indoor and outdoor environments at a center are examined carefully for hazards.

The staff of a center also needs to know about and check for fire safety, safe use of utilities, safe automobile travel, and water safety. Being prepared for emergencies includes training staff in first aid, equipping first aid kits, and planning and carrying out evacuation drills. Emergency numbers should be posted in all rooms and next to all telephones in a center.

Injuries are best handled by using correct first aid procedures. Staff members need to learn these procedures, which should also be posted in the center. Caregivers need to be able to give first aid for skin wounds, bites, burns, fractures, eyes, nosebleeds, fainting and unconsciousness, and choking. Other medical emergencies include allergic reactions, insulin reaction, and appendicitis. Injuries and emergencies are always documented in an injury report, and copies are provided to both parents and the child's doctor.

Children learn about safety in a child care center by being taught safety rules and being introduced to the roles of community helpers.

Terms and Concepts

Hazards	Impact-absorbing surfaces
Child-proofing	Car safety seats

Supervising adult   Insulin reaction

Evacuation drill   Appendicitis

Respiratory distress

Checking Your Understanding

1. What kind of accident is the major cause of injury and death in children under four?

2. What are the two most common accidents causing injuries in child care centers?

3. What dangers are particularly hazardous to infants, to toddlers, and to preschoolers?

4. Describe how adults can child-proof a home or child care center.

5. Choose one room of your home and crawl through it. Make a list of the potential hazards you find.

6. Visit a child care center or family day home. With the permission of the director, see how many hazards you can find and make a list of them. Compare your list with those of your classmates.

7. Visit a local pharmacy or drugstore. Using the list given in Illustration 8-1, price the items needed for a first aid kit. Compare your prices with those found by classmates.

8. Investigate various impact-absorbing surfaces that might be placed beneath climbing equipment and other outdoor play equipment. Evaluate each material for possible safety hazards. Compare the costs of the various materials.

9. Discuss ways to make sand play safe for children.

10. Evaluate a home or child care center for fire safety.

11. Visit a store that sells car safety seats and other safety equipment for use with young children. Check the equipment for possible hazards.

12. Make a list of rules that apply to supervising toddlers in a wading pool.

13. Get a copy of the floor plan for a building being used as a child care center. Plan appropriate exits and routes for evacuation drills.

14. Why do evacuation drills need to be practiced regularly?

15. Make a list of emergency phone numbers to post next to each telephone in a child care center.

16. Use activity resource books to find activities about community helpers. Make five cards for an activity card file.

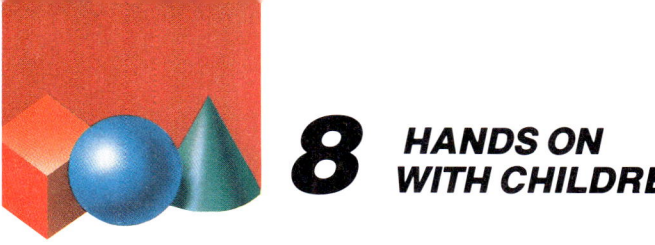

8 HANDS ON WITH CHILDREN

FIRST AID FOR CHOKING AND CPR

Before attempting these techniques, you should be trained by a qualified instructor. These procedures are demonstrated and practiced in special CPR classes.

FIRST AID FOR CHOKING

Infant. If an infant chokes and is unable to breathe, place the child face down over your arm with the head lower than the trunk. Rest your forearm on your thigh. Deliver four measured blows rapidly with the heel of the hand between the infant's shoulder blades. If the infant does not start to breathe, roll him or her over, face up, and give four compressions of the chest over the breastbone, using two fingers.

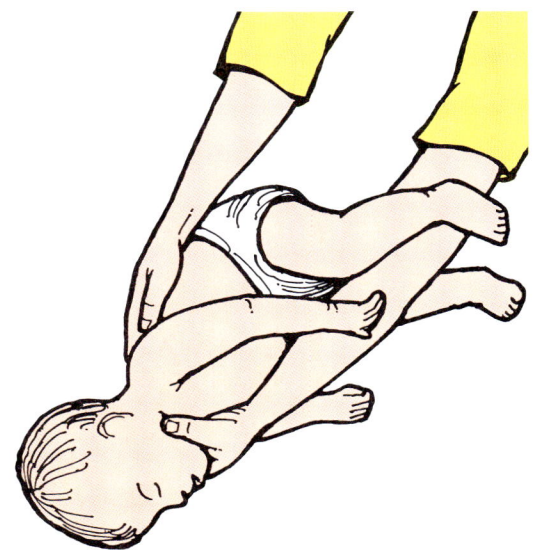

Larger child. Kneel on the floor. Drape the child across your thighs and deliver four measured blows on his or her back. Then, supporting the child's head, roll him or her onto the floor, face up, and deliver four chest compressions.

275

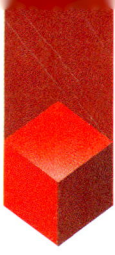

If the child does not start to breathe, open his or her mouth and place your thumb over the child's tongue. Wrap the other fingers of that hand around lower jaw. If you can see a foreign object that might be causing the child to choke, remove it with a sideways sweep of a finger of your other hand.

If breathing does not begin, transport the child to a medical facility as rapidly as possible.

CARDIO-PULMONARY RESUSCITATION (CPR)

Cardio-pulmonary resuscitation (CPR) is a technique used to help people recover from drownings, electric shock, and smoke inhalation. Every caregiver needs to have CPR training at least once a year from a medically approved instructor.

Infant CPR. Check to see if the child is conscious. Gently shake the infant and shout at him or her. If unconscious, call for help, then begin CPR.

Step 1   Check to see if the infant is breathing. If the infant is not breathing, check to see if any foreign object is causing the infant to choke.

Step 2   Clear the infant's throat, and wipe out any fluid, vomit, mucus, or foreign object that is in the mouth.

Step 3   Place the infant in the crook of your arm and tilt his or her head back enough to straighten the neck and lift the jaw. Or place the infant on a flat surface, straightening the neck and tilting the jaw by placing your hand under his or her neck.

Step 4   Blow gently into infant's nose and mouth. Give four quick puffs and check again.

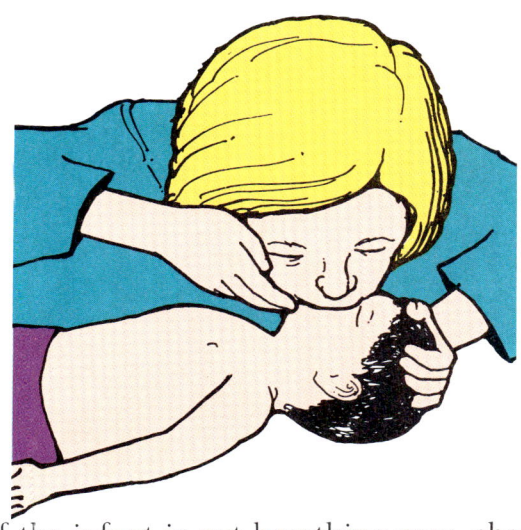

Step 5 If the infant is not breathing now, check the pulse by placing two fingers against the inside of the child's upper arm.

Step 6 If pulse is absent, use two fingers to depress breastbone between $\frac{1}{2}$ and 1 inch at level of nipples. Compress 100 times per minute. Also give 20 breaths per minute, supplying only enough air to move the infant's chest up and down. To give the compressions and breaths at the same time, blow on every fifth compression as shown below.

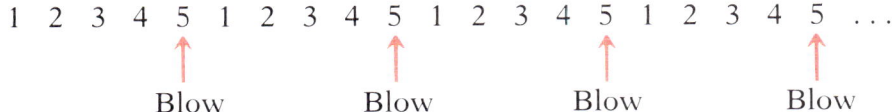

CPR for a larger child

Step 1 Check to see if the child is breathing. If the child is not breathing, check to see if any foreign object is causing him or her to choke.

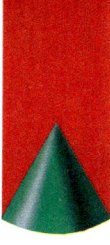

Step 2   Clear the child's throat, and wipe out any fluid, vomit, mucus, or foreign object that is in the mouth.

Step 3   Place the child on his or her back on a flat surface. Straighten the neck to open the airway, unless a neck injury is suspected. With your hand under the child's neck, lift the jaw.

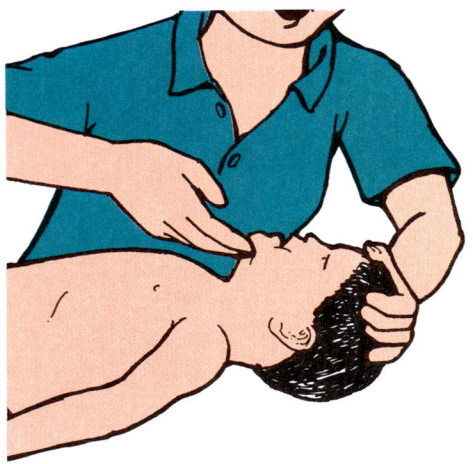

Step 4   Blow gently into the child's mouth with his or her nostrils pinched closed. Give four quick puffs and check again.

Step 5   If the child is not breathing now, check the pulse by placing two fingers against the inside of the child's upper arm.

Step 6   If there is no pulse, use three fingers to depress the breastbone 1 inch at level of nipples. Compress at 80 times per minute. Also give 15 breaths per minute, supplying only enough air to move chest up and down.

278

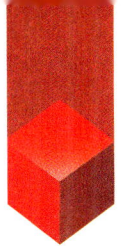

To give the compressions and breaths at the same time, blow on every fifth compression, as shown above.

Do not stop CPR until medical help arrives, the child begins to breathe, or you are absolutely exhausted and cannot go on.

Source: Techniques were adapted from "Choking/CPR," a chart published by the American Academy of Pediatrics and revised in January 1989.

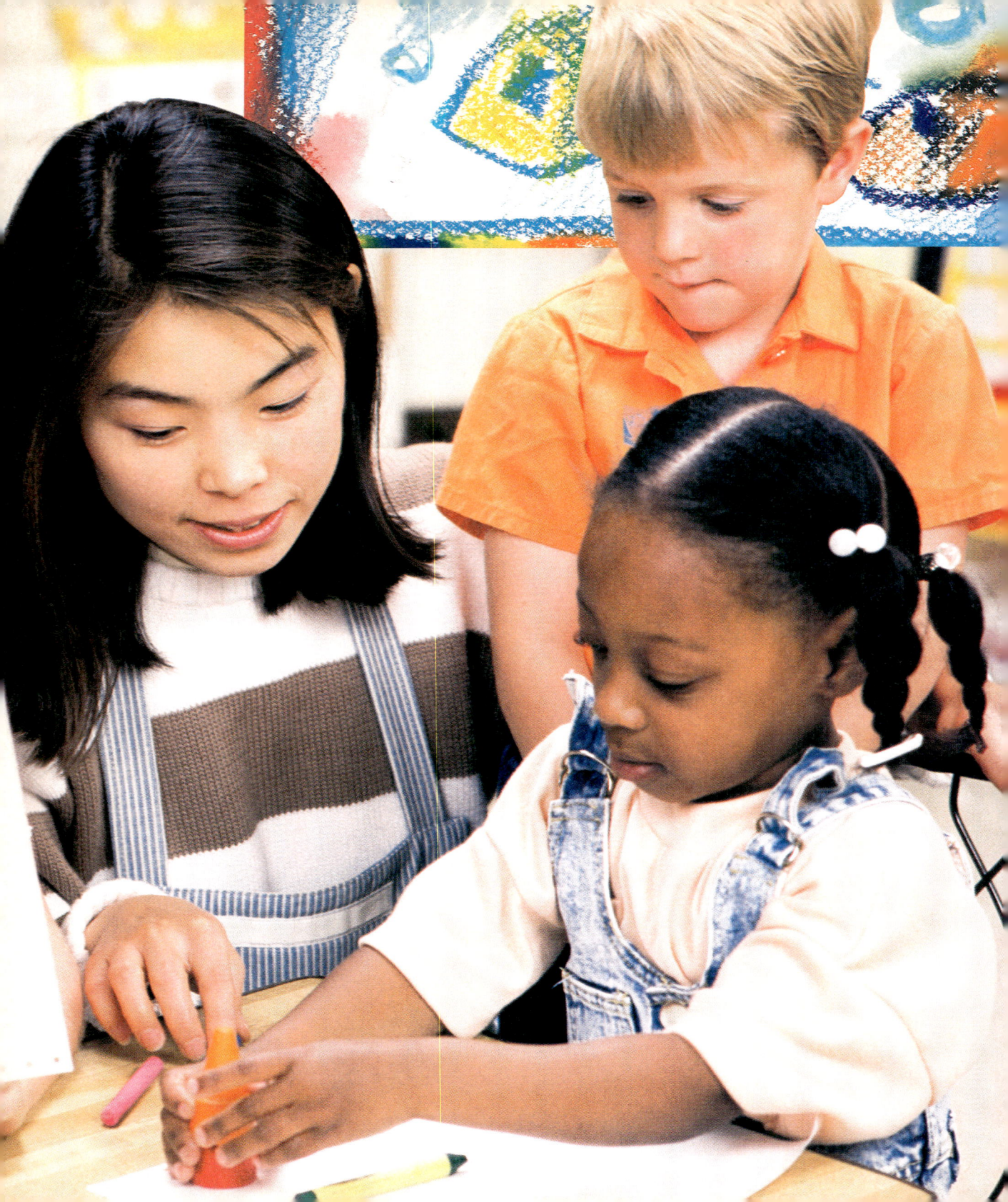

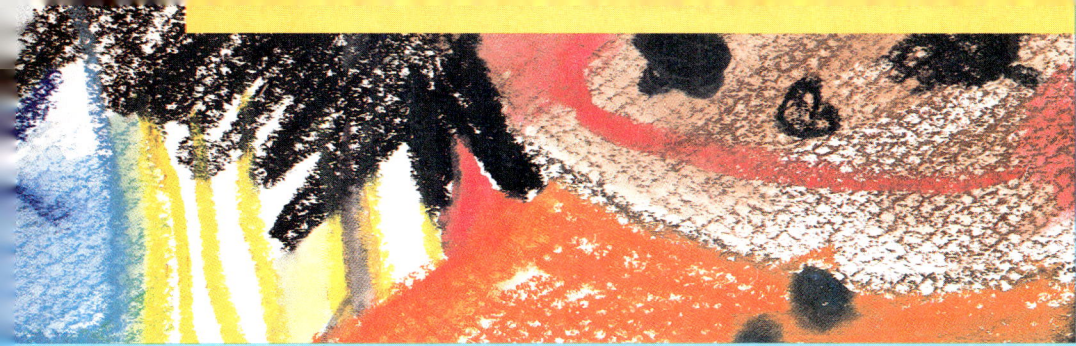

PART 3
Teaching Children

CHAPTER 9
Guidance, Discipline, and Abuse

OBJECTIVES

When you have finished this chapter, you will be able to

- Explain the guidelines for communicating effectively with young children
- Use the children's environment to provide indirect guidance
- Use positive statements to direct children
- Explain children's need for discipline
- Recognize signs of child abuse
- Explain how to report child abuse
- Demonstrate how to teach children self-protection skills

"Daddy, I want to paint!" Four-year-old Kristin pointed to three child-sized easels ready for young painters. The October sunshine, the clear, blue sky, and the brightly colored leaves formed a festive backdrop for the annual children's art fair that crisp Saturday morning.

"Sure, honey," he replied. Sam Cohen walked slowly at his daughter's pace, holding her hand. They stepped up to the awning where a colorful sign with a waving clown announced: "Easel Painting sponsored by La Casita Children's Center."

Mrs. Cisneros greeted Mr. Cohen, then stooped to where her eyes met Kristin's. "Would you like to paint this morning?" she asked.

Kristin nodded shyly, then hid behind her dad's arm. He bent down and put his arm around her. "If you want to paint a picture, I will sit close by."

Mrs. Cisneros slid a yellow plastic apron over Kristin's head to protect her clothing and allowed her to choose an easel. She showed her where the brushes and paints were. "Use the blue brush with the blue paint and the yellow brush with the yellow paint." She printed Kristin's name in the upper-left corner of the paper and showed Sam a chair near the easel where Kristin was painting.

Sam watched quietly while Kristin used first the blue paint and then the yellow to make lines, dots, and circles that became stick figures of her family. Sometimes the colors ran together or overlapped, forming various shades of green. "Why is Grandmother sick?" Kristin asked her dad.

"She has pneumonia, Kristin." Sam had been trying not to think about his mother's illness that morning. He was very concerned about her.

"Is Grandmother going to die?" Kristin asked.

Sam had not expected this question. "I don't think so." He reached out and put his arms around Kristin. "I would be very sad if she did."

"Me, too." Kristin took off her apron and handed it to Mrs. Cisneros.

COMMUNICATING WITH CHILDREN

Sam Cohen communicated well with Kristin. He listened to her and he spoke plainly and clearly when he talked to her. Too often parents and other adults do not communicate effectively with children. What makes good communication possible?

Listening to What Children Say

Listening is a skill that involves both hearing what the other person is saying and understanding what he or she is feeling. A good listener accepts what another person says even if he or she cannot agree with it. Hearing only part of what a person says is not good listening.

Listening to children requires a real interest in them and a desire to understand, because their speaking skills are limited. Parents who want to be good listeners start when their child is born to learn to listen for the different sounds of his or her cry. They listen attentively to the sounds of cooing and babbling, responding the best they can to their children's growing language skills. Parents who listen carefully more often create a desire to speak in their children. Language develops more rapidly in young children whose parents have meaningful conversations with them.

Parents and teachers need to listen for evidence of children's feelings. Sometimes what a child says and what he or she feels are not the same. Adults need to use words to help children identify feelings. When children say what their feelings are, they will be reassured that adults understand if the adults express those feelings using other words.

Good listening requires observation. Parents and teachers who really understand children watch their eyes, facial expressions, and body movements. Listening is an ongoing process. If parents want to listen effectively, they have to maintain their awareness of their children's needs, thoughts, and feelings. Hearing what a

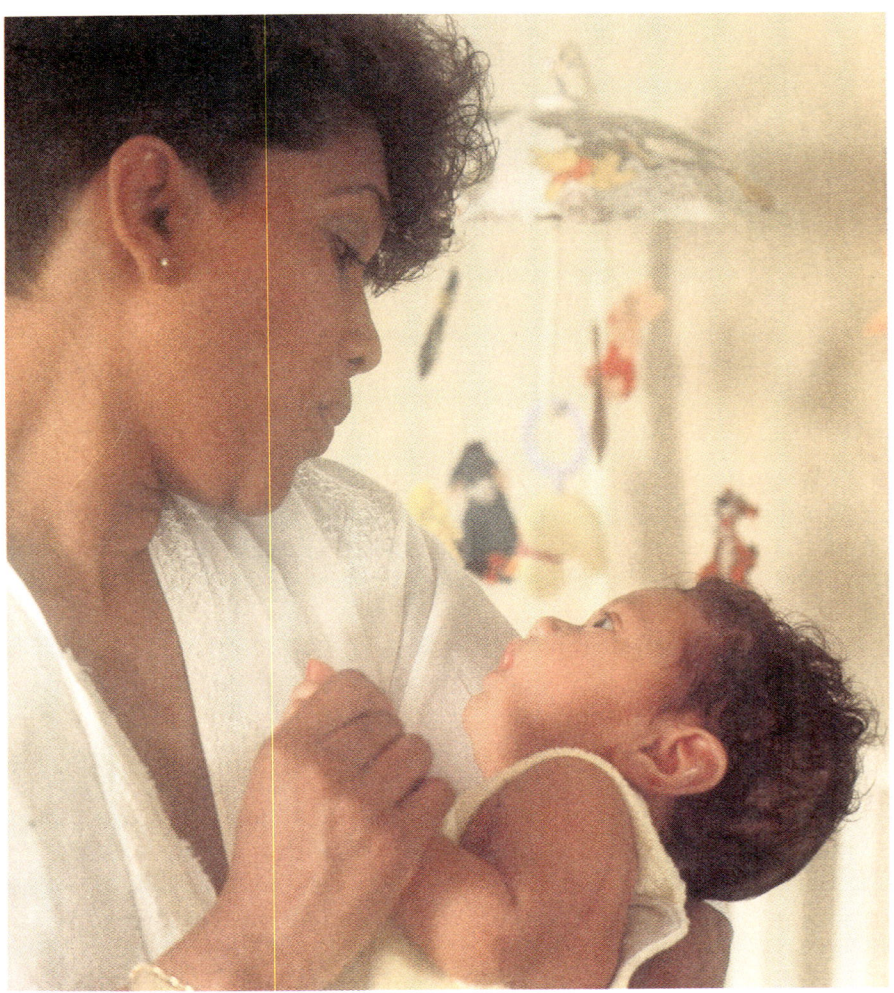

FIGURE 9-1 Listening attentively to infants' sounds and responding to them encourage language development.
Source: Superstock International Inc.

child has to say leads to understanding when it is accompanied by this kind of knowledge.

Speaking Clearly to Children

Good speaking is plain and clear. Words need to be said by adults so that a child can understand what they mean. The tone of voice an adult uses when speaking to a child also carries the message. Facial expressions and other body language should match the message as well.

When speaking to a child, use the following guidelines for better communication:

- *Position yourself so that your eyes are at the child's eye level.*

- *Get the child's attention.* Wait until the child's eyes meet yours to begin speaking.

- *Use clear words.* Use only the words needed to express what you want to say. Use words the child should understand. Make your ideas plain so that there is no question about what you mean.

- *Avoid talking about children to other people in front of them.* This makes a child feel like an object.

- *Avoid spelling words out to keep children from understanding what you are saying.* Go elsewhere to talk if you cannot say what you need to in front of a child.

- *Use correct grammar.* You are a language model for children.

- *Talk about appropriate subjects only.* It is not appropriate to talk about adult topics in the presence of children unless children ask questions about them.

- *Answer children's questions honestly.* Do not go beyond a direct answer to a child's question unless he or she asks other questions. Children often want only simple answers. Avoid giving detailed answers about adult topics.

Dealing with Children's Unacceptable Behavior

Children regularly test limits set by adults. Sometimes they misbehave because they have not been told what kind of behavior is expected. They need and expect adults to give proper guidance and to enforce rules.

When dealing with a child's unacceptable behavior, you need to follow one fairly easy guideline: *Speak about the child's behavior only.* Do not talk about his or her thoughts, wishes, ideas, or personality. Dr. Haim Ginott wrote about these ideas in a book entitled *Between Parent and Child.*[1] He said that when a parent gives guidance or disciplines a child, the parent communicates more effectively if he or she tells the child what behavior will be accepted and what behavior will not be accepted. That is, parents should make their standards for behavior clear.

If adults criticize or boast about a child's personality, wishes, thoughts, or ideas, the child draws his or her own conclusions about self-worth and self-importance. The conclusions are not always what the adults intended.

GUIDING CHILDREN

Adults guide children in two general ways: by controlling aspects of the environments in which children live and play and by telling or showing children what is expected.

Indirect Guidance

Indirect guidance means guiding children by controlling their circumstances. Mrs. Cisneros practiced indirect guidance by providing only a limited number of colors from which children could choose at each easel. A fenced-in yard is a form of indirect guidance because it sets boundaries for children's activities. Boundaries of all kinds need to be movable. As children grow and gain the ability to control their own activities, the boundaries will be expanded.

ALLOWING FREEDOM WITHIN LIMITS

As it is within a fence, all activity within established boundaries needs to be safe, acceptable, and right behavior. When adults establish appropriate and well-expressed boundaries, children have the freedom to choose within those limits. **Freedom within limits** is a way of defining behaviors from which children can choose freely as long as they obey the rules that apply to those behaviors. This form of indirect guidance builds strength and

[1]Haim Ginott, *Between Parent and Child: New Solutions to Old Problems* (New York, NY: Macmillan, 1965).

allows children to experience what it means to live in a democratic society.

OFFERING LIMITED CHOICES

The freedom to choose is important because it affirms the value of unique individuals. **Structured choices** are those limited to a set of alternatives, all of which are acceptable. For example, a structured choice is allowing a child to choose carrots or sweet potatoes as part of lunch.

Offering structured choices is a form of indirect guidance because the adult decides the limits of what he or she will accept, then offers the child an opportunity to choose within those limits. This is a form of boundary setting. It is important to set boundaries for children's choices because children need to learn that there are limits on behavior. Every society sets limits on behavior. Any young child growing up in a society has a need and a right to know what those limits are.

ALLOWING LOGICAL CONSEQUENCES TO OCCUR

One form of indirect guidance is to allow the consequences to occur when children make inappropriate choices. Rudolf Dreikurs was an educator and psychiatrist who first wrote about logical consequences.[2] **Logical consequences** are the events that would normally follow an action. For example, if a four-year-old spills tempera paint on the floor, he or she is given a sponge and a small pail of warm soapy water to help the teacher clean up the paint.

Allowing the logical consequences to occur is appropriate only when the child will not be injured. For example, if a child has been told not to touch the stove, the logical consequence would be to allow him or her to get burned. However, this might be considered abusive. Logical consequences should be allowed to occur only when they will help the child to see the results of behavior and are not dangerous to the child's health and safety.

Logical consequences are not supposed to make a child miserable. They are intended to point out the results of the behavior.

---

[2]Rudolf Dreikurs with Vickie Soltz, *Children: The Challenge* (New York, NY: Dutton, 1987 [1964]).

A gentle reminder of what the consequences are is often enough to prevent a repeat performance. For example, a teacher could remind a child who spilled paint before, "Keep the paint in the tray on the easel. You will have to clean it up again if it spills."

EXPANDING THE LIMITS ON BEHAVIOR

As children gain control over their behavior and meet the challenges provided within the specified set of boundaries, those boundaries need to be expanded. The challenges within the limits on behavior need to get just a bit tougher. In this way children are helped to continue to develop. Progress is also made toward helping them become responsible for themselves.

FIGURE 9-2   A child who throws clothes on the floor can be shown the logical consequences of the action—the clothes have to be picked up before playtime.
Source: © Laura Dwight

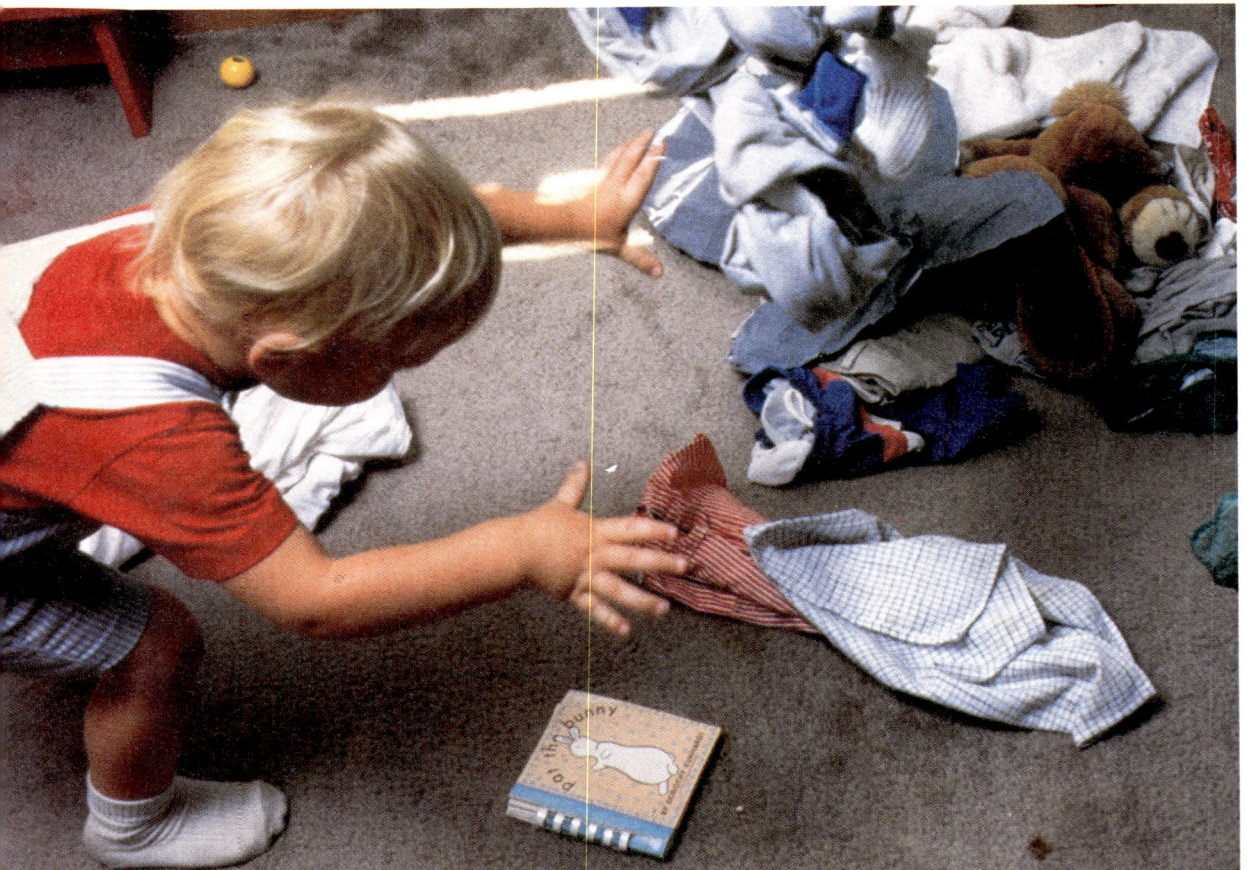

PROVIDING APPROPRIATE ACTIVITIES

An important part of guiding children is to know what they are capable of doing and providing the kinds of activities they need and are interested in. Expecting too much or too little of children often encourages unacceptable behavior.

GIVING ENCOURAGEMENT

Children need to know when they are moving in a positive direction. Adults who provide encouragement to children for their efforts give them a sense that the chosen direction is a good one.

Direct Guidance

Direct guidance is guiding children by telling and showing them what is expected. Boundaries for children may be physical, like fences, or they may be limits thought of by adults. When boundaries, or limits, exist in the mind of an adult, they must be communicated to children.

USING POSITIVE STATEMENTS

When adults set and enforce boundaries for children's behavior, they need to use positive statements. **Positive statements** are sentences that give children a direction to go in rather than telling them something they cannot do. For example, if a child is throwing sand, a teacher might say, "Don't throw the sand." But a more positive way to say the same thing is "Keep the sand in the sand box."

SETTING LIMITS

Adults have to decide what behavior will be allowed. Adults need to set only rules that are *necessary* and *important*. Children should be given encouragement in their activities whenever possible. Three kinds of decisions that must be made about the limits on behavior concern safety, values, and consideration for others.

What behavior is safe and what is unsafe? An activity or behavior that is safe for four-year-olds may not be safe for two-year-olds. When deciding about the safety, the adult has to analyze both the threat and the child's ability to handle danger.

What behavior is right and what is wrong? Small children understand right and wrong only as it relates to reward and punishment. A sense of right and wrong is not something that can be directly taught to very small children. However, adults, especially parents, need to make decisions about what kinds of values they want to emphasize. Then behavior that matches those values must be enforced consistently. For example, if parents want small children to learn not to get into purses, wallets, and other personal belongings, they should not let their children play in their personal belongings. If parents expect children to speak respectfully to adults when they are older, they need to stop children from "talking back" when they are small.

FIGURE 9-3 Playing in the water at the edge of the surf is safe for a young child only if an adult remains within reach.
Source: © Frederick Ayer/Photo Researchers Inc.

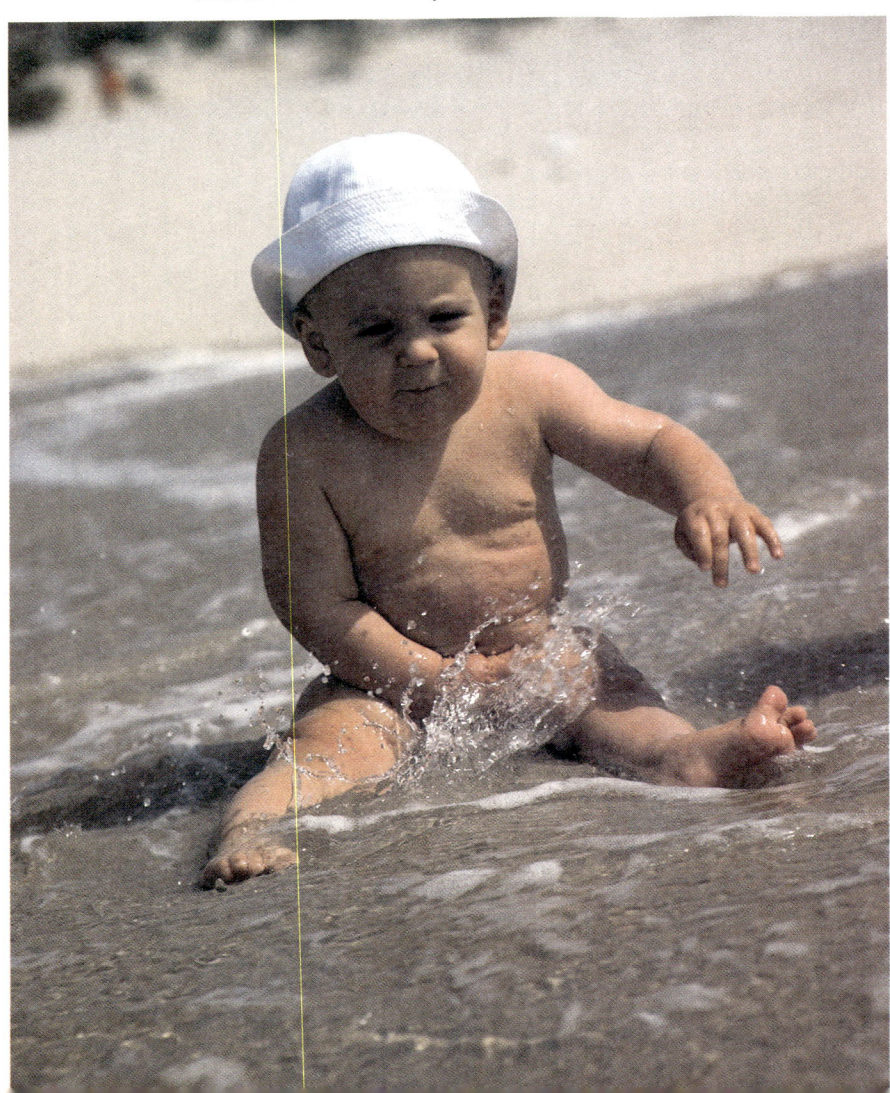

One way to decide what behavior is right and wrong is to consider what other people think. Another way is to consider the results of the behavior if it continues. If behavior is hurtful to other people or damaging to property, most people consider it to be wrong. If the behavior does not, or will not, hurt anyone or anything, then it can probably be allowed.

What behavior is acceptable and what is unacceptable? Sometimes there are behaviors that annoy a particular adult for reasons that have nothing to do with safety or values. For example, making smacking noises while eating annoys some people. Such behaviors are neither unsafe nor wrong, but if they truly annoy others, children need to be helped to learn to avoid them. This kind of limit on behavior is based on consideration for other people. Most manners fall into this category. As boundaries are expanded to allow a child more self-control, training in manners and social skills can be increased.

ENFORCING LIMITS

Limits that are clearly set in the adult's mind are easier to enforce. When a child crosses a boundary, or exceeds one of the limits that have been set, the adult needs to act. What actions are effective? The Hands On with Children feature at the end of this chapter deals with one way of enforcing limits.

Often adults spank children who behave in unacceptable ways. In many states the law prohibits teachers or caregivers from spanking children because it can be abusive. Should you spank a child who does not mind? The Something to Think About feature on the following pages deals with this issue.

REINFORCING DESIRABLE BEHAVIOR

When children behave in the way adults desire, they need to know they have done well. Praising children for their acceptable behavior makes them want to keep on acting in that way. Expanding the boundaries, or giving additional privileges, is another way of reinforcing desirable behavior. **Reinforcement** in this sense means strengthening a desired behavior by saying something positive or doing something the child will enjoy. With positive reinforcement a desired behavior can become a habit. It is important to remember to praise the behavior and not the child. The child needs to be accepted unconditionally.

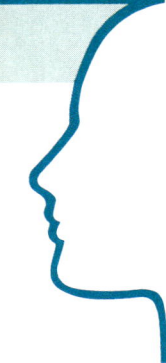

Something to Think About

Should Children Be Spanked?

It is against the law in many states to spank a child in a child care situation without written permission from the parents. Do you think this is a good policy? Laws about how parents handle children at home are less definite, although spanking that becomes abusive is covered by laws concerning child abuse. Should parents be allowed to spank their own children?

Both positive and negative effects are possible from spanking. Possible positive effects include the following:

- The child understands that he or she has broken a rule.
- The child understands clearly that the adult is interested enough to care about his or her behavior.
- The child may be less likely to repeat the behavior in the future.

These are some possible negative effects:

- The child may perceive that the parent is taking out anger or frustration on him or her.
- The child may learn that hitting is the way to solve problems or that authority is to be respected only if it can hurt you.
- If the parent is out of control, the result may be abuse and injury to the child.

Adults need to think about spanking before they get into a situation in which they have to take some kind of disciplinary action. Questions that adults need to consider include the following:

- Who should spank children?
- Should an adult spank a child if he or she is angry or frustrated with the child?
- Is the love tie sufficiently strong for the child to understand that the spanking is given because the adult cares?
- When does spanking become abuse?

- Will the child clearly understand why the spanking is necessary?
- Is there any other effective way to handle the situation?

Some authorities advocate a policy of no hitting at all when disciplining children. What are some strengths of this policy? What are some weaknesses? Is hitting the same as spanking? What do you think?

IGNORING UNDESIRABLE BEHAVIOR

Children sometimes do things simply to get adult attention. When adults do not give them the desired attention, they will often stop the undesirable behavior. In most cases, toddlers who throw tantrums are more likely to stop this behavior if adults ignore them. Ignoring is not an effective method for discouraging some behaviors. For example, if a child is biting another child, ignoring the behavior is not effective. Firm and immediate correction is necessary. Children need correction in many situations, and it must be given.

Teaching Social Skills

Young children can be taught simple manners, such as saying "thank you," taking turns, and helping to put away play materials. It is important to be sure that children are not being expected to perform actions because adults think they are cute but are learning common courtesy.

Being with other children gives children a chance to learn how to get along with other people. Playing and learning together give children many opportunities to cooperate and to work through conflicts. Teachers and parents help by planning activities that do not involve competition. Learning to work together, or cooperate, is an important skill for children to develop. Competition among preschool children causes conflict and can damage self-esteem. School-age children handle organized competition better than preschoolers do. If competition arises among young children, teachers and caregivers need to turn it into cooperative effort.

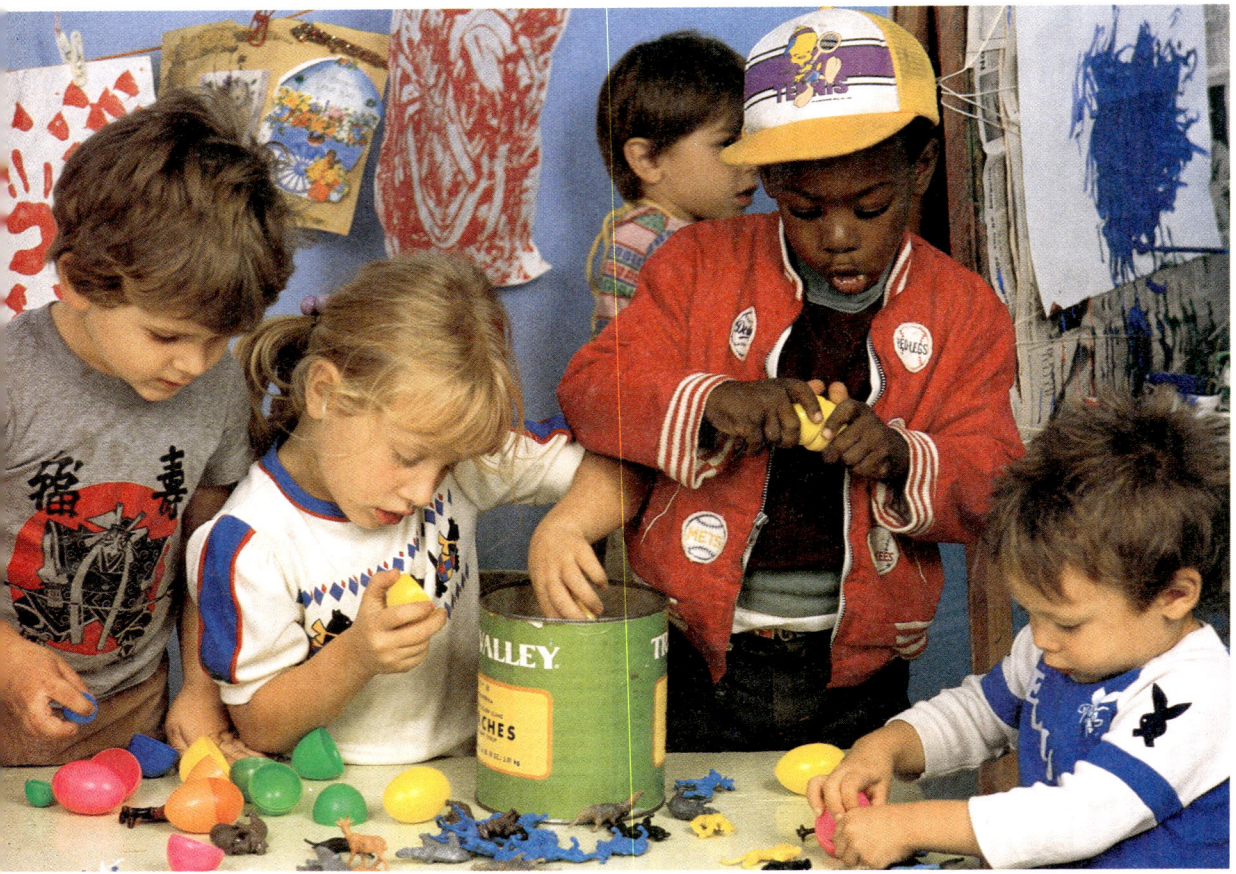

FIGURE 9-4   Learning to play together cooperatively is part of learning to get along with others.
Source: Judy Gurovitz/International Stock Photography

When children have conflicts, adults need to help them deal with them. Unless a child is being injured, however, adults need to avoid the temptation to solve children's problems for them. When adults solve problems for children, rather than helping them to work toward a solution on their own, they keep children from growing. This leads to social immaturity.

When conflicts occur among people, everyone concerned contributes to the problem. It is important that no child be made to feel as though he or she is the only one at fault.

Guiding Preschool Children in Groups

Guiding groups of children is a more demanding task than guiding one or two children. Indirect guidance is very important in group settings. An appropriate environment, a flexible and workable schedule, and developmentally appropriate activities are essential. It is also necessary that teachers know what the boundaries for the children are and how they will enforce them.

SETTING GROUP BOUNDARIES

Teachers in preschool classrooms must set and enforce limits. Rules that are commonly used with preschoolers include the following:

- Help put away play materials.
- Do what the teacher says.
- Use walking feet indoors.
- Use quiet voices indoors.

Some classrooms have additional rules. Rules for lining up to go to the bathroom and other activities are more effective with school-age children than with preschoolers.

ENFORCING GROUP BOUNDARIES

When children disobey a rule, they need to be given one clear warning. If they continue the unacceptable behavior, they need to have a time out. A **time out** is a few minutes spent sitting in a chair placed where the child can watch the other children play. Three to five minutes is usually sufficient and can seem long to the child. A teacher sits nearby and makes sure that the child stays in the chair for the full time. The child is not to leave the chair until the teacher tells him or her that it is time to do so. A prearranged signal, such as the bell of a timer, can be used to mark the time.

Before allowing a child to return to play, the teacher needs to remind him or her of the kind of behavior that is expected in the center. If the child continues the unacceptable behavior and a second time out is required, a note should be sent home to parents explaining what happened and what the teacher did. Parents should be asked to back up the teacher at home and encouraged to apply the rules followed at the center as much as possible.

BEING AWARE OF CHILDREN'S RELATIONSHIPS

Teachers need to be aware of the feelings that exist between children because those relationships affect how the group functions. When two children are close friends or have a major conflict, they can change the entire tone of the group.

GUIDING CHILDREN THROUGH TRANSITION TIMES

Periods of time between activities are called **transition times.** These times can be structured so that children have direction and purpose to their actions. Giving them tasks to perform or singing with them while moving from one location or activity to another allows fewer opportunities for undesirable behavior. Some activities useful for transition times are described in Chapter 12.

PROVIDING GUIDANCE WHEN CHILDREN ARE AWAY FROM THE CENTER

Walks and field trips present special problems because children are away from the center, where some boundaries are physical and all are familiar. Devices for keeping children safe and together become more important at these times. Children should always wear seat belts or be strapped into safety seats when traveling in cars or vans. A walking rope with a designated spot for each child to hold should be used during group walks. It helps to have an assigned color or even a name taped at each child's spot. Name tags attached to children's clothing will be helpful in the event that a child becomes separated from the group or teacher.

There should be enough adults to control the children. For control to be adequate, one adult is needed for every two toddlers or two older children when a situation involves any risk. One adult for every four or five children will be sufficient if risk is low. Parents and volunteers can be asked to help with supervision during field trips.

DISCIPLINING CHILDREN

Discipline is the purposeful enforcing of acceptable behavior with the goal of teaching children self-control. The disciplining of children is a skill of mature people. Parents and teachers who really care about children, who love them, will discipline them.

Leadership at a Glance

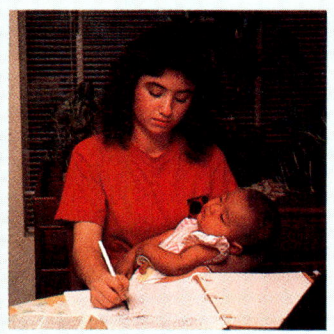

Source: © Jose Carrillo, Ventura, CA

James C. Dobson, Ph.D.

James Dobson is an authority on child development. He is especially well known for writing and speaking about discipline. He writes books, makes films, and does a weekday radio program, all designed to help families gain strength and raise children effectively. His most widely read book is *Dare to Discipline.*

Dr. Dobson served on the attending staff of Los Angeles Children's Hospital for seventeen years and has served on commissions dealing with issues concerning children and families under both Democratic and Republican presidents. These commissions have been concerned with missing and exploited children, juvenile justice and delinquency prevention, pornography, and prevention of teenage pregnancies.

Dr. Dobson is married and is the father of two children. He is perhaps best known for founding Focus on the Family, a nonprofit organization dedicated to preserving traditional Judeo-Christian values in families. You can contact this organization if you would like to know more about it:

Focus on the Family
Pomona, CA 91766

1-800-A-FAMILY

Discipline is different from punishment. **Punishment** is an action by an adult who is taking out feelings of anger or frustration on a child. Punishment is abusive and harmful to children. Punishment can be physical, mental, or emotional. People who punish children may make them behave in the desired way temporarily, but the goal of discipline is lost. Children who are punished are hurt, harmed, or crippled by the experience.

Children's Need for Discipline

Children develop in some ways if they are simply given the opportunity to develop. Physical skills develop if children have adequate opportunities to crawl, climb, walk, and run. In order to develop self-control, children must be taught. Children are taught both by giving them instruction and by providing a good example.

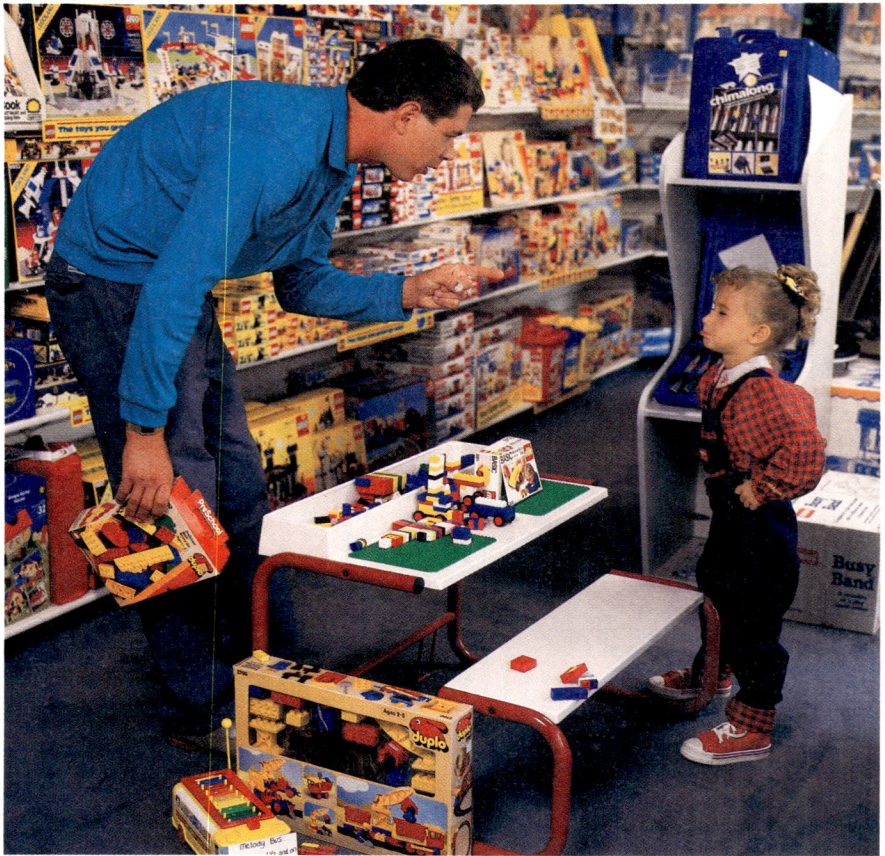

FIGURE 9-5 When children behave unacceptably, they need to be corrected firmly but lovingly.

When children go outside the limits set for them, they need and want correction. This correction has to be given with loving firmness if it is to be effective.

Responsibility and Authority

Responsibility and authority are balanced in parenting, just as they are in job situations. Parents are responsible for children, so they also have authority over them. They give the responsibility and authority to teachers or caregivers for part of the day. Responsibility and authority are realities that children will have to live with all their lives. They need to learn how to view authority and how to respond to it. They need to learn how to accept responsibility and how it is related to authority.

As children begin to take some responsibility for themselves, they earn the right to have authority over those areas of their lives. Good parenting and good teaching involve a slow and careful transfer of both responsibility and authority to the child. This transfer occurs in a series of many steps, starting at birth and continuing until full adulthood is reached.

Adults who give children more authority than they can handle are not being fair to the children. Those who do not allow children to accept responsibility may cripple the children and cause them to feel resentment.

The Goal of Discipline

The goal of discipline is to teach children self-control and self-responsibility and to teach them about authority. If discipline is just and fair and given with great love for the child, he or she will learn these lessons. If discipline is harsh and abusive, children are likely to learn to evade responsibility and defy authority.

CHILD ABUSE AND NEGLECT

Sam Cohen and his daughter, Kristin, had been gone only a few minutes when a four-year-old boy whose shirt and hair were dirty and jeans ripped walked up to one of the easels and started painting. Mrs. Cisneros stooped to his level, greeted him, and started to put an apron over his clothes.

"I don't want that!" he screamed.

Mrs. Cisneros replied, "You need to wear the apron so you will not get paint on your clothes." He didn't respond, but he allowed Mrs. Cisneros to fasten the apron over his clothes. She noticed a bruise on his arm in the shape of an adult's fingers.

For further information on child abuse, see James Mead, *Investigating Child Abuse*, 2nd ed. (R C Law & Co., 1987).

"Jake! Jake!" a young woman screamed as she approached the easels. "Get away from that paint!"

Mrs. Cisneros stood up and said to the woman, "It's all right. The paints are for the children to use. This must be your little boy."

"He's a brat! He never minds. He runs off. I'm just real sorry, ma'am." The woman had two smaller children with her. Thinking that she looked really tired, Mrs. Cisneros said, "It's all right. Maybe I could do something to help." She was concerned about the bruise on Jake's arm and about his mother's apparent inability to discipline him.

"No, I don't need any help. My mother raised me and my brothers, and we all turned out okay. Come on, Jake, that's enough. We gotta go now!" She reached for the apron and Jake jerked away.

"Don't mom! That hurts," he wailed. His shirt flew up when she pulled off the apron, exposing purple-, blue-, and yellow-colored skin. Mrs. Cisneros gasped softly.

"You look tired. Won't you sit down for a minute? I will send for something to drink," Mrs. Cisneros pleaded.

The mother hesitated, but Mrs. Cisneros's concerned expression reassured her. "I'm kind of tired. Okay—for just a minute," she said.

"I noticed a bruise on Jake's arm when I put his apron on a few minutes ago. How did he get hurt?" Mrs. Cisneros asked, trying to stay calm.

"He fell down. It ain't none of your business anyway," Jake's mother said. She started to leave.

"Just a minute," Mrs. Cisneros said firmly. "Sit down." Surprised by Mrs. Cisneros's firm and insistent manner, Jake's mother sat back down.

Mrs. Cisneros said, "Come over here, Jake." She turned him around where his mother could see his back and raised his shirt. "I think Jake has been abused."

The mother started to cry. "Please, ma'am, just leave us alone. There ain't nothin' I can do about it. His dad beats him and he beats me, too." For the first time Mrs. Cisneros noticed a bad bruise on Jake's mother's arm.

Mrs. Cisneros was working hard to contain her anger. "It is against the law to abuse children," she said firmly. "You don't have to put up with your husband's doing this. I'm going to get you some help."

Using children in hurtful ways to satisfy adult appetites or meet adult needs is the common element in all child abuse. A person who abuses a child is called a **perpetrator.**

Children can be abused in any way in which people can hurt one another. Researchers who study child abuse categorize it into four types: emotional abuse, physical abuse, sexual abuse, and neglect.

Emotional Child Abuse

Emotional child abuse is injuring a child mentally or emotionally. It is also called mental abuse. It may be inflicted intentionally or unintentionally by an adult. Any other person can be emotionally abusive to a child, but deeper injuries are usually inflicted by a parent. The deeper the human bonding, the more potential it creates for lasting injury. Teachers, grandparents, siblings, and other important persons in a child's life also have the potential to leave scars from emotional injury.

Emotional abuse can be difficult to prove when physical signs do not accompany it. Emotional pain is a part of all forms of

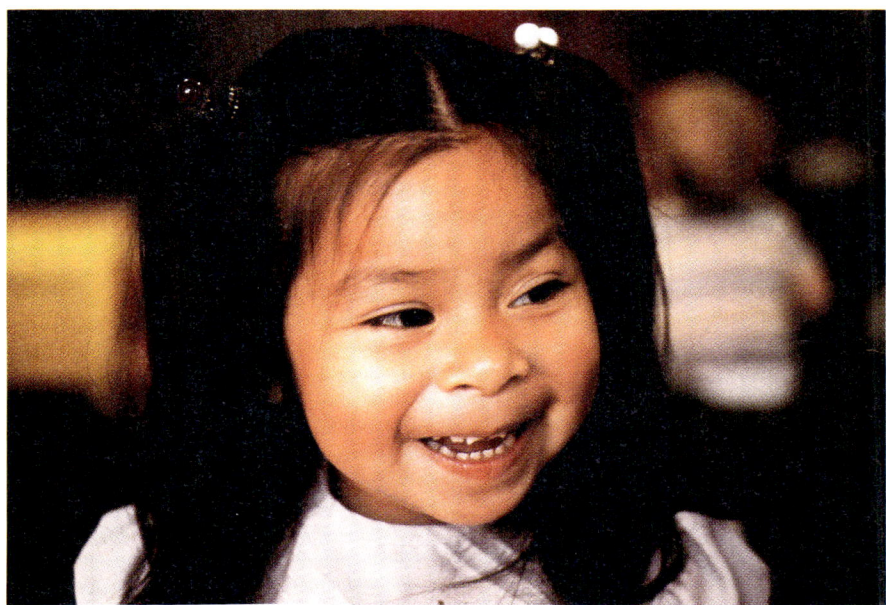

FIGURE 9-6 A child may show no signs of physical abuse but still be emotionally abused.
Source: March of Dimes Birth Defects Foundation

abuse. Being able to point to bruises, broken bones, burns, inadequate clothing, or poor health means that these signs are more likely to attract attention than the emotional pain children suffer. Yet it is the emotional effects of any kind of abuse that are often the longest-lasting and the most difficult to heal.

RIDICULE

Emotional abuse occurs when a child is ridiculed and his or her sense of self-worth is torn apart by an adult. Criticism of children's personalities, thoughts, feelings, and ideas belittles them. This kind of abuse is what Jake's mother inflicted on him when she called him a brat in front of Mrs. Cisneros. What Jake endured is mild compared to what many children face at home and sometimes in the classroom.

ABANDONMENT

Emotional abuse results when parents, or other significant adults, abandon children. The breaking up of a family makes children feel torn between their parents. The effects of feeling divided in this way can cause fear and insecurity for many years. A child who witnesses any family violence, whether or not it is associated with a break-up, suffers emotional abuse. When one parent kidnaps a child from the parent who was given custody, the child can feel torn between parents, confused, and insecure.

SELFISH PARENTAL LOVE

Parents create emotional problems for children by attacking the love bonds they have with other family members or other people. Adults who compete for or try to control children's love and affection cause them emotional pain.

Some parents play games with children's need for affection and love. Playing games in this sense means using children like objects rather than relating to them as persons. Parents who do this give and withhold love on a whim or based on the child's behavior, rather than loving the child unconditionally.

SUBSTANCE ABUSE BY PARENTS

Children who are abused more often than not have parents who abuse drugs or alcohol. When adults are under the influence of mind-altering substances, their attention is not truly on their children or those children's needs. When parents' needs are addressed first, children's emotional, and sometimes physical, needs are often neglected. As these children grow up, they often feel lonely and isolated.

Parents and other adults who abuse alcohol or drugs may be physically dangerous to children. Not only is it more likely that they will physically or sexually abuse children while they are intoxicated, but they may also cause children trauma because their own abilities are limited. For example, parents who drink heavily may injure their children in a car accident, accidentally start a fire in the house, or fail to detect a gas leak because of their condition. Using cocaine or PCP can also affect parenting skills. Mothers who take cocaine often abandon babies soon after birth. Parents high on PCP sometimes abuse their children badly.

Adults who abuse substances may stay away from children while they are under the influence of drugs or alcohol. Are children affected by adult behavior that occurs when they are not present? The Something to Think About feature on the next page discusses this question.

EXPLOITATION

A child's sense of self-worth is often destroyed when an adult exploits him or her. **Exploitation** occurs when parents use a child's talents, appearance, or abilities to make money or gain prestige or position for themselves without regard for the consequences to the child. Exploitation means that adults have abdicated their role as parents. **Abdication** is giving up one's responsibility and authority. Ways in which adults exploit children include the following:

- Requiring children to beg for money or using them to con or cheat other people

- Making children work for money and then taking it from them

- Getting children to pose for sexually explicit or revealing photographs or to perform sexual acts for filming (The pictures are usually produced and sold for profit. Sometimes they are used privately. The products of this exploitation are known as **child pornography.** Children's sense of self-worth is seriously damaged.)

- Selling children's talents or looks for adult gain (For example, entering children in beauty pageants or pressing them to perform either publicly or privately could be exploitive.)

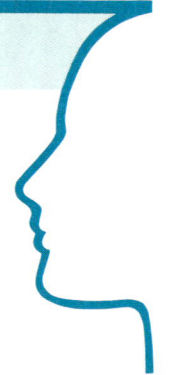

Are Children Affected by Adult Behavior They Don't See?

Adults tend to feel that what they do in private is their own business. Most people agree with this as long as what is being done does not interfere with other people's rights. But what about children? Are they affected by private adult behavior?

The law recognizes that some things adults do affect other people. For example, teachers, government workers, and most employees in private business are not allowed to come to work under the influence of alcohol because it impairs judgment and response time. In addition, teachers are an example to children and are not allowed to appear to be under the influence of alcohol when they are with their students.

What effect does parental drinking have on children? If parents abuse alcohol and drugs only when they are not with their children, are the children affected?

Being addicted to a substance of any kind means putting it above everything else. Getting the substance and using it become more important to an addicted parent than meeting children's needs. An addict thinks about getting and using a favorite substance even when he or she is sober or straight. What affect might this kind of thinking have on a parent's relationship with a child? If a child must compete with an unseen, unknown substance, what emotional needs might go unattended?

Does looking at pornography affect children as long as it is kept away from children? Does looking at sexually stimulating pictures or films create an atmosphere where abuse is more likely?

Are children affected by private adult behavior? What do you think?

Physical Child Abuse

Physical abuse is what most people think of when they hear the term child abuse. **Physical child abuse** is causing any non-accidental bodily injury to a child. Injuries may occur by burning, hitting, beating, grabbing, tossing, throwing, shaking, dropping, twisting, or kicking children's bodies. Injuries may be external (they can be seen when the child is examined) or internal (they are not visible).

EXTERNAL INJURIES

Injuries to the outside of the body are those most likely to be noticed by teachers and other adults who are not doctors or nurses. Over 70% of external injuries caused by abuse are between the neck and knees, on parts of the body that are frequently covered by clothing. How can you tell if an injury is accidental or is caused by abuse?

Bruises with a variety of colors may be caused by abuse. Bruises take on different colors, depending on how old they are. Bruises change color in the following order: from red and purple to blue, green, yellow, brown, and finally normal skin color. (On dark-skinned children it may be difficult to see the colors of bruises.) When the skin in bruised areas has all colors, this indicates that the child has been beaten or injured more than once.

A wound that shows the shape of something, such as a hand, a cord, a rope, or a fly swatter, may be due to abuse. Wounds that "wrap around" a child's body might have been inflicted with something flexible such as a belt, a cord, or a strap. A series of wounds of the same shape, especially around a child's hips and upper legs, may have been caused by hitting the child with a switch, a stick, or a wire hanger.

Broken bones, especially if arm or leg looks twisted, may be the result of abuse. Head injuries, especially those on more than one spot, may also be caused by abusive treatment.

Burns are sometimes inflicted on purpose. Caregivers can watch for burns that have the shape of an object, such as an iron, a coil on a stovetop, or a floor grate. Burns that have a distinctive shape such as a star or circle are sometimes caused by holding a child over a gas flame. Burns in which some of the skin in the middle is not burned, often found on the stomach or in the crease behind the knee or elbow, may come from holding children under hot running water. Deep, round burns, usually on the hands, face, or arms, may be caused by cigarettes.

Raw wounds around ankles or wrists may indicate that the child has been tied up. **Tethering** is the practice of tying children to beds, playpens, or other furniture to keep them from getting into things or making messes.

Bites, especially with adult-sized teeth marks, may be physical abuse.

INTERNAL INJURIES

Internal injuries from child abuse are often difficult to detect. Internal injuries affect a child's organs, including the kidneys, liver, heart, lungs, colon, or bladder. Both internal and external injuries may be suffered in the genital area.

Internal injuries may be caused by poisoning, which can be intentional or due to carelessness. Parents may poison children in an attempt to calm them down, by giving them sleeping pills or other drugs.

These are some symptoms that indicate that a child needs to receive immediate medical attention:

- Coughing up blood
- Nausea
- Blood in the urine
- Abnormal body temperature
- Swelling and tenderness

Caregivers also need to respond promptly to children's complaints of pain and reports of injury, especially if any of the above symptoms are present.

When parents shake or toss children, internal head injuries may occur. Symptoms of such injuries include the following:

- Nausea or vomiting
- Seizures or unconsciousness
- Muscle spasms
- Holding head in an odd position, such as turned to one side, or inability to lift head or turn it from side to side
- Dilated pupils (pupils remain large even in bright light)
- Visible spots or pools of blood in the eye

Child Neglect

Child neglect is failure to provide a child with adequate food, shelter, clothing, health care, and/or love. Some neglect of children is related to poverty, but it can happen in any family at any income level. What conditions surround children who are neglected?

POOR FOOD

Some neglected children do not have enough nutritious food to be healthy. They may be given enough food, but it does not contain the necessary nutrients. Children may be left to find ready-to-eat food for themselves out of containers. These foods include potato chips, sugar-covered cereals, soft drinks, candy, and sometimes alcoholic beverages. Even spoiled food may be consumed. In severe cases, there may be no food in the house and children may starve.

INADEQUATE SHELTER AND CLOTHING

Neglected children often live in filth. Bad living conditions may include urine-soaked mattresses without sheets, human and animal feces on floors or even on furniture, and signs of cockroaches, mice, and rats. The fixtures in kitchens and bathrooms may not ever be cleaned and weeks or months of garbage may be piled up. Water, gas, or electricity may be turned off or not working. Drains may be clogged. Any of these conditions is unhealthy for children.

Neglected children's bodily care is nearly always inadequate. Their skin is frequently dirty and has an unpleasant odor. Their hair is unwashed and uncombed. Their clothes usually do not fit and may be worn out and ragged. They often do not have adequate coats and shoes for the wintertime. The same clothes may be worn all year round.

POOR HEALTH CARE

Children who are neglected tend to have colds or diarrhea that does not clear up. They seem tired a great deal of the time. Medical problems they have go untreated. Cuts, burns, and bruises usually remain untreated.

EMOTIONAL NEGLECT

Children need unconditional love and appropriate affection. Those who are not given these can be considered to be emotionally neglected. Children whose needs are ignored do not sense their parents' love. Children who are loved only *if* they meet parents' expectations know that the love is not real.

The quality of interaction between parents and children who are emotionally neglected is very poor. The children do not thrive the way other children do. When this condition is severe during

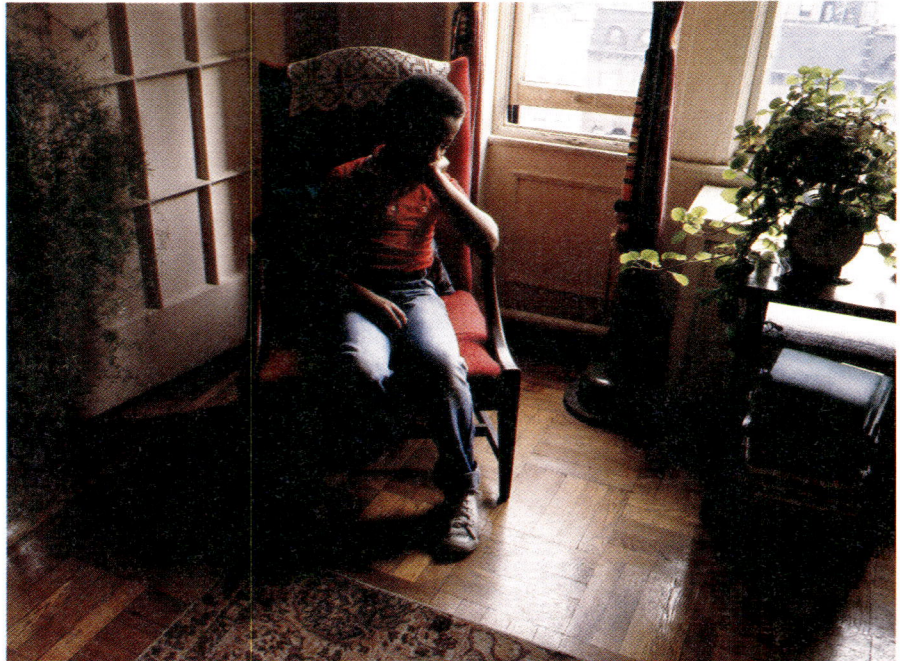

FIGURE 9-7   A child whose parents provide the nicest material things may still be neglected—by not receiving unconditional love or not sharing enough quality time with parents.
Source: © Bill Stanton/International Stock Photography

infancy, it is called failure to thrive (discussed in more detail in Chapter 10). If the infants are not treated, they can lose weight and eventually die. All children who are not loved fail to thrive in some degree. Some survive but their lives are seldom rich and full.

What are some signs of emotional neglect in children under six?

- The emotionally neglected child may not play.
- He or she may not be curious.
- The child may seek attention from teachers much more often than other children do.
- He or she may be very active or inactive for no obvious reason.
- The child may not cry when hurt.

- He or she appears to have no friends.
- The child may be aggressive, mean, or defiant.

CONFINEMENT

Parents sometimes lock children in confined places. This action is called **confinement,** or sometimes **closeting.** Parents confine children because they see them as troublesome, loud, or annoying or because they do not want them. Children who are confined are not allowed to walk or move about. Confinement results in emotional scars, developmental delays, and sometimes mental retardation.

LACK OF SUPERVISION

Adults can neglect children by pushing adult responsibility on them before they are ready to handle it. **Lack of supervision** occurs when children are left without an adult to watch and protect them from dangers. Children are sometimes left with other children or left alone without adequate knowledge of how to care for themselves.

Children who come home after school to an empty house and let themselves in are called **latch-key children.** Parents can help these children stay safe. Some suggestions are as follows:

- Inform a trusted neighbor that the child comes home after school and ask the child to check in with him or her before going in the house.

- Provide the child with the parent's telephone number at work and require the child to call when he or she is safely in the house.

- Provide emergency phone numbers and make sure the child knows how to use the phone.

- Put secure locks on doors and windows. Teach the child to lock the door from inside and *not* to answer the door under any circumstance.

- Provide children with nutritious food they do not have to cook; or if they are old enough, teach them to use appliances safely.

- Provide safe activities that can be enjoyed inside the house.

Sexual Child Abuse

Sexual child abuse is any action by which an adult uses a child for sexual purposes. It is far more common than most people think. It is estimated that one of every three girls and one of every ten boys are sexually misused in some way before they enter high school. It is the least reported and least treated form of child abuse.

Children can be sexually abused in many ways. They may be touched inappropriately in genital areas, exposed to adult nudity or sexual acts, raped, or seduced into participating in sexual activity with an adult. Most commonly the abuser is a parent, stepparent, grandparent, or older sibling. Ninety percent of the perpetrators are male. When a family member sexually abuses a child, it is called **incest.**

When a parent is sexually abusing a child, the other parent is often aware of the abuse and ignores it. Children who are sexually abused seldom recover from it without a great deal of professional help. Their lives may be ruined. They may feel lasting hatred for both parents, particularly the one who allowed the abuse to continue. Without help, they are likely to become abusive parents or to marry someone who will abuse them or their children.

PEDOPHILES

A **pedophile** is a person who has a sexual perversion and prefers children as sex objects. People with this problem often try to work with children so they can be around them. Children who are sexually abused by a pedophile usually know and like the person. Pedophiles may give children many gifts, asking for favors in return.

Some pedophiles are cruel. They torture or injure children while abusing them. This kind of pedophile is usually a stranger to children. Ninety-five percent of all pedophiles were sexually abused as children.

IDENTIFYING SEXUAL ABUSE

Some signs that a child is being sexually abused can be identified by teachers and caregivers. These include the following:

- Changes in habits or behaviors
- Running away
- Feeling unsafe at home
- Angry, aggressive, or hostile behavior

- Does not make friends
- Does not trust
- Has knowledge of sexual behavior beyond what is normal at that age level

- Babyish behavior
- Talks of suicide
- Takes, or wants to take, many baths

Physical signs of sexual abuse include the odor of semen on a child, tears or bruises in the genital area, and possibly difficulty urinating. Examination of a child's genital area should only be done by a trained professional in a medical environment. However, if a child complains of pain in the genital area or has difficulty walking or sitting, a teacher should ask if something has hurt the child.

The most important sign for a teacher of preschool children to be alert for is a child's talking about or reporting sexual abuse. Very few children make up stories about abuse, especially sexual abuse. *All stories or complaints about abuse must be taken seriously.*

Ritual Abuse

Children are sometimes victimized by parents and other adults during occult gatherings. A child may tell a teacher about being abused in this way. Sometimes the child will act out what happened during play or draw pictures about it. Those who work with children who have been abused in this way say that the pictures are often stick figures with a circle for the main body and very obvious sexual features. If a caregiver suspects that a child has been ritually abused, he or she should immediately report to a supervisor and to the children's protective services agency.

REPORTING CHILD ABUSE

Jake was being physically abused. Mrs. Cisneros could see the emotional scars as well. She sent one of her staff members to call the emergency number for the children's protective services agency while she talked with Jake's mom. When the social worker arrived, Mrs. Cisneros showed him Jake's bruises and described what she knew about the abuse case.

Laws Concerning Child Abuse

All states have laws concerning child abuse. The details of these laws vary from state to state. It is important that every child care worker know the law in her or his state. The law is often less clear about child neglect, but a caregiver has a responsibility to report clear cases of neglect.

REPORTING SUSPECTED CASES OF CHILD ABUSE

The law requires that any and all cases of suspected child abuse be reported to the agency for children's protective services as soon as a person becomes aware of the situation. It is preferable to report both by telephone and in writing. All cases of child abuse are considered to be only suspected until they have been properly investigated by a protective services case worker. Most states protect those who report child abuse from being sued as long as they do not knowingly file a false report.

When reporting abuse, it is very important to stick to the facts. The person reporting the case should describe the exact evidence of abuse that caused suspicion. Anything the child has told that person about the event or conditions related to the event also must be reported accurately.

The child's name, address, and telephone number and the parent's name, address, telephone number, and place of employment may be requested. If a medical examination is needed, the case worker may request the name of the child's physician. In a child care situation, the child's enrollment application may be the best source of this information.

The same procedures are followed whether a child care professional or a private citizen is reporting a suspected case of child abuse. Reporting a neighbor, friend, or relative can be difficult, painful, or even dangerous to an individual, but it is absolutely necessary to do if children are to be protected. Private citizens are legally required to report suspected child abuse and may be penalized by law if they do not, just as a professional may be.

PENALTIES FOR NOT REPORTING CHILD ABUSE

Both criminal and civil penalties can be imposed on people who are aware of child abuse and do not report it. The laws vary from state to state. In some states those knowing about child abuse and not reporting it can be held financially responsible for later injuries to or death of the child.

A Child Care Center's Policy on Reporting Abuse

Every child care center must develop a written policy regarding how child abuse is to be reported. The policy has to be

```
                      LA CASITA CHILDREN'S CENTER

               Policy Concerning Suspected Child Abuse


        All cases of suspected child abuse, no matter how severe, shall
   be reported immediately to the director. The center's intention in re-
   porting child abuse is to protect children and to provide help for
   parents.

        Failure of any staff member to report suspected child abuse or
   neglect, no matter how severe, shall be cause for dismissal or other
   disciplinary action.

        All cases of suspected child abuse will be turned over to the
   children's protective services agency for investigation. All cases are
   to be considered to be suspected, no matter how strong the evidence is,
   until the agency has investigated.

        The director will determine whether to contact parents or to
   allow the protective services agency to do that. Staff members are not
   to confront parents on their own.
```

ILLUSTRATION 9-1 This is an example of a child care center's policy on reporting child abuse.

in compliance with the law. A sample of such a policy is shown in Illustration 9-1.

If for any reason the director of the center instructs you not to report suspected child abuse or any other staff member tries to prevent you from reporting it, you have an obligation by law to report it on your own.

Help for Abusive Parents

Although all parents are potential abusers, most parents do not abuse children severely or continuously. What makes parents likely to be abusive? Some factors that may lead parents to abuse their children are as follows:

- Parents were abused themselves as children.
- They are under stress.

- They have inadequate knowledge about children.
- They discipline too harshly or unrealistically.
- They have unrealistic expectations for their children.
- They are inexperienced or very young.
- They had parents who were inadequate at parenting.
- They are unable to provide adequate food, clothing, and housing.
- They have poor self-esteem and frequently act impulsively.
- They have been through a recent crisis.
- They have few friends, or no support system.
- They move frequently.
- They do not know how to use community resources.
- They may be psychotic (only about 10 percent of abusive parents are).
- They want someone to love and take care of them.

In some families only one child is abused. In others all children are abused. Which children are likely to be abused?

- Children who are rejected for some reason
- Children whose bonding with the mother was delayed for some reason (such as prematurity, medical problems, or absence)
- Children who are resented because they brought changes in parents' lives or the family structure
- Children who are handicapped
- Children who require more of their parents' time
- Children who frustrate or embarrass parents

In most communities child abuse is a growing concern. Many organizations and agencies provide support or training for parents. These include churches, community colleges, protective services agencies, hospitals, and various volunteer organizations. In addition to local community resources, there are national organizations that will provide help and information. Some of these agencies are listed in Illustration 9-2.

ILLUSTRATION 9-2 This list gives addresses and telephone numbers of organizations that provide information about child abuse and neglect.

American Academy of Pediatrics
141 Northwest Point Road
Oakgrove, IL 60007
Telephone: 312-228-5005

For Kids Sake, Inc.
P.O. Box 313
Lake Elsinore, CA 92331-0313
Telephone: 714-224-9001

Henry Kempe National Center for Child Abuse
1205 Oneida Street
Denver, CO 80220
Telephone: 303-695-0811

National Center on Child Abuse and Neglect
Children's Bureau
Administration for Children, Youth, and Families
Department of Human Services
P.O. Box 1182
Washington, DC 20013

National Committee for Prevention of Child Abuse and Neglect
Suite 1250
332 South Michigan Avenue
Chicago, IL 60604-4357

Parents Anonymous
22330 Hawthorne
Torrance, CA 90505
Telephone: 213-371-3501

Investigating Reported Cases of Abuse

A case worker will investigate a report of suspected child abuse. In cases where it is appropriate, the person reporting is notified of the outcome of the investigation. Because of the heavy case load, not all cases are investigated immediately.

An investigation carried out by a protective services worker involves finding out about the child's environment and any history of child abuse in the family, getting a medical report when applicable, and having an interview with the child when appropriate. Evidence may also be taken from witnesses, if any. Professionals in the areas of education, medicine, psychology, law enforcement, and law are sometimes called in to give expert opinions.

If an investigation shows a child has been abused, the case worker has several options. The child may be left in the home with the case worker providing regular supervision. The child may be removed from the home and placed in foster care with or without parental rights to visit. Counseling and parenting classes may be required for the parents as a condition for leaving the child in the home or allowing her or him to return. The case worker may—when the situation is serious—file charges in court for the termination of parental rights. **Termination of parental rights** means removing a child permanently and legally from his or her parents.

TEACHING CHILDREN ABOUT SELF-PROTECTION ■

Children are on their own more than they were in the past. Neighborhoods are more dangerous. Children are in contact with more adults who may be dangerous to them. One way of protecting children is to teach them to protect themselves against abusive adults. Child care centers can help preschoolers protect themselves by teaching them the following rules:

- Do not talk to strangers.
- Ride only with your parents or someone they have given you permission to ride with.
- Lock the door and do not open it if your parents aren't home.
- Do not let anyone touch your private parts.
- If anyone does touch your private parts, tell someone you trust.

Children need practice saying no to adults who make inappropriate demands of them. To provide such practice, teachers can use a doll and point to places that an adult should not touch. They can ask the children to practice saying no assertively in such a situation. Of course, some children will use this skill in other situations. A skilled teacher or parent will simply explain to children what is and is not an appropriate time to tell an adult "no!"

The October morning had turned tense. Reporting child abuse was always difficult for Mrs. Cisneros. Jake's mother was angry with her for calling the case worker and at first refused to talk with him. When he explained that she was responsible for protecting her children from abuse and that she could be punished as well, she became more cooperative.

Jake was placed in foster care and his mother was required to attend parenting classes. His dad was charged with child abuse. Each week Jake's mother was allowed to visit him. In a few months he returned home with her, but the case worker continued to visit them to see that the abuse did not occur again.

Child abuse always made Mrs. Cisneros feel sad. Her concern was not only for the physical safety of the children but also for the tremendous emotional damage they were likely to have. She knew that she could not change the world alone, but by being a child care professional she was able to make some difference. That made it really worth the effort.

Summary

Communicating with children involves being able to listen to what they say and understand what they feel. It is also very important to speak clearly.

Adults guide children indirectly by providing them freedom to choose within limits and allowing them to experience the logical consequences of their actions as long as this does not injure or endanger them. As children gain control over their own activities, adults can expand children's limits. By providing developmentally appropriate activities and encouragement, adults can keep children moving in a positive direction.

Adults guide children directly by using positive statements, setting and enforcing limits, reinforcing desirable behavior, and ignoring some forms of undesirable behavior.

Teachers help preschool children develop social skills by teaching them basic manners, providing activities that are rich in opportunities for social interaction, and allowing them to solve as many of their own problems as they can.

Guiding children in groups is different from guiding them individually. Teachers need to set up simple, essential rules and inform children of them. Teachers need to use a fair and effective way of dealing with children who do not follow those rules. It is important for teachers to be aware of the interactions and relationships among the children in the classroom.

Discipline teaches children self-control and self-responsibility. Punishment is an adult's way of taking out anger and frustration on a child. Children need to learn how to view authority and how to deal with it. They need to learn about the balance between authority and responsibility.

Child abuse is categorized as emotional abuse, physical abuse, sexual abuse, and neglect. All forms of child abuse are sometimes linked to adult substance abuse. Emotional abuse involves ridicule, abandonment, selfish parental love, or exploitation. Physical abuse may involve external injuries that are readily seen or internal injuries that are more difficult to detect.

Child neglect usually involves insufficient or inadequate food, shelter, clothing, health care, or love. Neglected children may be confined or have a lack of supervision. Latch-key children are those who come home after school to an empty house and must care for themselves. They need basic survival skills to be safe.

A person who sexually abuses children is called a pedophile. If sexual abuse is perpetrated by a family member, it is called incest. Children who have been sexually abused often report that abuse to a teacher. Other signs of sexual abuse may be observed by teachers or caregivers.

Laws require that those suspecting child abuse report it. There are penalties for not reporting. The person reporting a case of possible abuse needs to supply facts and names and addresses whenever possible. In most states the law protects those who report abuse from being sued. Child care centers need to spell out procedures for reporting abuse within the center.

Help is available for parents who abuse children. Case workers who investigate reported cases of abuse deal with families in various ways, depending on the severity of the abuse. If it is necessary to remove a child from the home, a legal procedure called termination of parental rights is used.

Children can be taught to protect themselves from abusive adults. They need to learn to be careful and to say no when it is appropriate.

Terms and Concepts

Listening	Abdication
Indirect guidance	Child pornography
Freedom within limits	Physical child abuse
Structured choices	Tethering
Logical consequences	Child neglect
Direct guidance	Confinement
Positive statements	Closeting
Reinforcement	Lack of supervision
Time out	Latch-key children
Transition times	Sexual child abuse
Discipline	Incest
Punishment	Pedophile
Perpetrator	Termination of parental rights
Emotional child abuse	
Exploitation	

Checking Your Understanding

1. Describe how an adult listens effectively to a child.
2. Describe the kind of speech adults need to use with children.
3. How do adults speak to children when they wish to stop some undesirable behavior?
4. What guidelines should adults use to determine whether to allow children to experience the logical consequences of some action or behavior?
5. What is the benefit of using logical consequences?
6. How might expanding children's limits contribute to the development of self-control and self-responsibility?
7. Change the following to positive statements for guiding children's behavior:

    Don't throw the sand.
    Don't run indoors.

Don't yell indoors.
Don't take Jeremy's truck away.
Don't spill the paint on the floor.

8. How are indirect guidance and direct guidance alike? How are they different?

9. What must an adult decide when setting limits?

10. What steps does a caregiver need to follow when enforcing limits?

11. How can reinforcing acceptable behavior and ignoring unacceptable behavior contribute to good discipline?

12. Describe some basic manners that can be taught to preschoolers.

13. How is guiding children in a group different from guiding them individually?

14. Why is discipline important?

15. Why is learning to accept and deal with authority important?

16. What are some ways in which authority can be abused? Do you think people who abuse children misuse their authority?

17. What are some ways in which children can be emotionally abused?

18. How can you tell if children have been beaten or injured more than once by looking at their bruises?

19. How should a person go about reporting suspected child abuse?

20. Suggest some ways to teach children to protect themselves.

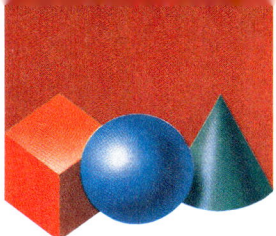

9 HANDS ON WITH CHILDREN

USING TIME OUTS TO ENFORCE LIMITS

Most adults discipline children too forcefully or not enough to be effective. Both ways are harmful to children. A logical and simple form of discipline that does not need to be abusive is having the child take time out. This is done as follows:

Step 1   If the adult can see the child, he or she can *use eyes and facial expression to say, "Don't do it."* Allow the child an opportunity to respond with acknowledgment or acceptable behavior. If a child does not respond acceptably the first time, the teacher or parent needs to act decisively and immediately.

Step 2   *Stop the behavior physically.* Adults can physically interrupt a child's behavior by placing a hand on his or her shoulder or by firmly, but painlessly, taking hold of the child by the hand or arm.

Step 3   *Calm the child down.* If the child is angry or aggressive, hold the child without hurting him or her until the child becomes calm.

Step 4   *Have the child sit and watch the other children play.* This period of sitting should last only a few minutes (from three to five minutes is usually enough). The purpose is to give the child a few minutes to think about why he or she is not playing.

Step 5   *Remind the child of the rule and allow him or her to return to play.*

CHAPTER 10
Infants

OBJECTIVES

When you have finished this chapter, you will be able to

- Identify appropriate routines and procedures to use when caring for infants in child care
- Help infants and parents handle separations due to child care
- Recognize positive skills for infant caregiving
- Set and enforce limits for infants
- Assist in maintaining a positive environment for infants
- Identify and demonstrate developmentally appropriate activities for infants
- Discuss the importance of talking with infants

Jayme had been home from the hospital for only six weeks when her parents placed her in child care. Her twin sister, Sarah, had come home three weeks earlier. Jayme and Sarah had been born prematurely and had stayed in the hospital for several weeks. Their mother returned to work to help pay the bills.

Jayme and Sarah were known as high-risk infants because they had medical problems that developed because they were born prematurely. Jayme's doctor placed her on a monitor so an alarm would sound if she stopped breathing while she was asleep in her crib.

La Casita was the only center in town equipped to care for high-risk infants like Jayme and Sarah. Caregivers in the infants' room had CPR certification, including training for infant and child CPR. An extra caregiver was assigned to help in the infants' room so that each child would have closer supervision. That made it necessary for Mrs. Cisneros to charge more for infant care than for that for older children.

The staff in La Casita's infant department had established very detailed caregiving routines and procedures. They kept careful records of the children's day and gave copies to parents daily. Sanitation was a major concern in order to protect the infants' health.

La Casita's staff members not only took care of the infants' physical needs but also provided them with **developmentally appropriate activities.** Providing such activities—ones that are suited to each child's needs and abilities—requires knowing how children grow and develop.

CARING FOR INFANTS' PHYSICAL NEEDS

Infants' physical needs include the need for food and sleep. Also, infants need to have their diapers changed and sometimes to receive medicine. To meet these needs, caregivers need to set up routines and follow procedures.

Routines, Records, and Schedules

One way of helping infants to develop the very important feeling of trust is to provide consistency in their environment. **Consistency** means sameness—that is, things are done the same way all the time. **Routines** are established times and ways of doing things that provide the children in child care situations with a sense of sameness and security. Caregiving routines include ones for rest and sleep, feeding, diapering, and giving medication.

Schedules are established in infant areas to assure that the caregiving routines are followed. A sample schedule for an infants' room is shown in Illustration 10-1. The schedule can be posted on a large chart or bulletin board on the wall of the infants' room. Color-coded index cards with children's names are pinned to the schedule in the appropriate places. Medication cards are put up and taken down daily. Other cards can also be changed or moved as infants' needs change. Caregivers cannot feed, diaper, and do activities with all children at the same time. Therefore, the schedule allows for doing these things in shifts.

An important part of the routine in an infants' room is keeping daily records. A sample form for keeping a child's daily record is presented in Illustration 10-2. A copy of the form is sent home each day with the child. Forms such as this one help the staff of a child care center communicate easily with parents. Writing down the times of events and amounts of medication or food, when important, gives parents a clear picture of their child's day.

Keeping accurate records requires organizing a place to store blank record forms and other supplies and writing down each event as soon as it occurs. Simple forms that are easy to read, understand, and use are most effective.

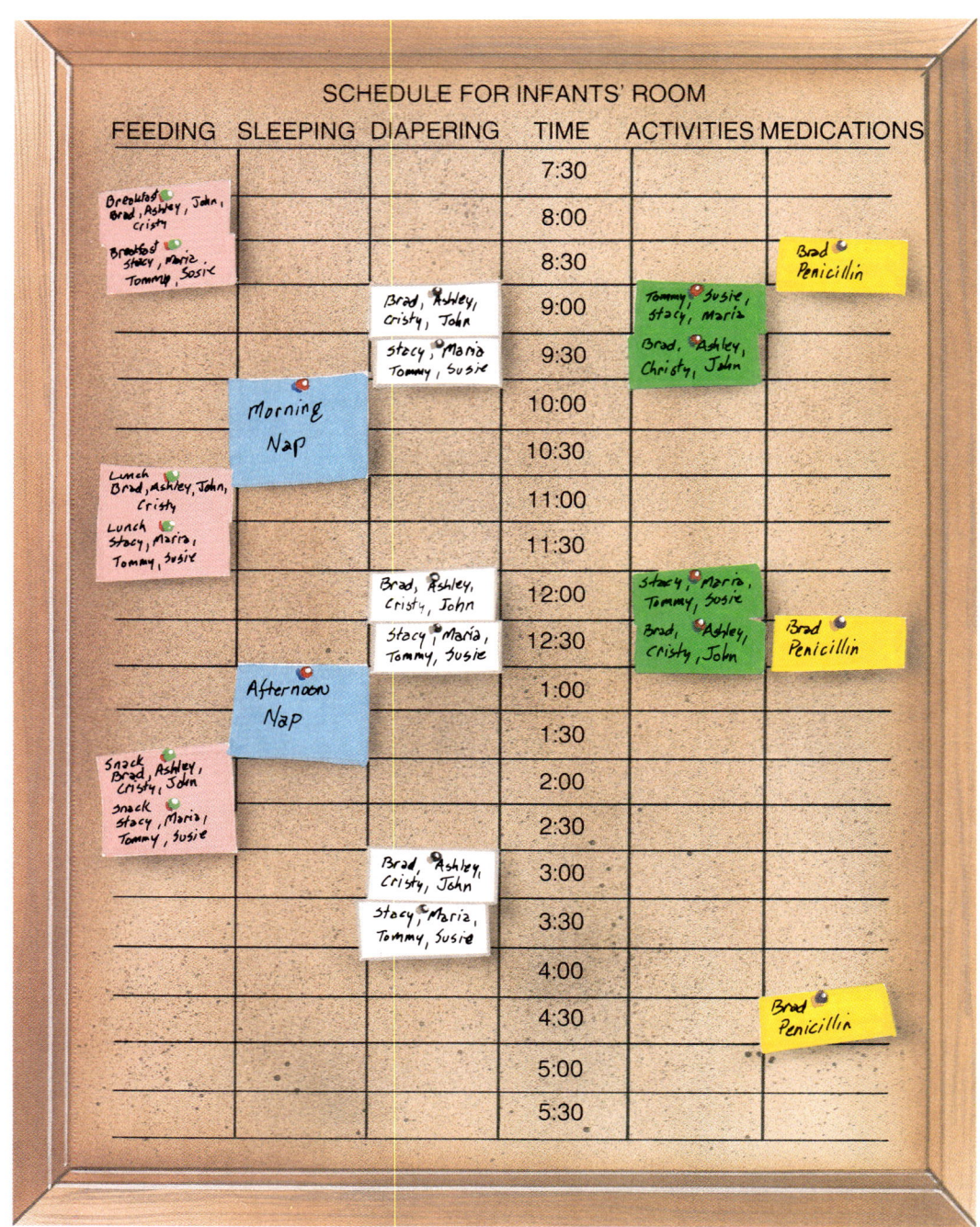

ILLUSTRATION 10-1 A schedule for an infants' room in a child care center can be posted on a bulletin board or a large chart.
Source: Courtesy of Odessa College, Odessa, Texas

LA CASITA CHILDREN'S CENTER

Infant's Daily Record Form

Infant's Name *Brad Thompson*   Age *4½ mo.* Date *1/28/91*

Current Diet *Infamil, rice cereal*   Medications *Penicillin (refrigerate)*

Special Instructions *none*

Comments *Brad has been fussy.*

D = Dry   W = Wet   S = Sleep   BM = Bowel Movement
Foods eaten, medications given, and activities are listed.

FEEDING	SLEEPING	DIAPERING	TIME	ACTIVITIES	MEDICATIONS
cereal *Infamil*			8:00		*penicillin*
		wet	9:00		
	nap		10:00		
	↓		11:00		
cereal *Infamil*	↓		12:00	*Rattles* *Talk*	*penicillin*
		BM	1:00		
Infamil	*nap*		2:00		
	↓		3:00		
		wet	4:00		*penicillin*
			5:00		

ILLUSTRATION 10-2 Caregivers can use a form like this to record daily events for each infant.

Procedures for Physical Care of Groups of Infants

Procedures are established techniques for carrying out necessary tasks in the most effective and efficient way possible. Procedures are developed for all caregiving routines and for many teaching techniques.

PROCEDURES FOR SLEEPING

New babies sleep most of the day. As they gain strength and become rested from the delivery, they sleep less and play more. If they get the kind and amount of rest they need, infants are pleasant to be with and have the energy they need for playing and being with other people. Infants sleep better if they are provided with the following:

- A firm mattress
- A fairly quiet place (some sound lets infants know they are not alone)
- Adequate ventilation
- Comfortable temperatures
- Comfortable and safe clothing and bedding

Each infant should be placed in a crib alone to sleep. A clean sheet is put on daily. If more than one infant uses the same crib, the sheet is changed and the mattress disinfected for each new occupant. Ideally a child care center should have as many cribs as infants so each sheet only needs to be changed daily.

Some infants need to be soothed in order to sleep. Some children have more difficulty settling to sleep than others. When young children do not feel well, they may need extra soothing. To soothe an infant to help him or her sleep, the following suggestions may be helpful:

- Wrap the infant snugly, but not tightly, in a receiving blanket. This will help most infants calm down.

- Hold the infant comfortably close to your own body. The rhythm of the caregiver's heartbeat is sometimes soothing.

- Speak in a calm, reassuring voice. As the infant relaxes, stop speaking.

- Rock with the infant, preferably in a comfortable rocking chair. If other infants are on the floor, be sure they are away from the rocker.

- Sing softly.

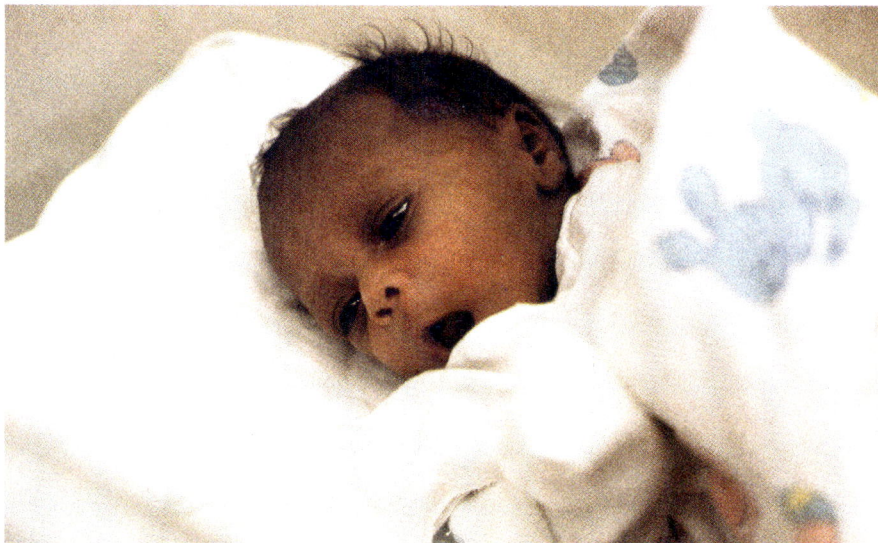

FIGURE 10-1 Infants need a lot of sleep, and they sleep better in comfortable clothes and surroundings.
Source: Bob Ohr for The Christ Hospital

■ Place the infant in the crib face down and pat or rub on the back until he or she falls asleep.

Caregivers record the time each baby falls asleep and the length of the nap.

Some infants fall asleep easily and others fight it energetically. A decision caregivers must make is whether to let an infant who is having trouble falling asleep "cry it out" or to settle him or her into sleep. Generally speaking, infants under six months should not be left to cry themselves to sleep. By six months some infants are ready to try settling to sleep on their own. An infant who is fussy but ready for sleep will generally fall asleep after only a few minutes of fussing. If it takes longer, the caregiver will have to decide whether the infant needs help settling down or is manipulating. Infants who cry instead of falling asleep may be overtired. If the infant needs help settling down, he or she is probably not mature enough to try the task alone yet. If the infant is trying to manipulate the caregiver, it is not good for either of them if this succeeds.

There is sometimes a risk that an infant may die suddenly while asleep. **SIDS** is an acronym for **sudden infant death syn-**

drome, a condition in which infants sometimes forget to breathe (usually while asleep). A **SIDS monitor** is a device attached to a pad placed under the infant. It sounds an alarm and flashes a small red light if the infant stops breathing while in the crib. A trained caregiver can apply infant CPR immediately and very often save the child's life. Unfortunately not all infants who are susceptible to SIDS are identified in time. And some parents cannot afford to pay for the monitor.

Caregivers need to watch infants carefully while they sleep. If a caregiver cannot see an infant breathing, he or she needs to check more closely. If an infant has stopped breathing, the caregiver must immediately start the procedure for infant CPR described in Chapter 8.

PROCEDURES FOR FEEDING

Most babies are bottle-fed in child care. The proper procedure for bottle feeding is as follows: Sit in a comfortable chair, cradling the infant in your arms. Allow the infant to suck $1-1\frac{1}{2}$ ounces; then hold the child in an upright position to burp. Continue feeding and burping until the baby is satisfied. Record the number of ounces consumed and the time.

Never prop a bottle! Infants can strangle or suffocate when drinking from a propped bottle. And, perhaps just as important, infants need the loving touch of a parent or caregiver during feeding. Touching is very important to young children's physical, social, and emotional development.

The primary food for most infants is milk. When adding solid foods, caregivers need to work with parents to determine what foods will be added and when. Caregivers need to keep careful records of the solid foods given, including the type of food, the amount eaten, and the time.

Some mothers are able to breast feed their infants in child care. Mothers will need a comfortable and fairly quiet place to sit while breast feeding. A high-quality child care center makes breast-feeding mothers as comfortable as possible.

PROCEDURE FOR DIAPERING

Diapers need to be changed as soon as they are wet or soiled. Allowing a child to wear wet or soiled diapers causes painful diaper rash. Changing diapers requires a procedure that protects the health of caregivers and infants. A sanitary procedure for diapering is given in the Hands On feature at the end of Chapter 1.

MEETING INFANTS' EMOTIONAL NEEDS

Newborn babies are nearly totally dependent on adults for all their needs. Adults must respond to their calls for help quickly, appropriately, and consistently. If an infant has a need and cries to get help, the more quickly the adult responds, the more secure the infant feels and the easier it is for him or her to learn trust. If an infant cries because he or she is hungry and an adult responds by trying to get the child to be quiet by playing with him or her, the infant's needs are not being met. If children are to be cared for emotionally, adults need to judge their needs accurately in order to meet them appropriately. Infants need adults to respond consistently—to respond every time they have a need and in similar ways.

The Importance of Attachment

When caregivers and parents respond to infants quickly, appropriately, and consistently, infants feel secure and develop a sense of trust. Infants become attached to adults who meet their needs in this way. **Attachment** is a sense of being closely connected to another person. Mary Ainsworth, Sylvia Bell, and others have demonstrated that infants about a year old who are attached to parents and caregivers use them as a secure base from which to explore.[1] Children who have the security to explore their world are able to learn. Early learning helps children to feel competent—to feel that they can handle themselves and their world. This confidence helps children build a sense of self-worth.

You can see that taking care of a child's early needs helps him or her to grow rather than to become spoiled. What is spoiling? The Something to Think About feature deals with whether infants can be spoiled.

Making Transitions Easier

Infants are usually more attached to parents than to caregivers. When parents bring infants, especially older ones, to child care, they sometimes cling to the parents and cry when left with the caregiver. **Transitions** are changes in situations, such as mov-

[1]Mary Ainsworth and Sylvia Bell, "Attachment, Exploration and Separation: Illustrated by the Behavior of One-year-olds in a Strange Situation," *Child Development* 41 (1970):49–67.
Mary Ainsworth et al., *Patterns of Attachment* (Hillsdale, NJ: Erlbaum, 1978).

ing from home to center and from center to home. Smooth transitions help reduce the possible negative effects of being apart for both parents and infants. The following actions by caregivers can help bring about smooth transitions:

■ Meet parents and child at the door, greet them, and invite them into the room.

■ Be pleasant. Make eye contact with both the infant and the parents.

■ Take the time to allow parents and infants to adjust to the child care situation at their own pace.

■ Take time to listen to special concerns and answer as honestly as you can.

FIGURE 10-2 Infants grow attached to those who respond to their needs—especially parents.
Source: Bob Ohr for The Christ Hospital

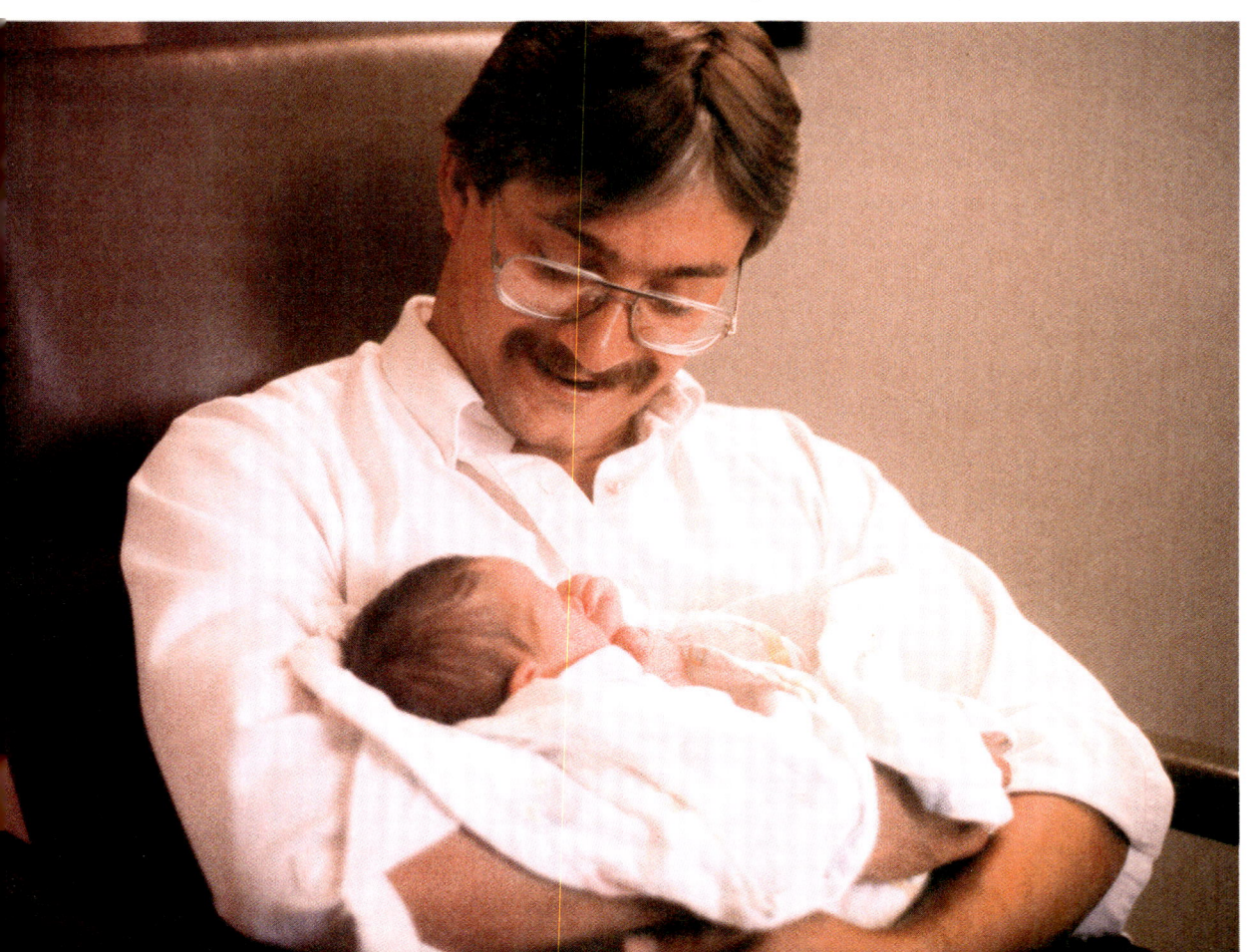

Something to Think About

Can an Infant Be Spoiled?

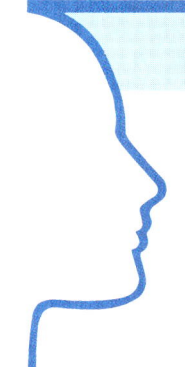

Spoiling is letting a child have anything he or she wants on demand. Manipulating adults in this fashion is not good for children. Spoiling begins when parents or caregivers do things for infants that they are capable of doing for themselves. Sometimes well-meaning parents and caregivers do so much for young children they have no challenges—no reason to grow and mature.

Spoiling is unfair to children because they gain the mistaken idea that they are the center of the adult's world. They may come to feel that they are worth more than other people. It can be really tough on them when they get older and find out that not everyone feels that way about them. They almost always lose respect for parents and other adults who have elevated them to this unrealistic position.

Babies who cry are not necessarily spoiled. Very small infants sometimes have colic. Colic is pain in the stomach or intestine that may be caused by adjustments to eating food when the digestive system is still underdeveloped. Some infants cry because of colic for most of their first three months. When parents do not understand why the infant is crying, they may not respond appropriately to his or her needs.

How do you decide when you are meeting an infant's needs and when you are spoiling him or her? Part of the art of caring for children is learning to discern the difference between a need and a demand. If you have responded to a child's cry and checked for all possible needs, further demands probably should be ignored. If a child seems extremely distressed, you may have missed some problem. If the child is simply angry, however, you probably need to let him or her work it out in a nonharmful way. It is not cruel to let an older infant or toddler cry for a little while if his or her needs have been met.

Very small babies only have needs; they do not know much about manipulating. Older babies learn that they can make things happen, including causing parents or caregivers to behave in certain ways.

Can an infant be spoiled? Does it hurt to spoil a baby? What do you think?

■ Encourage parents to say good-bye to the child, even if the child cries.

Infants usually become attached to caregivers, too. Allow infants to stay close to you for a few minutes until they are ready to let go and get into play.

Infants also need help making the transition to home at the end of the day. Caregivers who pass along to parents highlights of the day and any concerns help them orient their thinking and help make the end-of-the-day transition smoother for the infant.

Disciplining Infants

Only the very simplest procedures are needed to discipline infants. They include establishing routines, child-proofing the environment, removing infants from situations to prevent behavior, and allowing infants to work through their frustrations.

There is never any reason for an adult to spank an infant. Spanking an infant is child abuse. An adult who becomes frustrated or angry with an infant should get another adult to take over caregiving tasks for a while and take a break.

ESTABLISHING ROUTINES

Infants do not know how people arrange for eating, sleeping, bathing, and playing. When parents and caregivers establish routines, they help young children learn a structure for everyday things. Families and caregivers who set up and follow routines provide a predictable environment. This predictability brings security and control into an infant's life.

CHILD-PROOFING THE ENVIRONMENT

Child-proofing the environment was discussed in Chapter 8. Basically child-proofing means making a place safe for young children to be in. In terms of meeting infants' emotional needs, it also means creating an environment in which young children can make some choices without adults' having to constantly be saying "no!"

REMOVING INFANTS FROM PROBLEM SITUATIONS

When an infant has found a way to do something that is not desirable or acceptable, the best strategy is usually to get him or her away from the situation. An example is when an older infant is dropping food from a high chair. Rather than punishing the infant, simply remove him or her from the high chair, clean up child and chair, and end the meal or snack. Yelling or spanking will not improve the situation.

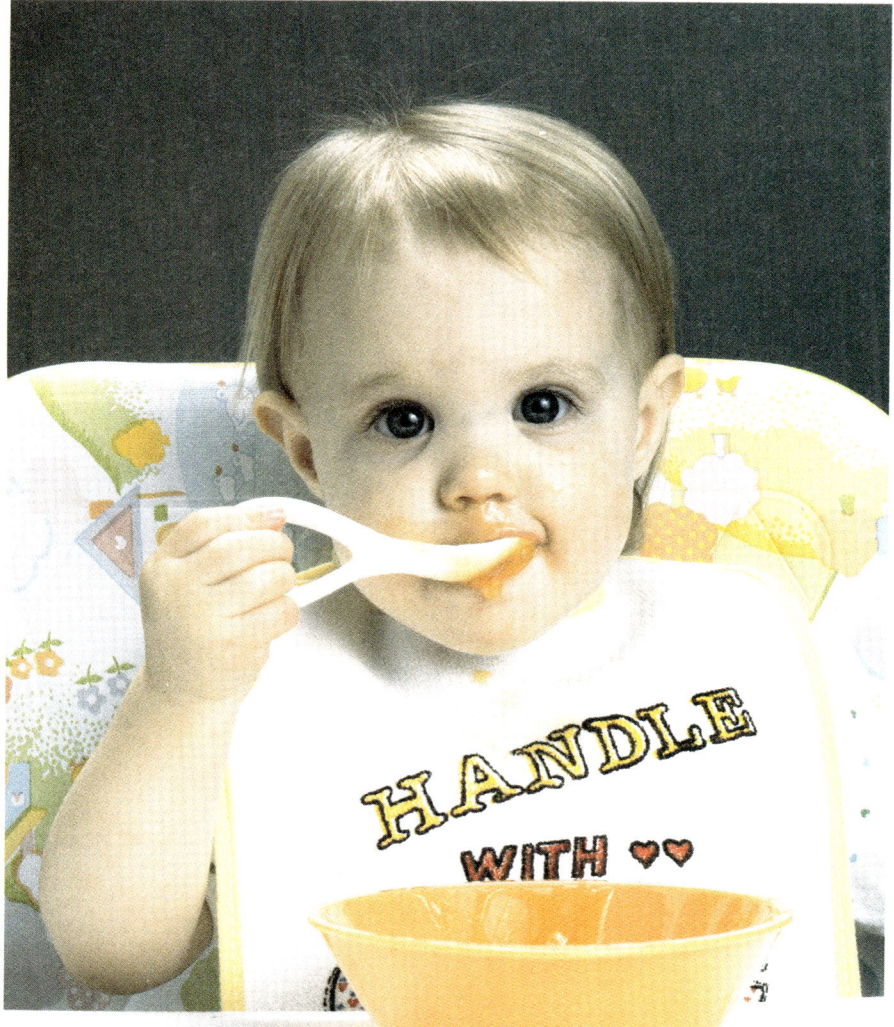

FIGURE 10-3   Infants should not be disciplined for being messy while trying to feed themselves. If they deliberately throw or drop food on the floor, they can be removed from the high chair.
Source: Gerber Products Company

ALLOWING INFANTS TO WORK THROUGH FRUSTRATION

When small babies cry, they have a need. As babies become older, they begin doing some things for themselves. Things babies between 6 and 12 months old can do usually include the following:

- Feed themselves with finger foods
- Move around
- Settle themselves to sleep
- Communicate their needs other than by crying

As with other new tasks, infants have to practice doing these things. Sometimes infants become frustrated by their unsuccessful efforts. When children cry from frustration, caregivers who have observed their efforts can decide whether they need to be left alone to work through a problem or need to be comforted.

Nonorganic Failure to Thrive Syndrome

Infants whose needs are met and who have love and a good environment do well, or thrive. When an infant does not thrive, either there is something physically wrong or there are problems in the baby's environment.

Dr. Gerald Powell of the University of Texas Medical School at Galveston has studied children who do not grow and develop normally when there is no physical cause for this failure. He calls this condition **nonorganic failure to thrive syndrome.**[2] Some infants begin to show symptoms of the syndrome between 6 and 12 months of age. Most commonly it is caused by poor communication between parents and infants. Poor communication is occurring when any of the following are true:

- Parents do not respond appropriately, quickly, or consistently to the infant's cries for help.

- Parents do not talk with their infant and listen to his or her sounds.

- Parents do not touch and hold the infant enough.

- No sense of attachment has developed between parents and child.

[2]Gerald Powell, "Failure to Thrive" (Workshop presented at 8th Annual West Texas Perinatal Conference, Odessa, February 1986).

Leadership at a Glance

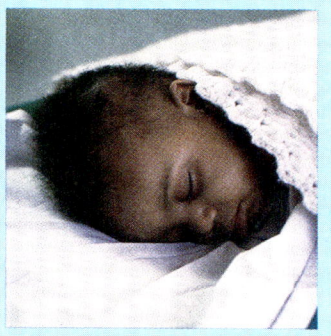

Source: Gerber Children's Center, Inc., a subsidiary of Gerber Products Company

Dr. Gerald Powell

Dr. Gerald Powell is a pediatrician who also teaches and conducts research on how well children grow and develop. He has focused on infants who do not develop normally when there is no apparent physical reason. These children do not eat as well, gain as much weight, or develop as well as expected. Dr. Powell found that these children sometimes do not grow well because they do not get enough loving attention from their parents or other important caregivers.

Dr. Powell teaches, studies, and works with children and their parents at the University of Texas Medical School in Galveston. He spends most of his day in a clinic seeing children who have nonorganic failure to thrive syndrome or who do not develop well because of the environment they live in. The information in this chapter about nonorganic failure to thrive syndrome is based on what Dr. Powell has learned.

If you choose a medical career in which you work with children, you may have opportunities to read some of the articles Dr. Powell has written about his research. His study and teaching clearly distinguish him as a leader to look to when learning about how to work with infants and young children.

SIGNS AND SYMPTOMS

The symptoms observed in an infant depend on how serious the problem has become. Most infants suffering from nonorganic failure to thrive syndrome have a majority of the problems described in the following paragraphs.

Physical symptoms. Infants with nonorganic failure to thrive syndrome tend to be shorter, lighter, and have a smaller head circumference than other infants their age. They often move their fingers more than their arms and legs. Infants who should be very active have posture like newborns with knees against their stomachs and hands held in a power sign. They avoid physical contact and sometimes draw back from caregivers. Many suck their thumbs very vigorously.

Emotional problems. Infants with this syndrome show little or no emotional response. They usually do not cuddle with caregivers. They seldom vocalize but may cry excessively—especially when approached by someone. They do not seem upset when their parents leave them with caregivers. They often have an expressionless face.

Mental development. Secure attachment and healthy interaction between infants and adults are highly important conditions for learning, especially during the first year. Infants with nonorganic failure to thrive syndrome tend to be behind in mental development because they do not have the essential communication with parents and caregivers.

Family characteristics. Children who develop this syndrome are often from families with problems, including poverty, lack of friends, a history of alcoholism or drug abuse, and a very disorganized household environment. Parents of these children are often depressed and may be sexually promiscuous or unfaithful. The father is often absent and does not help with child care when he is at home.

HELPING INFANTS WHO HAVE THE SYNDROME

Caregivers cannot change families. However, they can help infants with nonorganic failure to thrive syndrome. Caregivers can do the following:

■ They can encourage the parents to have the infant examined by a competent pediatrician. A children's doctor can tell whether the problem is physical or emotional and can provide help in either case.

■ They can work with the infant. Caregivers can work at making eye contact and talking to and listening to the infant. (See the Hands On With Children feature at the end of this chapter.) Most important, they can respond quickly, appropriately, and consistently to the infant's cries for help.

■ Caregivers can listen to the parents' problems, so they do not feel isolated.

■ Caregivers can provide information to all parents about nurturing and parenting skills.

Infants with this syndrome need at least one nurturing parent or caregiver. Dr. Powell states that nurturing parents tend to have a loving relationship with one another. They are securely attached to their child and have an unbroken relationship with her or him. They have high self-esteem. Nurturing parents provide stimulating interaction and parenting in their home.

Behaviors of adults who are nurturing include the following:

■ The parent or caregiver gives undivided attention to the infant. This attention makes the infant feel that he or she is the only person the adult is thinking about for the moment.

■ The caregiver or parent is goal-directed, that is, has intentions concerning the infant's growth and well-being.

■ The parent or caregiver clearly enjoys being with the baby. Adults who are obviously delighted to be with babies show it in their eyes, voice, and facial expressions. Babies sense the adults' pleasure.

■ The caregiver or parent understands the baby's cues, especially nonverbal ones.

■ The parent or caregiver knows the things an infant can do and recognizes the infant's potential for growth.

■ The caregiver or parent tests the infant's skills and urges him or her to try new things.

■ The parent or caregiver uses an exaggerated facial expression and voice when speaking to the infant.

■ The caregiver or parent lets the infant lead in play.

■ The parent or caregiver stimulates the infant to learn first in one way, then in another.

■ The caregiver or parent responds to the infant's attempts to communicate.

MENTAL DEVELOPMENT IN THE FIRST YEAR

Full-term, healthy newborns have a large number of abilities. Babies are able to identify their parents, or another primary caregiver, by two weeks of age. (The abilities of newborns were described in Chapter 4.) High-quality infant care is based on care-givers' understanding of the characteristics of infants and their growth and development.

Jean Piaget was a Swiss scientist who observed his own children daily and developed a theory of mental development.[3] He identified the first two years of life as being a time when learning occurs primarily through the senses and body movements. Piaget identified four separate levels of mental growth during the first year.

Mental Development in the First Month

Infants are born with reflexes that aid in survival and learning. They learn by experience. By three weeks of age, they know that sucking will stop hunger pains. They can focus their eyes, but eye muscles still need strengthening. When adults talk and listen to them, they can engage in primitive conversations.

Mental Development from the First to the Fourth Month

During this stage infants react to things they do themselves, such as shaking a rattle. They repeat actions just to get the results. They reach for things they see. They look toward sounds they hear and at things their hands are touching. If they see part of a familiar object, they will look for the rest of it. (For example, if an infant of this age sees a nipple, he or she will look for the bottle.) They begin to see the difference between what they do and the result of their actions.

Mental Development from the Fourth to the Eighth Month

Infants from four to eight months old repeat their actions because of the effect these have on objects outside themselves. They make noises with toys just to hear the sound; and they respond to music. They drop toys from a crib or high chair to watch them fall; then they look for the object that has fallen. They learn to crawl to get somewhere. Other people become more important to infants during this stage. They use their hands to explore faces. They play peek-a-boo with enthusiasm because they like to look for "lost" objects.

[3]Jean Piaget, *The Construction of Reality in the Child* (New York, NY: Ballantine Books, 1971 [Basic Books, 1954]).

Mental Development from the Ninth to the Twelfth Month

During this stage infants begin to be able to apply something learned in the past to a new situation. They do a great deal of imitating. They search actively for "lost" objects or people. They now know that an object they can no longer see does not cease to exist. They can also anticipate events that are not a result of their own actions.

LEARNING ACTIVITIES FOR INFANTS

Activities for infants have to be selected with an understanding of their abilities. What kinds of activities are suitable for infants? The following sections describe activities suitable for infants at different age levels.

Activities for Newborns

The infant's first month is spent learning who his or her primary caregivers are and getting oriented to the environment. What does Mom's face look like? What does Dad's voice sound

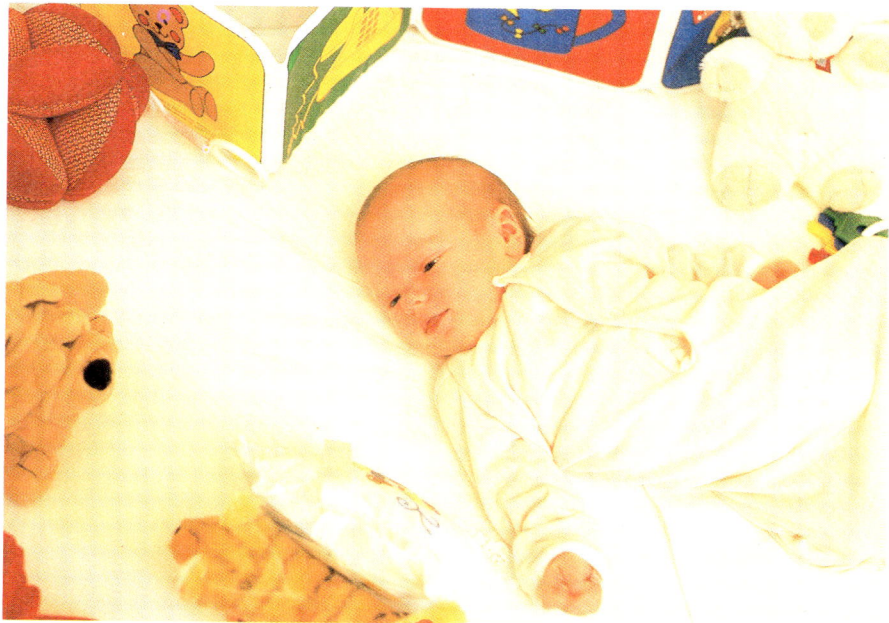

FIGURE 10-4   A variety of safe, colorful objects placed around an infant in a crib add interest to his or her environment.

like? How do I get the pain to leave my stomach? More than anything else, a newborn is learning how to survive.

Good activities for infants at this age include the following:

■ Face-to-face "conversations" with adults that are taken seriously by the adult but also are fun for both parties

■ Interesting but safe objects placed near enough for the infant to focus on (9–16 inches from the face)

■ Simple, brightly colored pictures with clear lines placed where the infant can see them easily

■ Objects moved slowly in the infant's field of vision so that he or she can track, or follow them with the eyes

■ Smiles from caregivers

Exaggerated facial expressions and vocal tones should be used with young infants. Since the world is new to infants, they need to have differences made clear. Most importantly, adults must listen to infant vocalizations and respond.

Activities for Infants Aged 1–4 Months

As infants become comfortable in their environment, they respond to any stimulus to their senses. They need to spend some time in safe places other than the crib, including the floor. A variety of sounds, smells, colors, and textures will excite the infant to learn.

Activities that allow infants at this age to cause a change in something they can see or hear are interesting. The following are some examples:

■ Rattles that sound when the infant shakes them

■ Crib mobiles that make sounds or move when they are kicked

■ Time spent by caregivers in talking to infants and listening to their sounds

■ Placing a large picture of the infant's family, shown with pleasant faces, near the crib

■ Frequently changing objects to look at (Things must be hung safely.)

■ A picture book of the infant and his or her family, caregivers, and playmates

- A mirror where the infant can see himself or herself move
- Recording the infant's voice and playing it back for him or her
- Saying the infant's name frequently, especially when talking to him or her

Activities for Infants Aged 4–8 Months

By the fourth month, infants need a clean and safe place to be on the floor during part of the day. Safe, clean objects to scoot toward lead to crawling.

The activities listed in the preceding section can be continued through the eighth month. In addition, balls begin to be a good toy at this age level and remain so for many years. Balls need to be at least two inches in diameter and should not be made of soft foam. Babies can choke on foam, and small balls can become lodged in an infant's throat.

Other activities for young children of this age include the following:

- Provide objects that make noise, that infants can cause to make sounds.
- Touch and name parts of the infant's body.
- Crawl with the infant.
- Sing simple songs to the infant.
- Point out the infant's image in a mirror.
- Allow the infant to explore your face with his or her hands.
- Play pleasant, simple music at a comfortable volume.
- Play peek-a-boo.

Activities for Infants Aged 9–12 Months

Caregivers can continue playing simple games such as peek-a-boo with infants as long as they enjoy them. New activities to add between the eighth and twelfth months include the following:

- Touch and name parts of the body (the caregiver's body)
- Add toys to bath time routine.
- Introduce the infant to new people, one at a time.

- Play mirror games with infant, using toys and hats.

- Say simple nursery rhymes.

- Get the infant to walk with you, holding onto your fingers.

- Give simple directions, one at a time. Allow the infant to respond. Praise his or her efforts.

- Use a singing voice to give directions.

- Make books for infants using sturdy fabric and a variety of colors and textures for pictures.

- Expand peek-a-boo to finding objects the infant sees you hide. For example, hide a favorite toy behind a screen. Let the infant see you hide it. Encourage him or her to look for it.

- Provide toys that allow the infant to put objects together, such as putting blocks into a container.

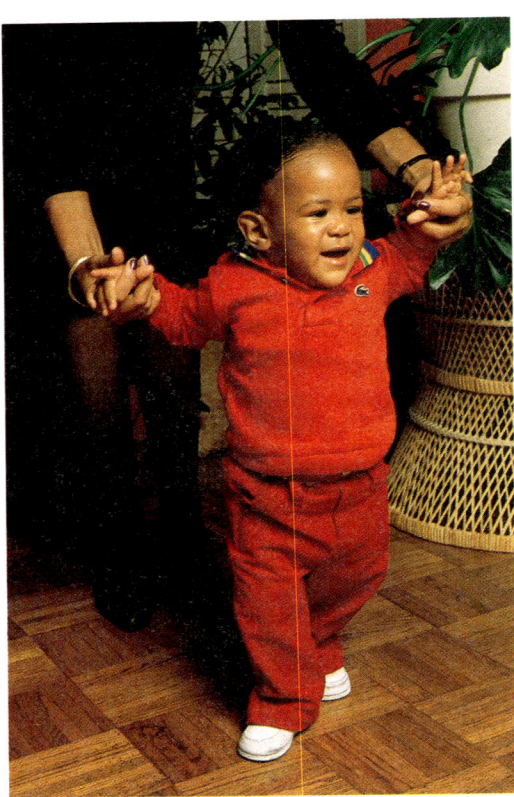

FIGURE 10-5
Older infants enjoy walking while holding onto an adult's hands.
Source: © *Mimi Cotter/International Stock Photography*

- Provide pots, pans, wooden spoons, measuring cups, empty boxes, and other safe objects to explore.

- Play give-and-take games, using a toy the infant can hold in his or her hand.

- Play copy cat, doing actions you know the infant can imitate.

Solitary and Parallel Play

Infants most commonly engage in solitary and parallel play. **Solitary play** is that in which the infant plays alone, without paying any attention to other children. **Parallel play** occurs when infants play side by side. They may vocalize and even take toys away from one another, but they do not cooperate with one another or develop games together. Books describing the details of games to play with infants are available.

THE CHILD CARE ENVIRONMENT FOR INFANTS

Infants learn from personal experience through their five senses and their own body activity. Being a good infant teacher involves learning how to set up a usable and stimulating environment. An effective learning environment for infants has many of the following features:

- It is child-proof, or safe to play in.

- It has a variety of colors that infants can see and enjoy.

- It has surfaces with a variety of textures, placed where infants can experience them. (Glass has a smooth, shiny texture. Carpet has a rougher, duller texture.)

- There is a variety of gentle sounds to hear. The most important of these sounds is the voice of the caregiver.

- There is a variety of pleasant things to smell. Fragrances and aromas should not be mixed but presented one at a time, perhaps only one each day.

- A variety of tastes are offered once infants begin to eat solid food.

- There is plenty of safe space in which to crawl and play, separate from sleeping, eating, and diapering areas.

- There are shelves infants can reach, where toys are kept.

- Some of the windows are low enough for crawling infants to see through.

- There is an area where infants can experience wet surfaces and objects safely.

- There is a place where caregivers can sit, relax, and rock an infant.

- There is an outdoor playground designed for infants that has all the features of the indoor play area.

Caregiving areas for infants include areas for sleeping, eating, and diapering. The sleeping area contains a crib for each infant in care. Sheets are changed daily. All cribs are visible to the supervising caregiver at all times. There is a storage area for each

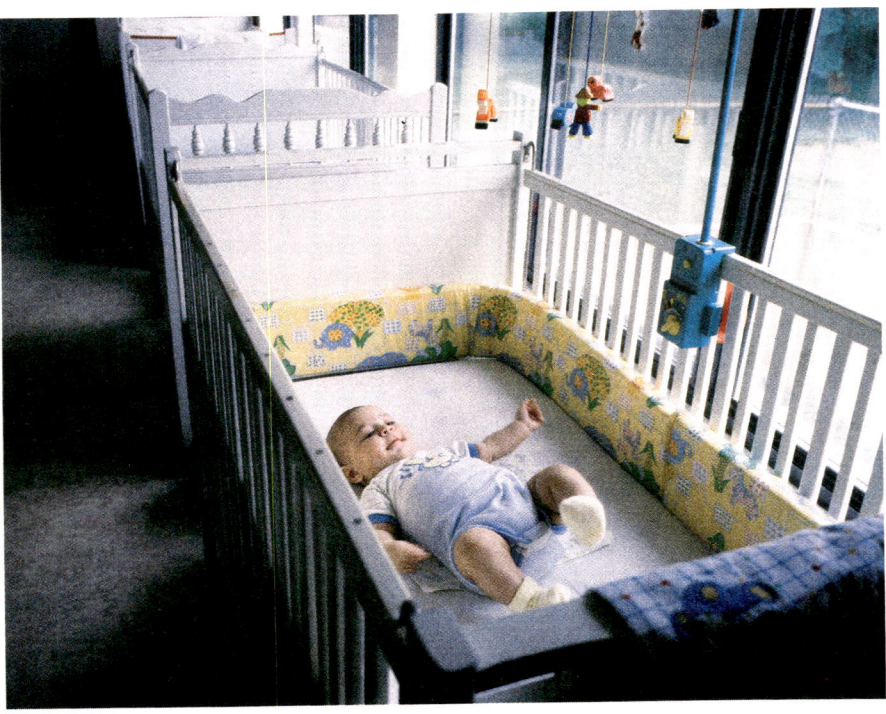

FIGURE 10-6   An ideal sleeping area for infants at a child care center has a crib for each child and a quiet and homelike atmosphere.

infant's diapers and other personal belongings. Nearby there is a quiet, soft space where caregivers and infants can rock, swing, or lie on the floor together. The overall feeling of the infant area is homelike.

Eating areas are set up to allow a caregiver to feed more than one infant at the same time. Necessary features of the infant feeding area include running water for cleaning and disinfecting utensils and surfaces, a lockable refrigerated space for storing infants' formula and medications, and a heat source for warming milk and food. Also needed is storage space for infants' food, utensils, and dishes.

The diaper changing area must be separate from the food preparation and eating area. It should have running water, a firm, flat surface that is easily disinfected, a place to store clean diapers, and a covered container for soiled diapers. A supply of disinfectant should be located where infants cannot reach it. A supply of clean, sterile cloths for cleaning infants' skin and lotion should be on hand.

The infants' room should have a space where parents bring infants and pick them up. There is often a bulletin board near the door that is used to keep parents informed of upcoming events or teach parenting skills. A space where daily infant records are kept is also needed.

THE ROLE OF THE CAREGIVER

Being a good caregiver for infants means learning how to understand their cries and bids for help. It means responding quickly, appropriately, and consistently to those requests. Being a teacher of infants involves understanding infants' capabilities and being willing to make the effort to be actively involved with them.

Supervising Infants in Child Care

It is impossible to say enough about the importance of staying aware of every infant in the room at all times. Infants can never be left alone. It takes only an instant for an infant to fall or choke. Fever can come on suddenly.

Nearly all states have established minimum standards stating how many infants can be supervised by one adult. Most states will not allow more than five infants per adult. Three infants per adult is the ideal maximum for a child care situation.

The large number of adults needed to supervise and care for infants, the cost of the liability insurance, and the special facilities needed for infant care make it very costly. Therefore, many centers do not offer care for children under two years. In most areas of the country there is a great need for more spaces to become available for infants in quality child care facilities.

Teaching Skills for Working with Infants

Good infant caregivers not only attend to the physical needs of the infants in their care but are great teachers as well. The single most important skill a good infants' teacher has is the ability to talk to and listen to her or his young pupils. Language skills develop very rapidly during the first year. Most of what an infant says is not verbally clear, but it does have meaning. Caregivers who listen to infants' attempts at language, who make eye contact as infants vocalize, and who respond as appropriately as they can to the expression in an infant's voice help infants mentally and emotionally.

Teachers who see infants as individuals, as people, who understand something of what it is to be human, are those to whom infants will form the strongest attachments. Teachers of this quality are a great example to young parents who are just learning how to guide children.

Good infants' teachers spend their time with the children rather than conversing about adult concerns with other caregivers. They believe the time they are investing is valuable to the children. They enjoy children as people, and they like their jobs.

The best teachers know that there is always more to learn about children—they seek ways to increase their knowledge. Caring for infants is more than just babysitting. It is a job for highly qualified professionals.

Sarah and Jayme were fortunate to be cared for at La Casita, where they not only were safe but also had many opportunities to learn. Being born prematurely might have become a handicap if they had been in a less well-planned environment. Instead they caught up quickly with children their age.

La Casita was good for Sarah and Jayme's parents, too. They were able to do their jobs without worrying because they felt the twins were receiving very good care.

Summary

Routines help children feel secure because things are the same every day. Keeping daily records helps caregivers communicate with parents. A schedule is a guide for caregivers to use in establishing routines.

Procedures are techniques for caring for infants in a consistent manner. Routines in infant care include ones for sleeping, feeding, and diapering.

Good caregivers meet infants' needs quickly, appropriately, and consistently. Infants become attached to parents and caregivers who meet these needs. Infants are disciplined through establishing routines, child-proofing the environment, removing them from potentially troublesome situations, and allowing them to work through frustrations.

Infants whose parents do not respond adequately to their needs and who communicate poorly with them may develop failure to thrive syndrome. There are physical, emotional, and mental signs of this condition. Infants with failure to thrive syndrome often come from families that have problems. Doctors and caregivers can help parents and children in most cases.

Infants' mental abilities have been identified by Jean Piaget. He pointed out four separate levels of mental growth during the first year. Learning activities for infants need to be based on these stages of developing mental abilities.

The environment for infants in child care centers also needs to be based on infants' physical and mental developmental abilities. Infants always need close supervision. The teaching skills of infants' teachers can make the difference in the quality of care provided.

Terms and Concepts

Developmentally appropriate activities

Consistency

Routines

Procedures

Sudden infant death syndrome (SIDS)

SIDS monitor

Attachment

Transitions

Nonorganic failure to thrive syndrome

Solitary play

Parallel play

Checking Your Understanding

1. What is the advantage of keeping a record of each infant's day in a child care center? Why do parents need a copy of their child's daily record?

2. Why are routines important in a child care center?

3. Why is it important to follow established procedures in a child care center?

4. How might you calm a small infant with a stomachache who has been crying for some time?

5. Why do infants' caregivers need to be able to do CPR?

6. What is the advantage of responding to an infant's needs quickly, appropriately, and consistently?

7. How can smooth transitions help an infant's day and evening go more smoothly?

8. List and briefly describe four ways of disciplining infants. Why is spanking not appropriate for disciplining infants?

9. Why is it important for infants' caregivers to be able to recognize the signs of failure to thrive syndrome?

10. How can a caregiver help an infant with failure to thrive syndrome at a child care center?

11. Discuss with your class ways in which infants' mental growth occurs. Why is it important to understand stages of mental growth when planning activities for infants?

12. Describe a good child care environment for infants.

13. Write a paragraph describing activities infants' teachers can provide.

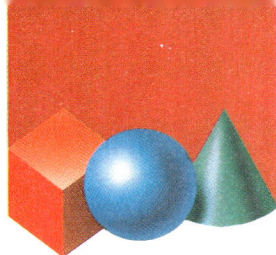

TALKING WITH INFANTS

Good conversation is like dancing with someone who dances well. One person leads, the other follows; then perhaps the leader and the follower trade places.

Daniel Stern has studied mothers and infants while they are sharing and enjoying conversations in which both are very involved. He observed that they sometimes work together much like dancing partners. Mothers watch and listen while infants vocalize. When the infants stop, they look into their mothers' eyes. The mothers then begin to talk to the infants. They raise the pitch of their voices and place their faces close enough to keep the infants' attention. Infants respond by looking intently at their mothers and producing coos and squeals. When the infants are ready to talk again, they move their eyes away from the mothers' faces and begin to vocalize. When the infants become tired of the conversation, they stop vocalizing and will not look back at the mothers. The mothers then stop the conversation.

What do these observations reveal about how to talk with infants?

Babies want to be talked to. What do you talk to an infant about? You can talk about anything that is going on around the two of you. Tell him or her about parents and other family members. Talk about the activities in the center. Ask about his or her day and listen for an answer.

If at first you feel foolish because of what other people may think, remember that they do not know the capabilities of infants as you do. Remember, too, that infants are delighted and are learning an incredible amount from you.

The most important part of having a conversation with an infant is thinking of him or her as a small, growing person with something to say. Think about how nice it is when people listen to you. With a little practice, talking to infants can be one of your favorite things to do.

CHAPTER 11
Toddlers

OBJECTIVES

When you have finished this chapter, you will be able to

- Assist toddlers in learning self-care skills
- Assist young children in dealing with being away from parents
- Discuss the qualities of good supervision of toddlers
- Describe guidance techniques that help toddlers develop personal strength and self-esteem
- Work and play at a toddler's pace
- Describe good environments for toddlers
- Identify developmental strengths and abilities
- Identify developmentally appropriate activities for toddlers
- Set up a learning environment for toddlers

Kim Liu smiled and looked into Bradley's eyes as she stooped to greet him. "Good morning, Bradley." Bradley buried his head in his mother's skirt, then peeked shyly at Kim.

Kim asked, "Would you like to come climb with Joey and Kristie?" She stretched her hand toward him and waited for him to respond.

"No!" he replied, stepping behind his mother once again. She finished signing him in and stooped to say good-bye. He began to whine, "I wanna go with you today!"

"I'm sorry, Bradley. I have to go to work. You have fun playing with Miss Liu and the children." She kissed his cheek and placed his hand in Kim's.

Kim Liu was a high school student who helped at La Casita as part of a course in child care she was taking. She was surprised to see Bradley so upset about being left. Usually he came right into the room and began to play. Today was different. Kim put her arms around Bradley and said, "Say good-bye to Mommy."

"I wanna go with Mommy," Bradley cried.

"I know," said Kim, "but Mommy has to go to work. Sit here with me until you feel more like playing." Bradley sobbed and reluctantly waved good-bye to his mother. He stopped crying but stayed close to Kim Liu for several minutes. Before long he was ready to join the other children in play.

PHYSICAL AND EMOTIONAL CARE OF TODDLERS

Developmentally, children are classified as toddlers from the time they begin to walk, which is usually around the first birthday, until they can walk and talk fairly well, often by the third birthday. In child care situations toddlers are often divided into two age groups: those between 12 and 24 months old are called toddlers and those between 24 and 36 months old are called twos.

These children need caregivers who understand the unique developmental challenges facing this age group. Children between one and three move from babyhood to childhood. They learn and accomplish many things. Learning can be accompanied by frustration and anger. Teaching and caring for small children in this age group require skill and patience.

Self-Care Skills for Toddlers

One-year-olds begin to do things for themselves, and twos begin to be good at it. Development of self-care skills is essential for a child's sense of self-worth and growing sense of autonomy. **Autonomy** is the ability children develop to assert and care for themselves and to learn to stand for what is important to them.

Children who master self-care skills feel good about themselves and want to keep learning new and more complex tasks. A skilled caregiver can find ways to help young children extend these learnings in a safe way.

Self-help activities enable young children to gain control over their own lives a little at a time. Adults who establish adequate guidelines and provide positive discipline help children learn self-control.

Self-care is an important issue for toddlers. They want to do things for themselves. Their bodies may not work as efficiently as they want them to. The result can be a great deal of frustration, which sometimes results in a temper tantrum. (Temper tantrums are discussed in more detail later in this chapter.)

One-year-olds can begin to do things such as wash their own hands, undress and dress, get out play materials and return them to a shelf with adult guidance, and learn toileting.

Two-year-olds will continue to do the things they have done as one-year-olds, but they will get better at it.

They can wash their hands with much less help. They enjoy helping to wipe off tables and other surfaces with sponges.

Dressing skills improve and are used in dress-up play as imagination strengthens. Practice with simple fasteners becomes a favorite activity. Clothing that features easy-to-reach and easy-to-use fasteners is a good investment in helping children develop autonomy.

FIGURE 11-1   Toddlers begin to learn and practice self-care skills, such as getting dressed or undressed.
Source: © Laura Dwight

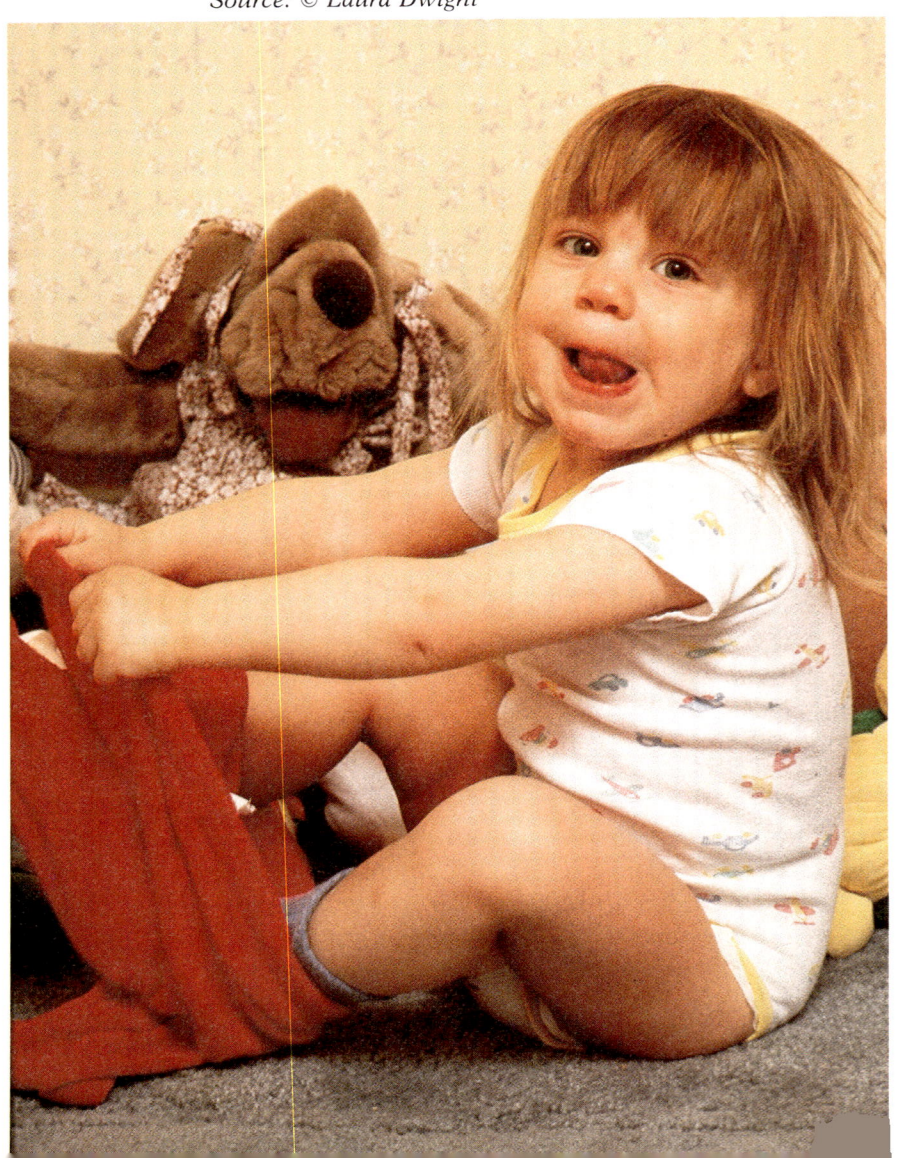

Caregivers will need to remind and encourage twos to put away play materials when they are finished. Twos can accomplish this task with little help if they have had practice.

Although most children have mastered basic toileting skills by age two, some are still working at it when they are nearly three. Occasional accidents can be expected when two-year-olds are not feeling well, when they are very involved in play and forget about toileting until it is too late, or when they are stressed because of changes in their personal lives.

Helping Toddlers Adjust to a Child Care Situation

Toddlers sometimes have a difficult time adjusting to child care. Those entering child care for the first time may have a particularly hard time leaving the security of home. Caregivers can help young children make the adjustment in the following ways:

- Encourage the parent to talk about staying at the center before the child arrives, especially the first time.

- Encourage the parent to arrive early enough to give the child time to adjust before the parent has to leave.

- Encourage the parent to tell the child good-bye as he or she leaves.

- Help the child say good-bye to the parent. If necessary, gently hold the child so the parent can leave.

- Calmly assure the child that the parent will return later that day.

- Get the child involved in an activity. If the child seems sad, stay close.

THE FIRST DAY OF CHILD CARE

The parents should visit the child care facility with the child the day before he or she is to be left there. A visit of 30 minutes to an hour is usually enough. It is helpful if, on a child's first day at the center, at least one parent can stay for the entire time.

Most one-year-olds and many twos will cry and cling to their parents every day for a week or more. Most of them recover within a few minutes after the parents leave. It is usually best to talk calmly with the parents and let them know what to expect. Discuss with them how you can work together.

SEPARATION ANXIETY

Small children grieve when they are first separated from parents. An entire day away from their parents and home seems to them to be a very long time. Most small children suffer some fear of being abandoned. When they must be separated from their parents, they sometimes experience **separation anxiety,** which is a general feeling of fearful insecurity about being away from parents.

Toddlers who have been in child care most of their lives may go through a period of time in which they resist being left. This may be caused by a change in the staff, by some other unsettling experience in the child's life, or by feelings of wanting to be with parents rather than caregivers. Caregivers need to be patient during this period and allow children the opportunity to work through their feelings.

Attachment to Caregivers

Once small children begin to trust and feel secure with the adults who care for them at a child care center, they begin to feel somewhat attached to those adults. As the children become secure, they begin to feel free to play and explore the environment in the classroom and outdoor area. Play and exploration lead to learning.

One- and two-year-olds love to learn. They are like dry sponges near water, soaking up every new piece of information. Play and exploration are the ways in which they find information to learn. When they are securely attached to parents and caregivers, they play more freely and learn more.

Getting Along with Other Children

ASSERTIVENESS AND LEARNING TO SHARE

An important lesson in learning to get along with people is learning to assert and defend yourself. Toddlers typically say "mine" when they have a toy and another child tries to take it. They can hold on tight and may hit to defend their right to keep a toy.

Adults who do not know children's growth patterns are sometimes alarmed when toddlers do not share. Sometimes these adults may try to force sharing. Children cannot learn to share until they learn to have and keep something for themselves. Most toddlers seldom share voluntarily. It is a good practice to keep more than one of the same toy on hand so small children do not have to be made to share. When one toy must be used by more than one child, an adult can help the children take turns. They may protest, but they are not made to feel guilty for not sharing. Taking turns is an adult-guided activity; sharing starts with the individual child.

Another way toddlers assert themselves is to say *"no!"* Although this can be very frustrating for parents and caregivers, learning to say no is an important skill. Adults need to learn to work around toddlers' tendency to say no without starting a confrontation. The following suggestions may be helpful:

■ Avoid asking toddlers questions that require a yes or no answer.

FIGURE 11-2 Toddlers' developing assertiveness leads them to have trouble sharing things.
Source: © Laura Dwight

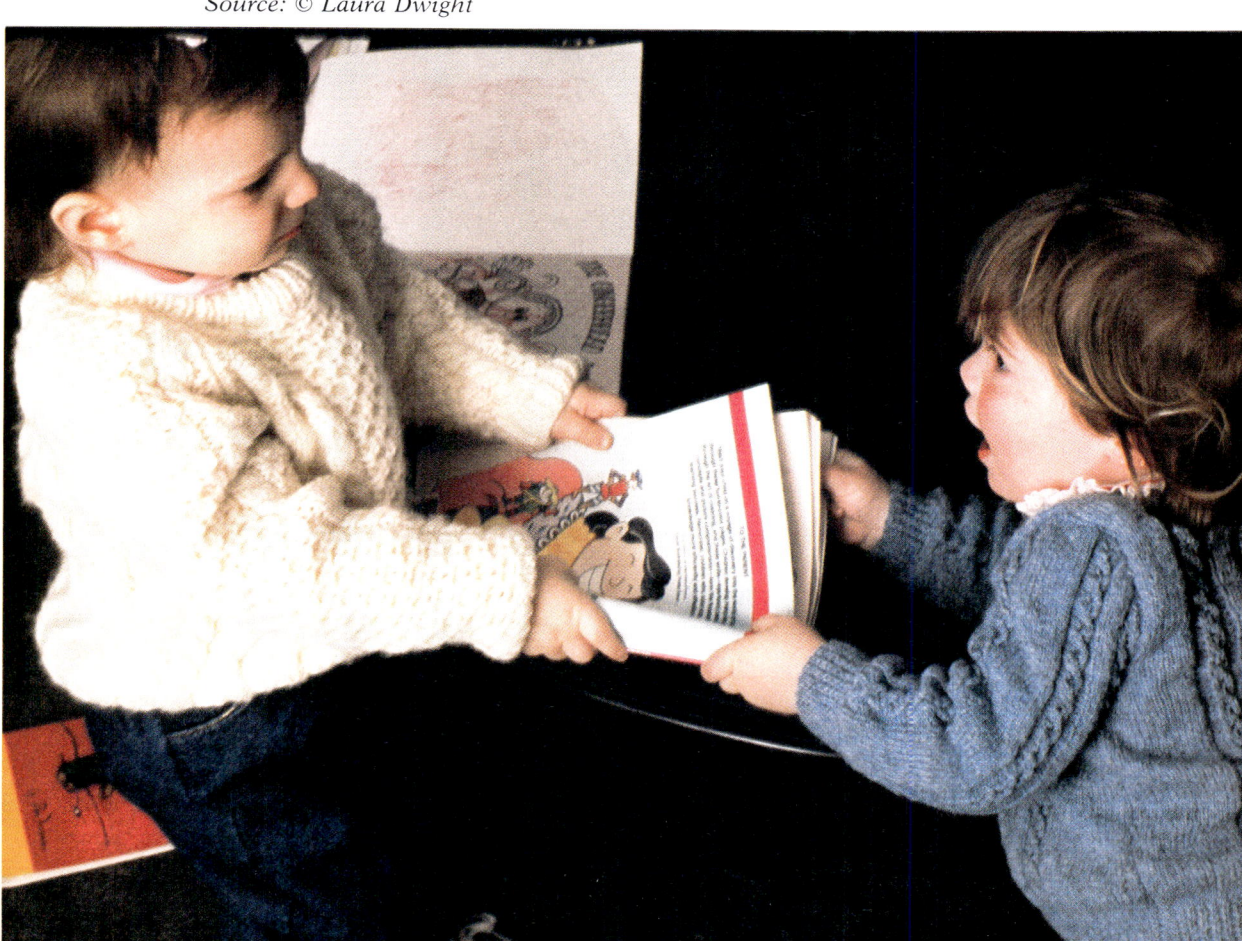

- Give a child a limited choice when possible, for example, by asking "Do you want to wear your red shirt or your blue one?"

- When there is no choice, do not offer one. For example, when a caregiving task has to be done, such as wiping faces after lunch, do not ask children if they want to have this done—simply do it.

- Expect and accept normal toddler behavior.

STEPPING IN BY ADULTS

When young children begin to injure one another or when one child bullies another, adults need to step in. Simple corrective action involves separating the children and then telling them what behavior is expected.

GUIDING TODDLERS

Guiding one- and two-year-olds requires some skill. Caregivers have to adapt to the children's pace, supervise their activities closely, and use appropriate guidance techniques.

Pacing Schedules to Fit Children's Needs

Small children are learning about how the world is organized. With established routines there are predictable times of day when children can depend on certain things happening. When eating, sleeping, toileting, and outdoor play occur at about the same times each day, small children learn to trust the people in their environment.

Small children have no understanding of time. They may be aware that adults are often in a hurry, but they have no way of understanding what makes them act that way. Exploring and learning have to be done at children's pace, which is different from that of adults. It takes a child time—more time than an adult—to figure out how balls fit into round holes or how the pedals on a tricycle operate. Small children learn best when they have as much time as they need and support for their learning. However, children need adult guidance to pace themselves.

Schedules in a child care center have to be designed to fit the needs of children. Most centers schedule mid-morning and mid-afternoon snacks and a noontime lunch. Some centers provide breakfast. Small children need a mid-morning rest and an afternoon nap. Playtime is scheduled so that periods of active play, such as outdoor play, are followed by quieter play, such as fingerpainting. Caregivers need to watch children carefully for signs of tiredness or hunger. Playtimes, snacks, and rest periods can be scheduled, but hunger, tiredness, and interest in play cannot be. Schedules should be flexible enough to accommodate the needs of the children.

Providing Close Adult Supervision

Toddlers are beginning to develop some sense of risk and danger, but they are unable to control their environment or to make sound judgments.

They require *constant and alert* adult supervision. The one absolutely necessary ingredient in their environment is close supervision by watchful adults.

Toddlers' curiosity exceeds their caution and self-control. They can climb onto and fall from an amazing variety of surfaces. They can crawl into smaller spaces or on top of higher places than most adults expect. They can get fingers, legs, or the entire body stuck in spaces adults cannot reach. They may try eating or drinking just about anything.

Some toys can be unsafe for toddlers. Part of adult supervision is providing them with safe toys. Desirable features of toys and play equipment are listed in Illustration 11-1, along with examples of safe toys for this age level. Toys for older children do not have play value for toddlers and can be dangerous for them.

Using Appropriate Guidance Techniques

Guidance techniques used by those caring for toddlers include giving encouragement, singing reminders, offering a choice, providing clear directions, and handling tantrums.

GIVING ENCOURAGEMENT

Toddlers need adults to give them encouragement and positive attention—to cheer them on. Adults who gently remind and encourage small children about toileting and other self-help skills are far more effective than those who push and yell. Toddlers, even more than other people, hate to be pushed. They resist.

SINGING REMINDERS

Toddlers tend to cooperate when reminders are sung rather than spoken. Try making up words about self-help activities to

ILLUSTRATON 11-1   Toys should not have unsafe features and should be suitable for the age level of the child.

Features of Safe Toys for Toddlers

- No sharp edges
- No sharp points
- No small parts (nothing under $1\frac{1}{4}$ inches in diameter)
- No strings more than 12 inches long
- Does not make loud noises
- Has no pinch points (where small fingers could be pinched)
- Is flame-retardant

Good Toys for One-Year-Olds

- A safe riding toy that will not tip over and is foot-propelled
- Large balls
- Things that fit one inside another, such as nesting cups
- Books with stiff pages (not cloth ones)
- Simple construction blocks, such as cardboard blocks
- Objects to carry other things in, such as suitcases and wagons
- Small, simple dolls (about 10–12 inches high) that can be carried around and can be easily washed

Good Toys for Two-Year-Olds

- Simple puzzles with pieces that match the shapes of the picture (one piece is a hat, another the coat, and so on)
- Dolls
- Beads to string
- Pegboards
- Objects to carry other things in, such as purses and lunch pails
- Mathematically sized blocks
- A tricycle that is pedal-propelled
- Safe trucks
- A climbing structure that allows children to climb, crawl into and over, and hide under
- A sturdy, simple dollhouse with simple furnishings
- Objects that encourage children to talk to one another, such as toy telephones
- Objects that encourage children to pretend

This list was adapted from material presented by Burton White and Mike Meyerhoff at conferences at The Center for Parent Education, Houston, Texas, February, 1983.

familiar tunes. For example, you might sing words like these to the tune of "Row, Row, Row Your Boat": "Put, put, put your dolls, put your dolls away. Nancy and Donnie and Kristie can help put the dolls away."

Small children are fascinated by the rhythm of singing. If caregivers follow the sung reminder with the motions being called for, such as helping to pick up, children nearly always follow the example happily and move on to other activities.

GIVING A CHOICE

Toddlers often respond positively to a guidance technique called **structured choice.** Structured choice means giving a child an opportunity to act with autonomy while following the adult's leadership. For example, if you want a child to brush his or her teeth with toothpaste on the brush, ask this question: "Do you want to squeeze the toothpaste tube, or do you want me to do it for you?" You have to be willing to accept the child's choice and allow him or her to follow through with the decision. Structured choices give children an opportunity to succeed; succeeding helps a sense of self-worth to develop.

GIVING DIRECTIONS CLEARLY

Give directions one step at a time. Give small children enough time to follow the directions. Physically guiding them is sometimes helpful. Provide an example. Show toddlers what you are asking them to do. Do the action with them.

HANDLING TEMPER TANTRUMS

Temper tantrums can be ways of venting frustration; but they can become manipulation when children learn they can use them to get desired results. How does an adult respond to a toddler's temper tantrum?

Usually tantrums can be ignored. It is important that a child not get any reward or benefit from throwing a tantrum. Attention of any kind from an adult can cause a repeat performance.

Some children become so frustrated and angry when they throw a tantrum that they may lose control and begin to cry uncontrollably. If a child is unable to calm down, an adult may need to help. Sometimes simply sitting the child on your lap while staying very calm and quiet yourself has a calming effect. Wiping the child's face and hands with a cool, damp cloth may help.

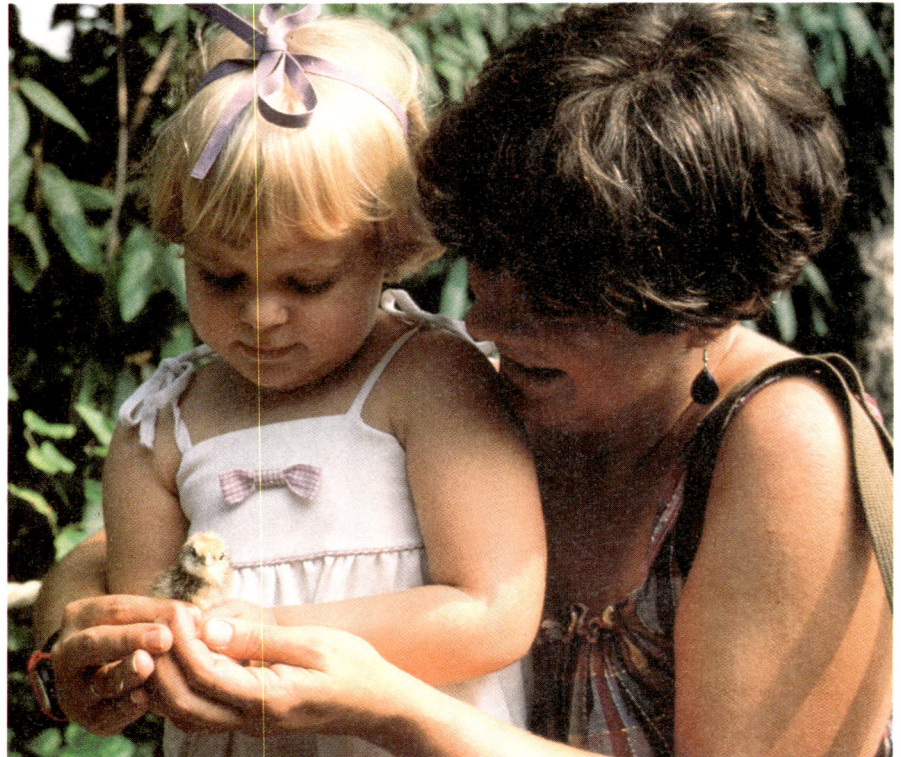

FIGURE 11-3   It is helpful if an adult shows a toddler how to do something, for example, how to hold a baby bird gently.
Source: Courtesy of the Cincinnati Zoo and Botanical Garden

The adult's task is to stay very calm and in control of himself or herself and to help the child regain self-control after a reasonable period of time. The skills involved in doing this include learning to tell whether the child is frustrated and angry or just being manipulative and learning how to determine whether the child can get over the tantrum alone if ignored or needs help to calm down.

If a child begins to throw objects, remove the objects. If the child begins to bang his or her head on a hard surface or to injure himself or herself in any other way, simply move the child to a surface that will not cause injury. The necessary adult behavior is *to stay calm and maintain self-control*. It is also important to realize that you cannot *make* the child stop. You have to create circumstances that will allow him or her to regain self-control—with dignity intact.

It is a mistake for an adult to respond to a child's frustration and anger by becoming frustrated and angry with the child. An adult who hits, yells, or stomps off is out of control. If you do these things, you place yourself on the child's level and are no longer acting as an adult.

THE CHILD CARE ENVIRONMENT FOR TODDLERS

Quality child care centers have rooms for toddlers that are spacious, safe, and easy to supervise. At least part of the space is scaled to children's size. These environments offer challenging opportunities to climb and run, interesting places to explore, and many chances to learn self-care skills. Such rooms are arranged to fill the needs of small children.

Designing the Environment for Self-Help

When children's rooms are scaled to their size and equipment and furniture are selected with their developmental abilities and needs in mind, the environment encourages self-care. Such an environment contains certain self-help features specifically designed for one- and two-year-olds. These allow young children to learn to wash their hands, dress themselves, put away play materials, and use the toilet.

HAND WASHING

Self-help features for hand washing include a child-height sink or a safe step stool to reach the sink, easy-to-use mild soap, warm water (not over 120°F), and easy-to-reach towels. A caring adult helps by supervising and teaching.

UNDRESSING AND DRESSING

Small children often begin learning to dress themselves by undressing themselves. Removing one's pants often goes along with learning to use the toilet. Adults can help children learn dressing skills by choosing clothing that has easy-to-use fasteners and by allowing them to try to work the fasteners. It takes time and patience to allow a child to help dress himself or herself. Therefore, adults need to allow unhurried time for dressing whenever possible.

When children undress themselves during the day, adults need to help them put the clothing back on. Some children go through a period when they want to change clothing frequently during the day. This increases the amount of laundry. Caregivers can supply comfortable dress-up clothes and encourage children to try dressing up as a substitute for changing clothes. Children will enjoy trying on adult clothes, hats, and shoes. Child-height mirrors, hooks, and shelves for storage of the dress-up clothes should also be provided.

PUTTING THINGS AWAY

Small children need an organized environment. To learn to put play materials and other things away, they need a place for everything. Things they use should be kept where they can find them and help put them away.

TOILETING

A chart for identifying times when children are likely to need to use the toilet is a useful tool for caregivers in helping children develop toileting habits (see Chapter 7). A toilet or toilet seat that fits a small child in a way that he or she can manage helps in developing self-care skills. It is important to allow enough time to use the toilet at the child's own pace.

Planning for Play

Toddlers spend most of the day in solitary play (playing alone) or parallel play (playing beside and aware of another child but not actually playing with the other child). By their second birthday most small children begin to play close by one another in similar ways and with the same toys. This kind of play is called **associative play.**

One- and two-year-olds learn more by doing than from words. They experiment, spending many hours trying new things and learning from both successes and failures. These times of play are also times of learning about other people, especially about their peers. **Peers** are people of similar ages or interests. Learning to get along with others often involves conflict as well as learning to give and take. Other values of play are listed in Illustration 11-2.

ILLUSTRATION 11-2   Children receive these benefits from play.

- Play gives children the chance to learn by doing, the way they learn best.
- Play gives children the chance to see how what they have learned relates to what they know.
- Play helps children learn how learning works.
- Play helps children learn about how the world works.
- Play helps children handle their emotions.
- Play can help children to relax.
- Play can help children learn to enjoy playing.
- Play helps children to appreciate the arts.

Adapted from Helping Young Children Develop Through Play *by Janet K. Sawyers and Cosby S. Rogers (Washington, DC: NAEYC, 1988).*

Pre-reading Features of the Environment

An effective way to help small children know where to put toys and other play materials is to place an outline of each object on the shelf or wall space where the object is kept when not in use. Children can learn to match the shape of the object with the object. Matching helps children recognize the shape as a symbol for the object. This skill is a beginning for later reading.

Names of objects and toys clearly printed in correct printscript are an important feature. A printscript alphabet is shown in Illustration 11-3. Uppercase (capital) letters should be used only at the beginnings of sentences and of names of people and places. Toddlers are not yet ready to read words, but learning that they mean something and seeing them printed correctly is a pre-reading activity.

Posting children's names in correct printscript on their belongings and personal space and telling them that that is how their name is written helps them learn that their name has a symbol. If children make pictures or collages to take home, print their names in correct printscript in the upper left-hand corner of their papers. The upper left-hand corner is the place on a page where eyes start when reading.

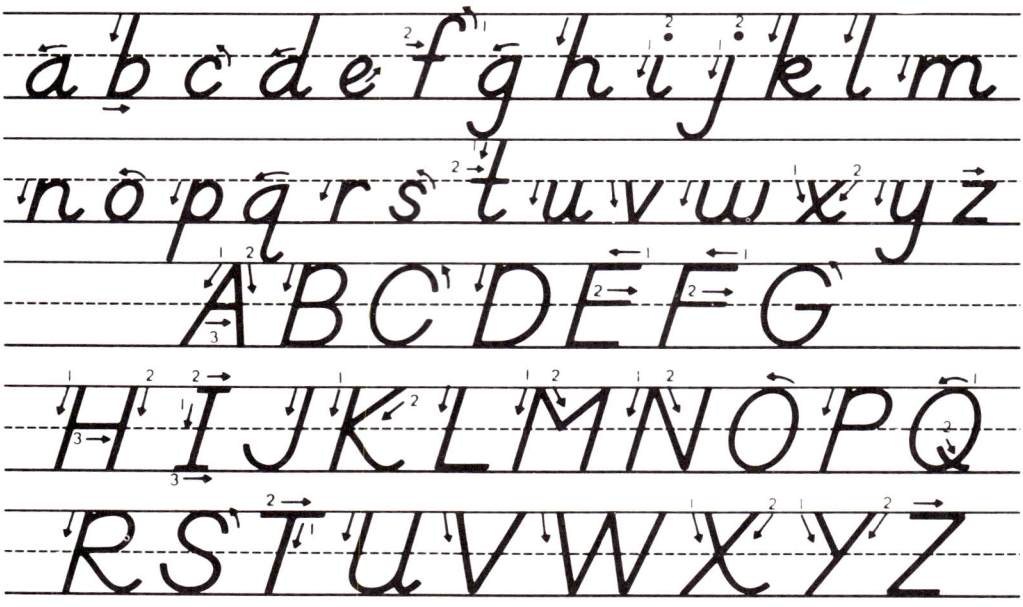

ILLUSTRATION 11-3   Teachers of young children can use this printscript alphabet. *From D'NEALIAN® HANDWRITING by Donald Neal Thurber. Copyright © 1987 by Scott, Foresman and Company. Reprinted by permission.*

Adults in the Child Care Environment

Small children need adults to support their play. Adults help most when they allow learning to go on without interruption, except when necessary to prevent injury. Adults who step in to show a child how to do something "right" rob the child of the opportunity to learn for himself or herself. In a sense this shows a lack of respect for the child. The adult assumes that the child needs help, but the help often interferes with the learning process. Ultimately this kind of caregiving will lower a child's self-esteem.

Adults aid children's play in positive ways when they do the following:

- Provide activities and materials that challenge children to learn new skills

- Arrange children's space and schedule so that play is not interrupted unnecessarily

- Provide simple props to stimulate imagination (such as objects from children's homes)

- Let children choose their own activities and play as long as they are interested

Features of the Physical Environment

Toddlers need a large play area with a great deal of room to run. More challenges are added to the room as toddlers grow. It should be possible to supervise the children from any place in the room. Barriers to keep toddlers in one area of the room need to be low.

The following features are important aspects of a toddlers' room in a child care center:

- A structure that allows children to climb, slide, roll, jump, and crawl through, under, and over it. It can have gradual slopes, 6-inch steps, tunnels, low platforms, and a variety of textures and colors.

- A structure or part of a structure that allows a rocking motion, for example, a rocking boat, rocking chairs, a swinging bridge, or a very large ball for rolling

- Water in manageable amounts, for example, in dishpans or bowls with sponges or manually powered mixers, or mixed with sand

- Pathways and symbols (such as stop signs) for riding, pushing, and pulling toys

- Self-help features including outlines of shapes marking where materials are stored. Storage for coats and other personal belongings that is low enough for children to reach encourages self-help as do sinks and toilets low enough for children to use with little help.

- Room to move both indoors and outdoors

- Barriers and boundaries that provide indirect guidance for children during play

- A wide variety of colors, shapes, textures, smells, and sounds, including a variety of soft and hard surfaces for play

- Soft surfaces for comfort, for cushioning the impact of falls, and for absorbing sound

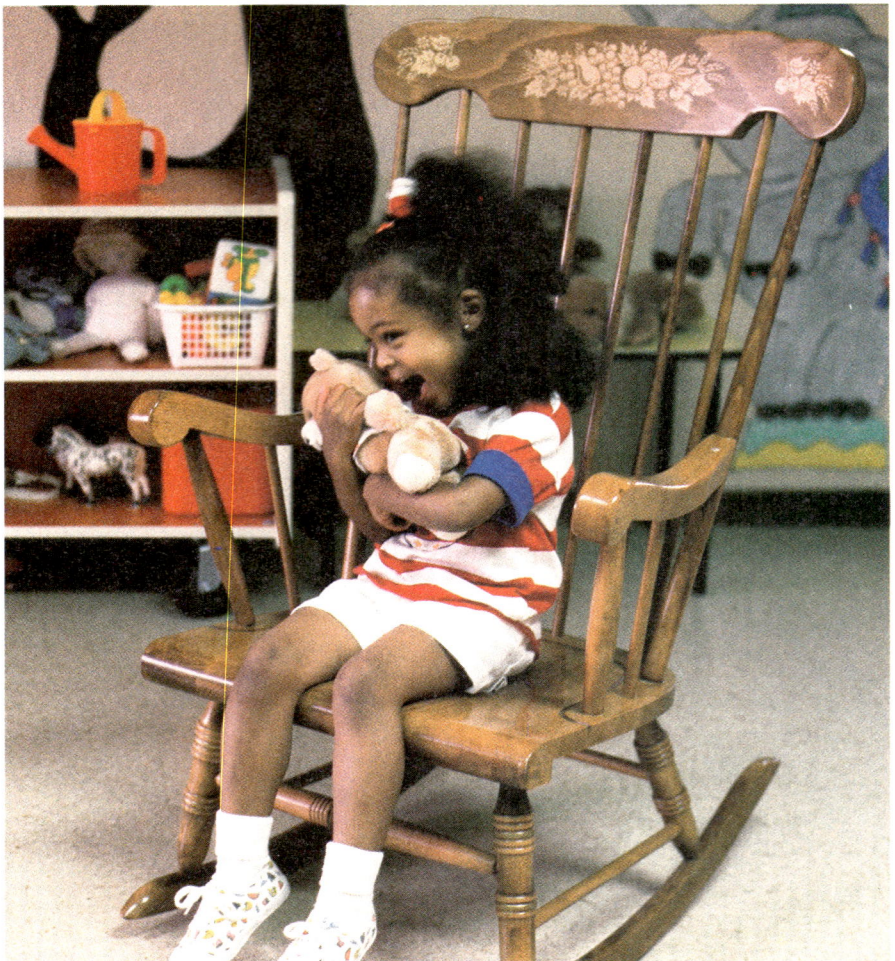

FIGURE 11-4 A rocking chair or some other structure that allows a rocking motion is a recommended feature of a room for toddlers at a child care center.

■ A quiet corner to give children a place to rest quietly or be alone for a few minutes. This area must be easy to supervise.

■ Child-sized furnishings and spaces, for example, chairs and tables small enough for children's feet to touch the floor

LEARNING ACTIVITIES FOR TODDLERS

Children between one and three learn by playing. They can play quietly.

Activities for Physical Development

Physical development is encouraged by play that uses large and small muscles and by movement to music.

LARGE AND SMALL MUSCLE DEVELOPMENT

Toddlers play actively using their large muscles. They like to climb, crawl, jump, slide, carry, throw, kick, run, and walk. They investigate space by crawling inside, outside, around, onto, and over objects. They love to move and especially enjoy having the rhythm and melody of music to encourage their movement. Balancing, somersaulting, and tumbling are fun for them, too.

They like to play with water, sand, mud, rocks, and other creative materials. They like to dump, pour, and sprinkle. They

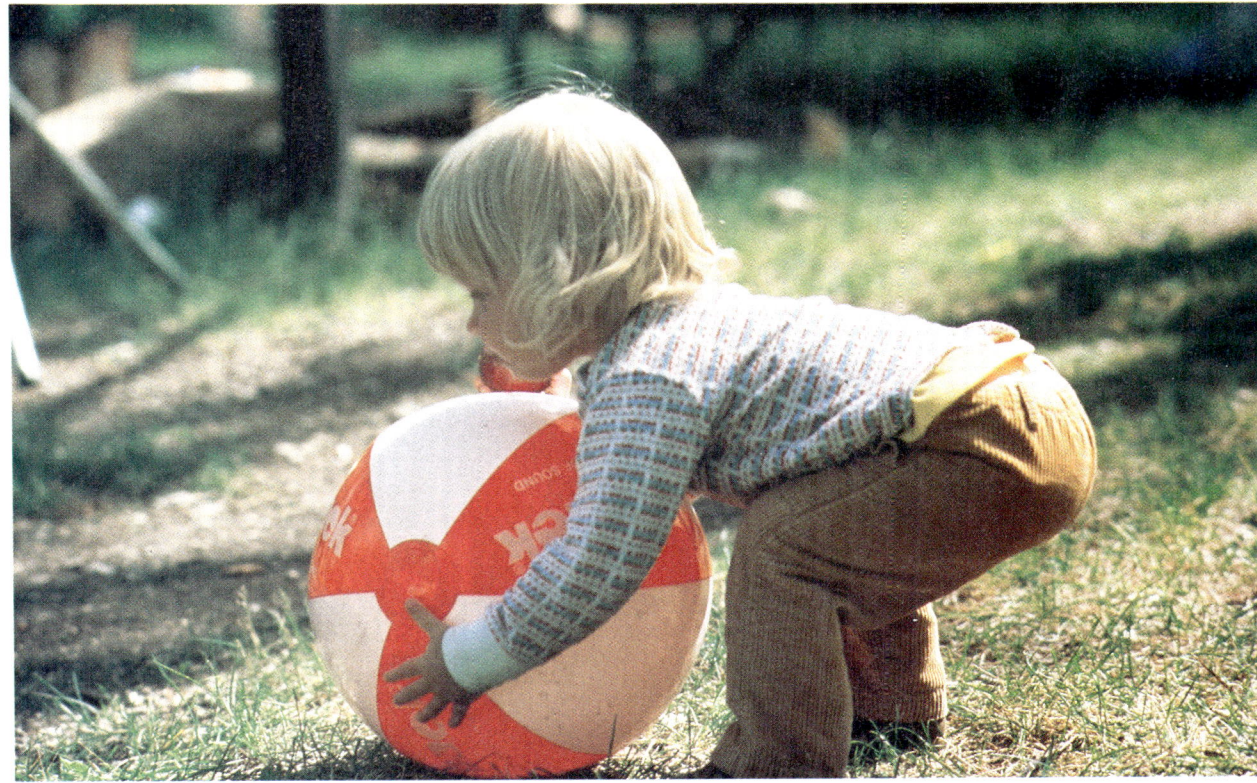

FIGURE 11-5 A large ball encourages toddlers to throw, carry, run, and so on. They enjoy such active play.
Source: North Dakota Tourism Promotion

enjoy exploring the use of art materials such as blank paper, crayons, markers, scissors, brushes, and paint. They concentrate while exploring materials and playing with blocks, puzzles, and other toys that exercise their small muscles.

Toddles like to watch and then to help. They are able to help with tasks much better than doing them alone.

MUSIC AND MOVEMENT

Small children enjoy music. They tend to bounce and dance to a simple beat. They can be led in very simple movement activities by the words of a song. **Movement activities** are those designed to get children to move and exercise various parts of their bodies. Many good records and tapes are available for children to enjoy.

Activities for Language Development

Toddlers need to talk about what they are doing. They need adults who listen to their attempts at language. Nursery rhymes and finger plays are favorite activities for toddlers. They love to sing, to mimic, and to experiment with language. They like to hear simple stories, especially ones about when they were babies.

SONGS

Sing to young children. Ask them to sing along with you. Do not expect the tune to be exact. Choose songs that have a simple, easy melody. Begin with one- and two-line songs. As children learn to enjoy songs, you can increase their length to four lines.

Sometimes adults ask children to perform. Do you think this is a good idea? The Something to Think About feature considers this question.

STORIES AND BOOKS

By the time children are 18 months old, most of them enjoy simple stories. They especially like ones about babies and families. Stories should be very short and uncomplicated.

It is best if books for small children are sturdy, so they cannot be torn easily. If books are used as toys, children will not understand their use or value, so an adult needs to be with children when they look at books.

Toddlers usually enjoy looking at a book with an adult. Talking about the pictures and pointing to the pages helps them to

Something to Think About

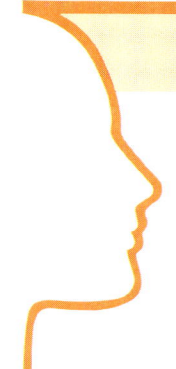

Should Small Children Perform?

When friends or relatives visit, children are often asked to perform in some way—to sing, play, or dance. Proud parents want to show off what their growing children can do. Is performing helpful for young children?

Some people say yes, it is helpful. They believe that performing in front of adults will make children confident. They feel that if children can get a head start in this way, they may have a better competitive edge.

Other people believe that performing is harmful to young children. They feel that having children perform is using them like objects and not thinking of them as persons. They feel that it is exploiting children to teach them songs or dances to do before groups of parents or other people. They feel this is especially true if children are being paid for performing, as in the case of child actors.

How does performing affect young children? Some children are confused and do not know what is really going on. Some adults think this is cute. Other children feel embarrassed because they feel their performance is inadequate. Their self-esteem may be damaged.

Children who learn to be at ease in front of an audience sometimes experience the power that comes with being a star—even locally. That power can give them an unrealistic view of their place among people.

Teaching children to sing, do finger plays, or dance does not have to be teaching them to perform. It can be teaching them to experience and enjoy the activity for itself.

Should children be taught to perform? What do you think?

---

enjoy books. Adults can tell a two-year-old about the story as the child turns the pages. Most children are three and four years old before they begin to enjoy having stories read to them.

Toddlers enjoy talking with puppets. Puppets can be used to help toddlers develop language skills. The Hands On with Children feature at the end of this chapter discusses how to present puppets to young children.

NURSERY RHYMES AND FINGER PLAYS

Small children are fascinated with rhythm and rhyme because they are learning language. Children's natural interest in nursery rhymes and finger plays makes these activities good opportunities to encourage language development. Four lines is a good length for the poems first used with toddlers. Short stories can be told in rhyme form to interest children.

Teachers using nursery rhymes and finger plays need to know them well before introducing them to the children. As with songs, it is the experience of hearing the rhyme and later saying it that is important.

MIMICKING

Children learn language by copying the speech of people around them. Toddlers enjoy it when adults make sounds they can copy and then the adults repeat the sounds. When one- and two-year-olds mimic adults, they are experimenting with sounds and language.

TALKING AND LISTENING

Between the ages of one and three, people learn to say and use more words than during any later two-year period in their lives. The more toddlers can use language, the better they will learn it. Using language means talking. Just like the rest of us, toddlers talk when someone will listen. A very important teaching skill for any teacher of toddlers is being an attentive, interested listener.

Speaking is called **productive language.** It is called that because people produce it. Another kind of language skill is called **receptive language.** Having receptive language means being able to understand, or receive, what someone else says. Children have much more receptive language than productive language. They develop receptive language when adults talk to them so that they can understand.

One important technique in helping small children develop receptive language is to give them practice in following simple directions. Teachers of small children spend a great deal of time giving simple directions, such as these:

"Hand me the book."
"Give Jimmy the ball."
"Put your hands in the water."

Once children follow simple directions readily, they can be given directions that involve two steps, such as these:

"Hand me the book, then go get your coat."
"Give Jimmy the ball, then go get the big red one."
"Put your hands into the water and find the rocks."

The older and more experienced children become, the more complex the directions given to them can be.

Activities for Mental Development

One- and two-year-olds want to learn. The world is new to them. They absorb information at an amazing rate. Most of their learning is through discovery. One of the important reasons for making a learning environment safe is so that small children will feel free to experiment and discover. They try out their ideas in their play. They learn what works and what does not. This process is sometimes called **trial-and-error learning.**

Part of trial-and-error learning is learning about what causes things to happen. Children are fascinated by activities that enable them to see a cause-and-effect relationship. Cause-and-effect activities include punching keys on an old typewriter, ringing a bell, blowing bubbles, playing rhythm instruments, and flushing toilets.

Learning activities for toddlers change as they grow. The following indicates activities that are challenging for young children during three periods:

- *Children between 12 and 18 months of age* love to play hide-and-seek games with objects, to find out what is inside, under, or behind something. They are very curious. They use objects in new ways and try new ways of reaching goals.

- *From 18 to 24 months old,* children learn much more language. They begin to pretend, to do and say things from memory, and to recognize familiar symbols.

Leadership at a Glance

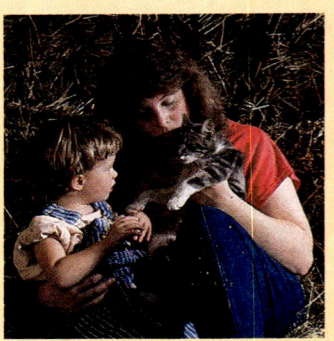

Dr. Burton White

How infants and toddlers learn best has been the focus of studies led by Dr. Burton White at the Harvard Graduate School of Education. While studying preschools and Head Start programs, Dr. White noticed that some three-year-olds were well developed and others had to struggle. He started trying to find out what made these children different. He found that the way parents teach babies and toddlers makes a big difference in how well they learn.

Dr. White concluded that parents are a child's first and most important teachers. Since 1978 he has devoted time and expertise to developing professional support services for the family as a learning environment. Recently he has worked on a project in Missouri concerning new parents as teachers.

Dr. White has written many books, the best known of which is *The First Three Years of Life.* He is the director of the Center for Parent Education. Many of Dr. White's ideas are included in this chapter. If you would like to learn more about the importance of parents as a child's first teachers or about how children under three learn, you can write to this address:

Center for Parent Education
55 Chapel Street
Newton, MA 02160

■ *Children between 2 and 3 years of age* begin to develop simple reasoning skills. However, their reasoning is not completely logical because they can only think about one part of something at a time. They make up their minds about how things are based only on their own experience; they do not yet know how to look at something from someone else's point of view. They believe the world is the way they see it and can be no other way.

There are four learning tasks young children work at mastering. These are classifying objects, putting objects in sequence, exploring spaces, and understanding time.

ACTIVITIES ABOUT CLASSIFICATION

Classification means sorting objects into categories by their features. How are things alike, and how are they different? Many teaching materials are available to help young children develop the ability to classify objects by similarities and differences. A simple one is the shape box that allows children to match a triangular block to a triangular hole and so on.

FIGURE 11-6   Playing with a shape box helps toddlers develop the ability to classify objects.
Source: © Suzanne Szasz/Photo Researchers, Inc.

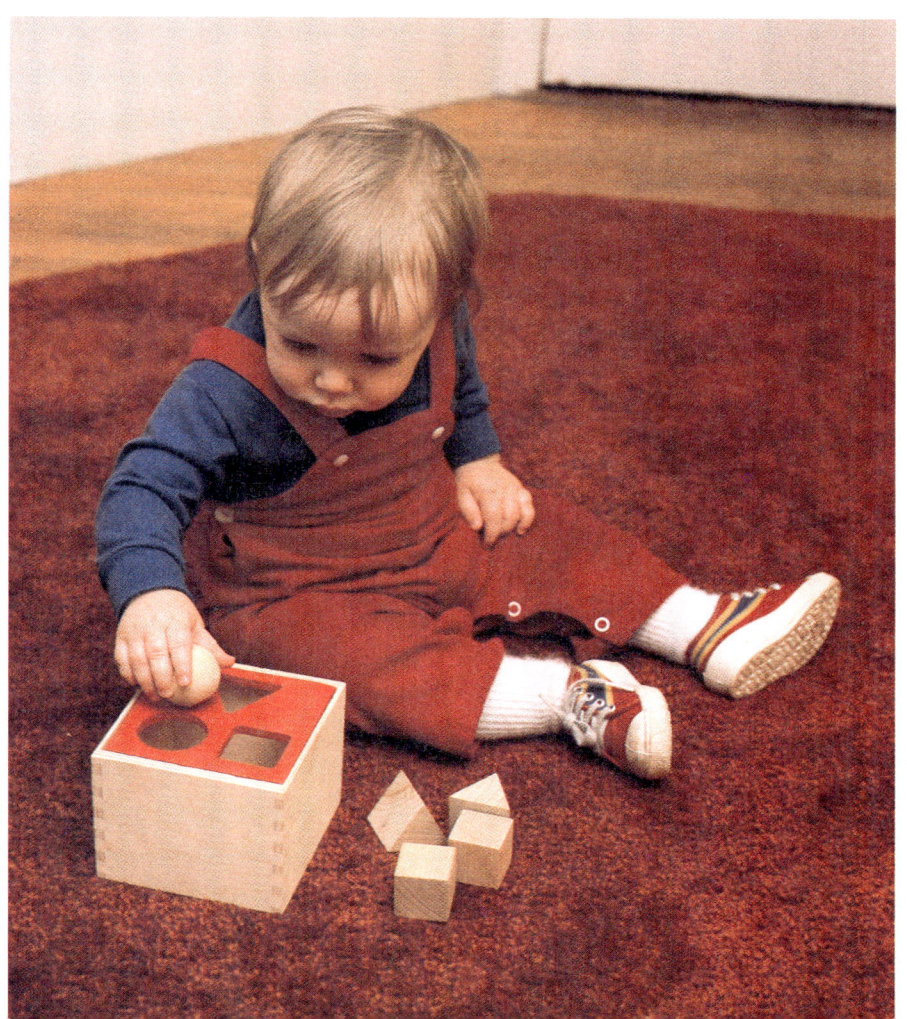

Classification activities involve sorting and matching. Shapes are usually the easiest and first features for children to match. It is important for caregivers to use words to help toddlers identify the same and different features of objects. When children experience differences such as warm and cool, hard and soft, light and dark, the caregiver uses words to help them define the differences. Talking about the differences and similarities of objects, actions, and experiences helps language develop.

ACTIVITIES ABOUT SERIATION

Seriation means arranging things in an orderly sequence. Which things are bigger or smaller, louder or softer? Activities based on such questions are a beginning to understanding the comparisons that are later a part of learning math. Good teaching of toddlers includes many experiences and much conversation comparing sizes and amounts of things. As children grow and build on these experiences, they will be able to put more complex groups of objects or experiences in order.

ACTIVITIES FOR EXPLORING SPACES

How do spaces work? What is inside, under, over, outside, and around? How big is this space, and how do I fit into it? Small children learn to understand space by exploring many spaces of different sizes. A good environment for toddlers provides a variety of spaces that can be safely explored.

ACTIVITIES FOR UNDERSTANDING TIME

What happens before lunch and what happens after lunch? What do we put on before we go outside? When will mommy pick me up? Small children ask many questions about how time is organized. Schedules and routines help them to begin to understand time and how it works.

Planning Activities for Toddlers

Establishing the environment, the routines, and the schedule for child care of toddlers provides a framework for planning activities. Each day teachers need to plan activities that promote children's physical, language, and mental development and that fit naturally into their play. It is important to plan activities so that new ideas are brought into the children's experience. When teachers do not plan, they forget to do new and interesting things with the children. Planning techniques are discussed at length in Chapter 12.

Summary

Physical care of toddlers centers on helping them to learn self-care skills. Emotional care involves helping toddlers adjust to the child care situation, understanding their attachment to caregivers, and helping them to be around other children.

Guiding toddlers requires developing routines and schedules that allow children to do things at their own pace. Constant, alert adult supervision of toddlers is necessary. Guidance techniques that work well with small children include providing encouragement, singing reminders, giving a choice when possible, giving directions clearly, and handling temper tantrums calmly.

Good environments for toddlers are structured to support self-help and play activities. The environment should include pre-reading features and adults who work well with toddlers. The physical environment for toddlers is adapted to their developmental skills and needs.

Learning activities for toddlers include ones that promote physical, language, and mental development. Mental tasks for young children include learning to classify objects, to put them in order, and to understand space and time. Planning helps to bring a constant supply of new and fresh activities into the toddlers' classroom.

Terms and Concepts

Autonomy

Separation anxiety

Structured choice

Associative play

Peers

Movement activities

Productive language

Receptive language

Trial-and-error learning

Classification

Seriation

Checking Your Understanding

1. What self-care skills can toddlers learn? How are two-year-olds different from one-year-olds in self-care abilities?

2. If you were the primary caregiver in a toddlers' room, what instructions would you give to parents about bringing a child to the center for his or her first day?

3. What is the advantage of toddlers' being securely attached to caregivers?

4. Why is it very difficult to teach toddlers to share?

5. When do adults need to allow young children to work out their own problems? When do they need to step in?

6. Why are routines important in taking care of toddlers?

7. Why is it hard on young children to be rushed?

8. Describe the kind of adult supervision needed for toddlers.

9. Name four guidance techniques appropriate for using with toddlers.

10. Briefly summarize the main ideas that guide the handling of temper tantrums by toddlers.

11. Explain how to set up an environment that enables toddlers to learn the following self-help skills: hand washing, dressing, toileting, and putting things away.

12. How is play related to learning?

13. Name three pre-reading features that can be included in the toddlers' room.

14. Describe the role of adults in the child care environment for toddlers.

15. Use the ideas presented in the section about the child care environment for toddlers to design a toddlers' room, with the help of your classmates and teacher.

16. Find five activities for physical development, five for language development, and five for mental development of toddlers. Put each activity on a 4-by-6-inch note card. With the help of your teacher, set up an activity card file and add to it regularly.

17. Learn five finger plays that could be used with toddlers and share them with your class.

18. Explain how a teacher who is a good listener helps children learn to talk.

19. The years between the first and third birthdays are very important for children's language learning. Why do you think it is considered important that *all* adults who work with young children model good language at all times?

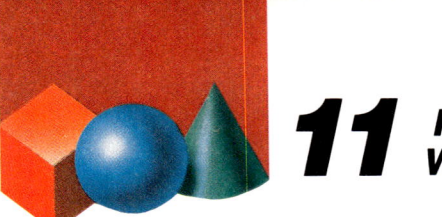

USING PUPPETS WITH TODDLERS

Toddlers, especially two-year-olds, are drawn to puppets. A puppet held in a teacher's hand where the child can see how it is being operated is the most effective kind. Since children are learning language, a puppet whose mouth moves with the words is very helpful in increasing their language skills.

Children can become engrossed in puppets and what they are saying. Puppets can be used to make a story more interesting, to draw a child into conversation or an activity, or to encourage children to help with clean-up or participate in routines.

Only puppets who represent friendly characters are acceptable for young children. Occasionally a child is afraid of puppets. Children need to be allowed to meet and talk to puppets when they are ready, and not be forced to do so.

Puppets can be made from scrap materials or old socks. Children enjoy colorful puppets with mouths that move. One form of puppet that children also like is the glove puppet. A small figure is placed on each finger of a glove. The teacher puts the glove on to tell a story and wiggles each finger when that character is speaking or doing something.

Once a puppet is made, it is given a name, a personality, and a voice. That name, personality, and voice stick with that puppet just as they do with a pet. In a sense the puppet can become a member of the class.

Young children sometimes pull or hit at puppets—this should not be allowed. Puppets need to be used out in the open for toddlers and twos. Later, in preschool, puppet shows can be presented behind a stage.

CHAPTER 12
Preschoolers

When you have finished this chapter, you will be able to

- Summarize the tasks of caregivers or teachers in the physical and emotional care of preschool children
- Describe the role of play in learning
- Identify key experiences for preschool learning
- Name the learning tasks preschoolers master through play
- Identify activities that help children develop mental skills
- List curriculum areas for preschool children
- Describe the four main types of learning centers in preschools
- Set up a learning center or activity area
- Explain the steps in planning a curriculum for young children
- Describe methods of teaching preschool children
- Describe methods of evaluating children's progress

"Justin, it is your turn to tell us what you're going to do during playtime today," Ms. Martinez said quietly. She laid her hands in her lap and listened attentively to four-year-old Justin.

"I'm going to the carpentry table to build something," Justin said eagerly.

"Tell me about what you are going to build," Ms. Martinez suggested, encouraging Justin to expand on his plan.

Justin looked across the room toward the carpentry table, then up toward the ceiling. "I'm going to make a car for my dad," he replied.

Ms. Martinez smiled warmly. "What tools do you plan to use?"

"The hammer and the glue," he said thoughtfully.

"Good!" Ms. Martinez said, encouraging him again. He was the last of the children in her small group to plan playtime. Looking around the circle, Ms. Martinez said, "You may all go to the learning centers now."

Ms. Martinez watched Justin as he found his way to the carpentry center. He would need careful supervision. She believed challenge was important for preschoolers, but she felt responsible to manage the amount of risk she allowed them to experience. She had set up her classroom at La Casita to give her nearly five-year-old preschoolers opportunities to think and create. She believed that challenging them would encourage their growth and give them the personal strength they would need to succeed later, in kindergarten and beyond.

PHYSICAL AND EMOTIONAL CARE OF PRESCHOOLERS

Child care for three- to five-year-old children involves achieving a balance between physical and emotional care and learning.

Challenge versus Safety

Small babies live in a totally protected environment where they can depend on caring adults to satisfy their needs. As they grow, they become able to do more and more for themselves. Adults need to present growing children with challenges that require them to make some effort. Challenges usually involve risk. One important task for caregivers of preschoolers is providing stimulating challenges without too much risk. Children's safety needs to be considered when challenges are presented.

Adult Supervision of Preschoolers

Preschool children continue to require constant adult supervision. They can get involved in a dangerous situation while an adult's back is turned for only a few seconds. When child care environments have been child-proofed and children have been given positive guidance concerning safe play, adult supervision is an easier task.

Self-Care Skills for Preschoolers

By age three, children who have been learning self-care skills continue to practice them and learn others readily. In any child care situation, however, there are children who have not been taught much or anything about self-care. With these children teachers have to begin at a more basic level to help them learn self-care skills.

Helping Preschoolers Manage Emotions

Children experience most of the emotions adults do. Infants and toddlers express their emotions without restraint. Their emotions tend to be general in nature. Preschoolers' emotions become more specific. Children of this age also begin to gain some control over how they express their feelings. They have an increasing number of ways to cope with strong feelings.

Fear is a powerful emotion for preschool children. They are afraid of abandonment and bodily harm. Sometimes children express fears directly, by verbalizing them. Because children's productive language is still limited, however, they sometimes need adults to help them express fears and other emotions. Sometime during their fourth year, children's fears become more specific. Scary stories in books or on television may cause nightmares. Sometimes sounds or shadows in the night frighten children.

How can adults help children handle fears? The following suggestions may be helpful:

- Be truthful with children without adding unnecessarily to their fears.

- Avoid presenting scary stories or allowing children to watch scary television shows.

- When children are afraid of something, help them to see the real situation. Fear tends to diminish when children see the way things really are.

- Prepare children for new experiences by letting them know ahead of time what to expect.

Developing Personal Strength and Getting Along with Others

When children develop personal strength, they feel good about themselves. Children develop this strength by meeting challenges and solving problems.

Getting along with other children is an important skill for preschoolers to learn. A child's sense of personal strength and feelings about himself or herself affect how well he or she will get along with people. The way children get along with others affects how they feel about themselves. Children who feel good about themselves are more likely to get along well with others. Children who feel rejected by other children usually do not feel

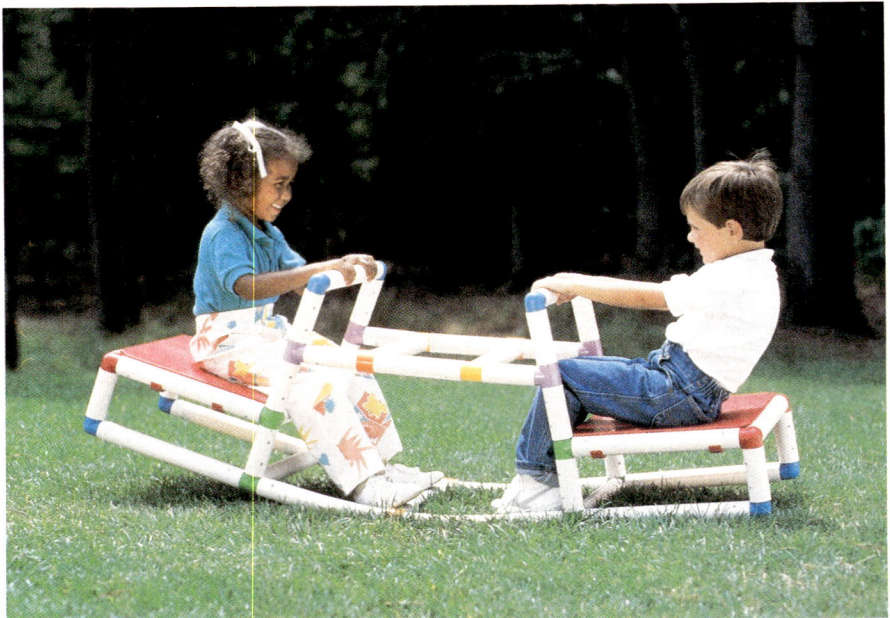

FIGURE 12-1   Getting along well with other children makes preschoolers feel good about themselves—and that makes
it easier to get along with others.
Source: © 1988 PlaySkool Inc., A Division of Hasbro, Inc.

good about themselves. Feelings of rejection can sometimes be
associated with rebellion.

In the preschool classroom a curriculum aimed at developing
both a sense of self-worth and good social skills is very important.
In what ways does the curriculum help preschoolers with these
developmental tasks?

PROVIDING CHALLENGES

Preschoolers need manageable risk. They need to try activities
at which they can succeed with some effort. They need many
opportunities for success. Challenges must be neither too easy
nor too difficult if they are to be effective.

ALLOWING CHOICE

When children are allowed to choose activities suited to their
own interests, they feel a sense of affirmation. **Affirmation** means
acceptance as a person of worth. It is not based on performance.

ENCOURAGING SELF-RESPONSIBILITY

Preschoolers can be expected to participate in self-care activities to the degree that they are able. This may mean determined encouragement by a teacher from time to time.

PROMOTING CREATIVE EXPRESSION

A good preschool curriculum provides children with opportunities to express their own thoughts and ideas in appropriate ways rather than conforming to adult ideas. Learning centers designed to promote creative expression include areas for music, blocks, carpentry, art, dramatic play, sand play, water play, and gardening.

ALLOWING CHILD-INITIATED PLAY

Play in which children lead and adults expand and encourage adds to each child's sense of worth and personal strength.

PROVIDING OPPORTUNITIES TO PLAY WITH OTHERS

Playing with other children requires practice in learning to share and negotiate. Survival skills are developed when observing adults allow children to solve their own problems so long as there is no injury. Children who can defend themselves and who develop personal strength tend to feel good about themselves. Other children tend to respect them and therefore like them more.

ALLOWING CHILDREN TO SOLVE THEIR OWN PROBLEMS

Whether children play alone or with others, they use mental skills when they are allowed to solve their own problems. The adult's role is to allow the child to explore solutions to the problem independently, as long as this is safe and not too frustrating to the child. When adult guidance is needed, the adult should ask questions that lead the child to find his or her own solution. The questions should be phrased so that they encourage the child to think about the problem one step at a time.

HOW PRESCHOOLERS LEARN

Children learn mostly from experience. They experience things with their senses and through their movements. As they play, they try out their ideas and succeed or make mistakes. This process is called trial-and-error learning.

Children also learn from hearing adults explain things in words. Mostly what they learn from being talked to, however, is language and how to use it. Telling a child how seeds grow is not nearly as meaningful to him or her as providing an opportunity to plant seeds, care for them and water them, and watch them

FIGURE 12-2 Learning from experiences is the best way for pre-schoolers to learn. Planting seeds and seeing what happens is more interesting and memorable than being told about plant growth.
Source: USDA photo

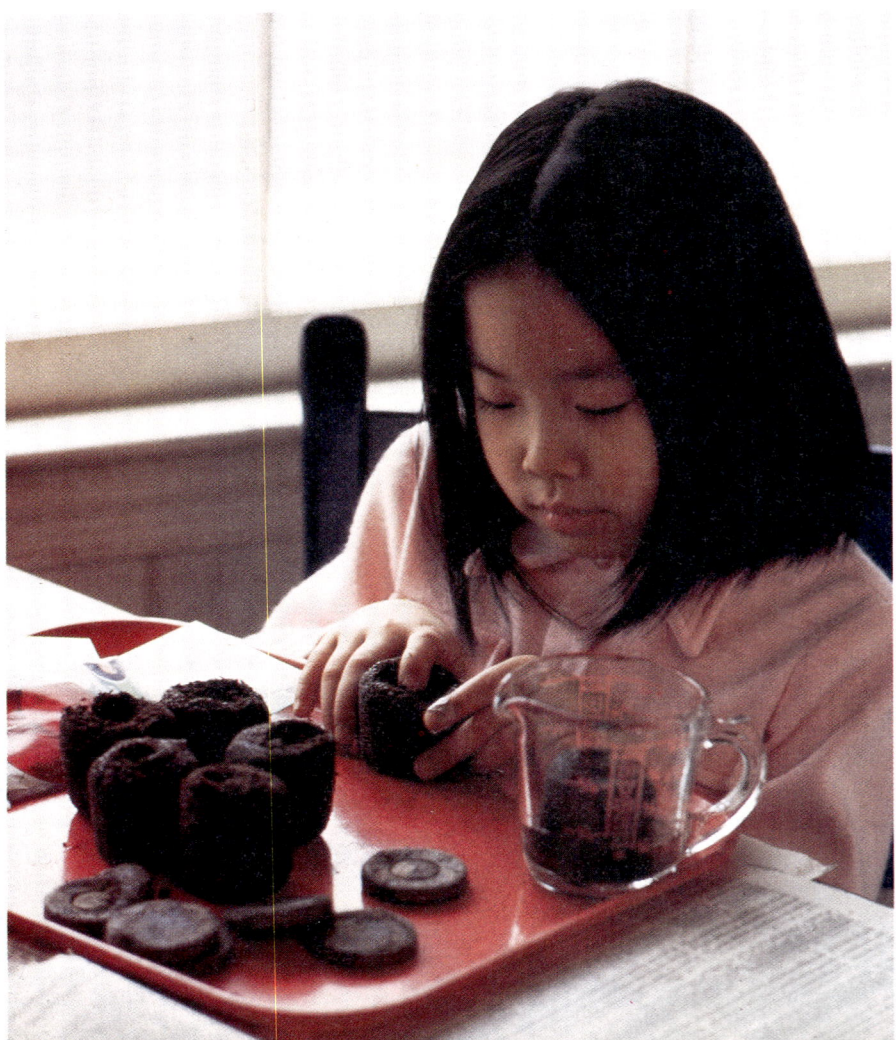

grow. Once children have experienced the way something works, they are ready to talk about it. They may even learn more from such conversation, but only if it takes place after actual experience.

Play and Experience

Effective programs for preschool children are based on providing experiences because children learn best through their own experiences. After they have had a sufficient number of experiences, they are able to learn from verbal instruction.

ACTIVE AND PASSIVE LEARNING

Active learning occurs when children learn by experience, by doing. When they actively participate with materials or people, they learn as they experience. An example of an activity that promotes active learning is block play. Children directly experience some of the laws of physics and basic math concepts.

Passive learning occurs when a child is not actively involved, but just absorbs information. Classroom lectures and watching television are situations that allow only passive learning. The Something to Think About feature considers this aspect of television watching as well as some other effects.

High/Scope Educational Research Foundation teaches preschool teachers to plan for and lead children in active learning. Active learning is fostered by providing children with opportunities and motivation to interact with people and materials.

PLANNING AND REVIEWING PLAYTIME

One way of actively involving children's minds in their play is to help them plan their play and later review it. Helping preschoolers plan their playtime gives them an opportunity to think about events that will happen in the immediate future. This helps them expand their thinking skills. When playtime is over, talking about what they have just done helps children use thinking skills to think back to the immediate past. As children talk about playtime, teachers can plan for activities for the near future that include children's ideas. Talking about the past and future also helps children get a grasp of how time works.

Planning is usually done in small groups of no more than fifteen children. Teachers give each child an opportunity to say what he or she is going to do. Teachers enable the children to

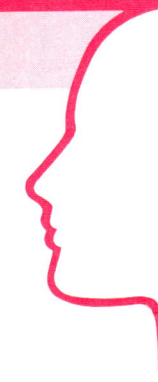

Something to Think About

How Much Television Is Too Much?

Can children watch too much television? Is television harmful to children? Answering these questions requires some background information concerning children and television.

How does watching television affect children's physical development? The time children spend watching television is an inactive period. They get little or no physical exercise and often consume a great deal of junk food.

Is the passive learning from television as effective as active learning? Learning from watching television is passive. Children watch and hear, simply absorbing and not processing or using effectively the information they accept. Only by participating actively and using materials are children likely to develop their thinking skills and a sense of autonomy.

How does television affect language development? Although some well-planned and well-designed programs do provide opportunities to experience language, they cannot respond to the individual child's attempts at producing language. Only by talking and interacting with people do children practice speech and gain competence in language use. Excessive television watching can limit these opportunities.

How does television affect relationships? When watching television, children are not interacting with people. Only by interacting with people can children learn to negotiate with others and to assert themselves. Some television programming presents relationships superficially.

How does television affect values? The wide range of values presented on television can be misleading and disturbing. Preschoolers especially need adult help to separate fantasy from reality. Violence is presented mainly for its dramatic effect, and its outcome is seldom dealt with in the long run. Some values presented on television do not support family strength and are in conflict with some families' religious or social values. Adult programming may not be appropriate for children because it may present situations they do not have the skills to handle emotionally.

What about children's programming? Cartoons and other programs designed for children are not necessarily safe viewing, since some present very violent actions and superficial relationships. Some programs are specifically designed to present some very positive, helpful values and to help children develop language skills.

Should children be allowed to watch television? How much? What is an adult's responsibility concerning children's television viewing? What do you think?

---

plan by helping them to learn the names of learning centers, to learn where materials and toys are kept and how they can be used, and to learn to make choices. When a child has a difficult time choosing, a teacher can offer two suggestions and let the child select the one that has greater appeal.

Once all the children have expressed their plans, teachers let them begin to play. If a child finishes with what has been planned, the teacher encourages him or her to plan something else to do.

When playtime is over, children help with clean-up and then sit down together to talk about their play. Reviewing can be done during a short time set aside for that purpose or during a snack. When children have the opportunity to talk about their play, they are practicing mental skills. Thinking about what has happened and talking about it can strengthen children's memory. Planning and reviewing give playtime more meaning and help to make it more productive than it would otherwise be.

LEARNING TASKS FOR PLAY

The learning tasks that play supports continue to be important during the preschool years. These tasks help children continue to develop their thinking skills in the areas first identified by Jean Piaget:

- Classification—thinking about how things are alike or different

- Seriation—comparing features of objects (such as larger or smaller, smoother or rougher, and lighter or darker) and arranging the objects in order (such as from shortest to tallest)

- Number—comparing amounts and numbers of things and counting objects

- Space—discovering how things fit together, seeing how objects or people look from different viewpoints, rearranging objects to see how they change, observing how people and objects move through space, and discovering ways to describe distances (such as near and far)

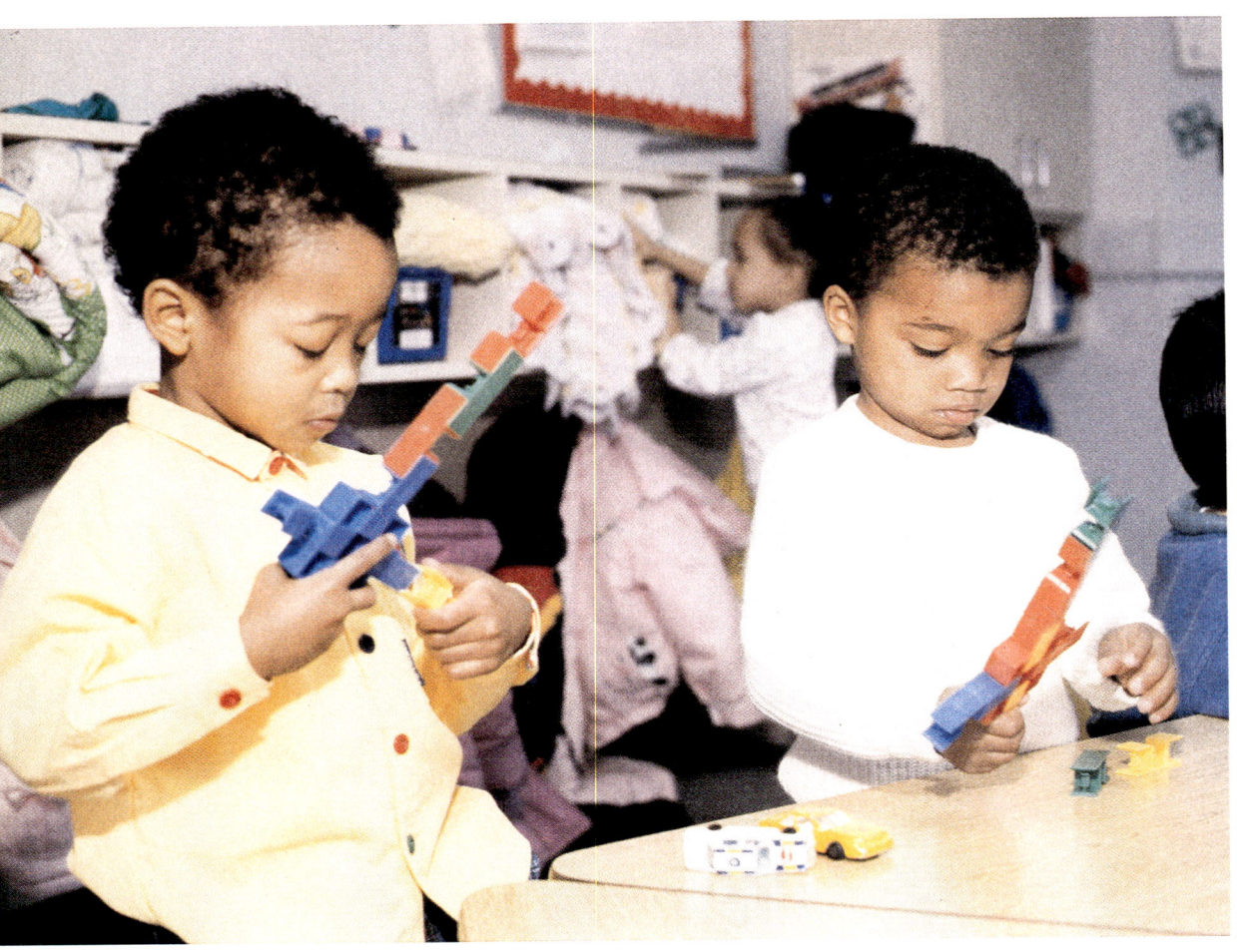

FIGURE 12-3 Toys consisting of parts that connect to form many possible structures develop preschoolers' ability to think about space.
Source: Gerber Products Company

- Time—developing an understanding of how events are ordered (for example, what comes before or after what we are doing now) and how fast or slowly things move, talking about past and future events, using words to describe time, and planning and following through with plans

KEY EXPERIENCES

Key experiences are ones that are basic to children's development and active learning. They are based on the learning tasks for play described above and are intended to help children with **developmental tasks,** the things they need to accomplish in order to develop. Illustration 12-1 lists key experiences for four- and five-year-olds identified by Dr. David Weikart and his staff at High/Scope Educational Research Foundation.

Developing Mental Skills through Play

As children play actively, they are developing and sharpening their mental skills. These skills include perception, memory, reasoning, and creativity.

PERCEPTION

Perception is the ability to absorb new information through the senses—sight, smell, taste, hearing, and touch. As children experience objects, materials, and people in their environment, they study features and classify them in order to understand them. Children need many opportunities to experience a wide variety of new things in order to sharpen their perception.

MEMORY

Memory is basically the storing in one's mind of experiences and information to use at a later time. **Short-term memory** is a person's ability to remember specific information for a short period of time. **Long-term memory** is the ability to recall information after a long time. To put information in long-term memory, a child has to rehearse it, that is, to run it through his or her head and relate it to something that is already there.

It takes time to build experiences into one's memory. During the first two or more years of life, the child organizes many experiences so that a way will be developed to allow memories to stick in the mind. Most people do not remember much from their

ILLUSTRATION 12-1 Key experiences for four- and five-year-olds can be divided into five general categories.

Key Experiences in Active Learning

- Exploring actively with all the senses
- Discovering relations through direct experience
- Manipulating, transforming, and combining materials
- Choosing materials, activities, and purposes
- Acquiring skills with tools and equipment
- Using the large muscles
- Taking care of one's own needs

Key Experiences in Using Language

- Talking with others about personally meaningful experiences
- Describing objects, events, and relations
- Expressing feelings in words
- Having one's own spoken language written down by an adult and read back
- Having fun with language: rhyming, making up stories, and listening to poems and stories

Key Experiences in Representing Experiences and Ideas

- Recognizing objects by sound, touch, taste, and smell
- Imitating actions
- Relating pictures, photographs, and models to real places and things
- Role playing and pretending
- Making models out of clay, blocks, and so on
- Drawing and painting

Key Experiences in Developing Logical Reasoning

CLASSIFICATION

- Investigating and labeling the attributes of things
- Noticing and describing how things are the same and how they are different; sorting and matching
- Using and describing something in several different ways
- Describing what characteristics something does *not* possess or what class it does not belong to
- Holding more than one attribute in mind at a time (for example, identifying something that is red and made of wood)
- Distinguishing between some and all

SERIATION

- Comparing (bigger/smaller, heavier/lighter, louder/softer, longer/shorter, and so on)
- Arranging several things in order according to some dimension and describing the relations (the longest one, the shortest one, and so on)

NUMBER CONCEPTS

- Comparing number and amount (more/less, same amount; more/fewer, same number)
- Comparing the numbers of items in two sets by matching them up in one-to-one correspondence (for example, checking whether there are as many crackers as there are children)
- Enumerating (counting) objects, as well as counting by rote

ILLUSTRATION 12-1 (cont.)

Key Experiences in Understanding Spatial Relations (Space) and Time

SPATIAL RELATIONS

- Fitting things together and taking them apart

- Rearranging a set of objects or one object in space (folding, twisting, stretching, stacking, or tying) and observing the spatial transformations

- Observing things and places from different spatial viewpoints

- Experiencing and describing the positions of things in relation to each other (in the middle, beside, on, off, on top of, over, above)

- Experiencing and describing the direction of movement of things and people (to, from, into, out of, toward, away from)

- Experiencing and describing relative distances among things and locations (close, near, far, next to, apart, together)

- Experiencing and representing one's own body (how it is structured and what various parts can do)

- Learning to locate things in the classroom, school, and neighborhood

- Interpreting representations of spatial relations in drawings and pictures

- Distinguishing and describing shapes

TIME

- Planning and completing what one has planned

- Describing and representing past events

- Anticipating future events verbally and by making appropriate preparations

- Starting and stopping an action on signal

- Noticing, describing, and representing the order of events

- Experiencing and describing different rates of movement

- Using conventional time units when talking about past and future events (morning, yesterday, hour, and so on)

- Comparing time periods (short/long, new/old, young/old, a little while/a long time)

- Observing that clocks and calendars are used to mark the passage of time

- Observing seasonal changes

Source: David Weikart, Young Children in Action *(Ypsilanti, MI: High/Scope Press, 1975). High/Scope Educational Research Foundation.*

early years because that is a time of getting the mind ready to remember.

REASONING

Reasoning is the mental process used to figure out how the world operates and to organize information in a way that makes it useful. Reasoning includes the ability to think logically. Thinking logically involves making judgments, comparing characteristics of one object or situation with those of another, solving

Leadership at a Glance

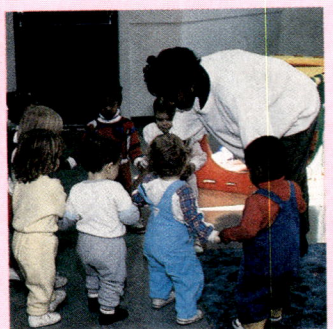

Source: *Gerber Children's Centers, Inc., a subsidiary of Gerber Products Company*

Dr. David Weikart

Dr. David Weikart is an educator who began his career working with both handicapped and normal children. In 1970 he founded High/Scope Educational Research Foundation for the purpose of studying what curriculum and teaching methods would be most effective for children from infancy through adolescence. He and his colleagues used what they learned to develop a curriculum based on children's being actively involved with both people and materials.

Dr. Weikart writes articles and books about effective teaching. He speaks in the United States and other countries, presenting workshops about the High/Scope curriculum and training teachers to use it with children. He frequently testifies before congressional committees on early education and related issues.

Dr. Weikart is best known for a long-term study on the effect of high-quality education on the growth and development of young children. He is recognized as a leader among those who teach young children.

To obtain more information about the High/Scope curriculum, materials, and training, you can write to this address:

High/Scope Educational Research Foundation
600 North River Street
Ypsilanti, MI 48198-2898

problems, evaluating situations accurately, and making effective decisions. Preschool children have limits on their ability to reason.

CREATIVITY

Creativity is the ability to form original ideas from experiences and to express them in a unique way. Creativity is a way of tapping a child's imagination. Preschool children have a strong need to practice thinking creatively and expressing themselves in creative ways.

The Role of Play in Preschool

Preschoolers' days are consumed by play. They like to pretend. Pretending helps them accept reality—they interpret what happens to them and give it meaning. **Imagining** is an important mental skill for children to develop.

A good early childhood program is based on the developmental needs of young children and is implemented through **developmentally appropriate practices.** That is, teachers provide opportunities for play and learning that are suited to the abilities of the children. Since each child develops at his or her own rate, what is appropriate for one child may not be appropriate for another. Illustration 12-2 presents a summary of developmentally appropriate practices for preschool teachers.

ILLUSTRATION 12-2   These teaching strategies are developmentally appropriate for preschoolers (four- and five-year-olds).

- The curriculum is presented mostly in learning centers and through play activities.

- Learning centers are set up for children to play individually or with a few other children. Children are expected to play cooperatively.

- Children choose projects or play activities from those set up in the environment by the teacher.

- Learning materials and activities are as real as possible and are directly related to children's lives.

- Teachers accept that there may be more than one right answer to a question or problem.

- Teachers move among the children, asking them questions and offering suggestions. They encourage children to play with the materials. Sometimes they encourage more complex thinking.

These teaching strategies are adapted from guidelines found in Developmentally Appropriate Practice in Early Childhood Programs Serving Children From Birth Through Age 8, *edited by Sue Bredekamp and published by the National Association for the Education of Young Children, 1987.*

Effective preschool environments provide experiences that meet children's needs and encourage learning in all of the following areas of development:

- Physical development is advanced by activities that improve large and small motor skills.

- Mental development is enhanced by activities that stimulate imagination and that help children to develop an understanding of space, time, classification, and seriation.

- Language development is encouraged by activities that give children opportunities to practice listening to and producing much language.

- Social development is fostered by activities that provide children with opportunities to enjoy other children and to learn to negotiate ways of getting along.

- Emotional development is fostered by activities that provide children with opportunities to develop personal strength and a sense of self-worth.

- Spiritual development is enhanced by activities that provide opportunities to develop a sense of the meaning of life.

THE CURRICULUM FOR PRESCHOOLERS

Ms. Martinez outlined a curriculum based on the guidelines that Mrs. Cisneros set for La Casita. Then she refined the plans to suit the developmental needs of the children she would be teaching. The curriculum includes all the experiences teachers plan for and provide to children so they can learn and develop. The preschool curriculum is also designed to promote individual growth and positive relationships. The curriculum for preschool children focuses on these goals:

- Developing physical skills
- Developing language skills
- Learning concepts in math and science
- Learning to enjoy beauty (aesthetics)

Developing Physical Skills

Children want to run, play, and use their muscles. Doing so helps them grow physically and develop motor skills.

GROSS AND FINE MOTOR SKILLS

Children develop strength and coordination through active play. Gross motor skills are improved through the use of the large muscles of the arms and legs. Activities such as climbing, running, jumping, throwing, and dancing provide an opportunity for large muscles to develop. By using the small muscles in the hands and fingers, children develop fine motor skills. Building with blocks, working puzzles, spreading cheese on crackers, and forming clay are some of the activities that encourage small muscles to develop. **Manipulative activities** are ones designed to strengthen and coordinate small muscles in the hands. (In this context manipulative means "done with the hands.")

COORDINATION

Coordination is the ability to use several muscles together to accomplish a goal. For example, stringing beads requires coordinating the small muscles of the hands and fingers to get the end of the string through the hole in the bead. Activities that require children to use more than one muscle or set of muscles to accomplish a task help to develop coordination. Activities that encourage coordination include practice on a balance beam, stringing beads, and placing pegs in pegboards.

MOVEMENT

Activities can be planned that encourage children to use their large muscles. Movement activities are designed to strengthen and coordinate large muscles. Music is an excellent way to encourage children to move. Safe, sturdy, and challenging climbing equipment also encourages movement. Obstacle courses can be set up that invite children to climb, crawl through spaces, and find their way around.

Developing Language Skills

Children understand ideas before they have the words to talk about them. They understand language before they can use it. Understanding the meaning of what others say is receptive language. Being able to express ideas in a meaningful way is productive language. Children can use receptive language before they can use productive language. How do each of these develop?

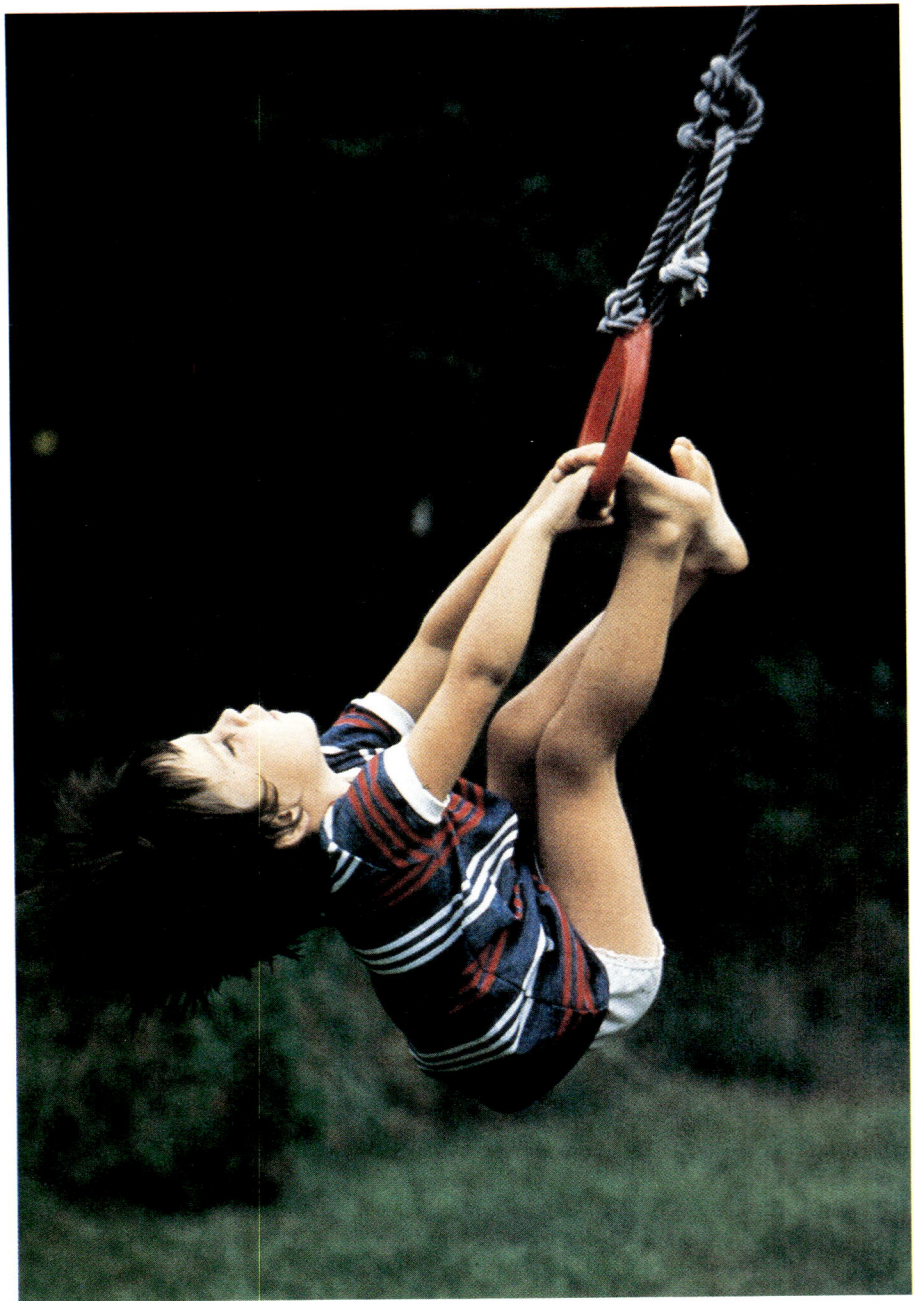

FIGURE 12-4 Gross motor skills and coordination are well developed in some preschoolers.
Source: © Suzanne Szasz/Photo Researchers, Inc.

LEARNING TO LISTEN

Children's receptive language develops when they hear a great deal of clear language spoken directly to them by an adult or older child. Speaking to a child in a way that implies that he or she is a person who can understand encourages receptive language to develop. Children who are around adults who do not believe children hear or understand adult speech do not develop receptive language as readily. Talking when children are around or letting them watch educational programs on television may add some to their vocabulary, but will not teach them language skills as effectively as having someone who is willing to invest the time to talk with them individually.

Receptive language also develops when adults give children simple directions and allow them time to carry them out. At first directions need to be given one at a time. For example, an adult might say to a toddler, "Hand me the ball." Once children have learned to respond to such simple directions, more complex directions can be given. For example, an adult might say to a preschooler, "Go get the ball from the shelf in your room and give it to Dad." This is a two-step direction. Once a child masters two-step directions, he or she can be given three-step ones, and so on.

LEARNING TO SPEAK

When children use language and experience other people's reactions to their use, they learn. Adults can help by listening carefully to children and responding to what they say. Most children speak slowly when they are learning to talk, so it takes time to listen. Some adults do not think children have anything important to say, and they do not really pay attention to children's speech. Children sense when this is true, and they tend to talk less to those adults.

Writing down what children say is one way to encourage them to use language. Preschool teachers can encourage children to talk by writing down what they say about their feelings, their family, things that happen to them, something they wish for, or something they saw. Teachers may also write down what children say after listening to stories or watching puppets. The written words are read to the children and posted where they can look at them.

When you write down children's words, be sure to use correct printscript. Preschoolers need to see clear letters if they are to learn to recognize them and write them correctly.

PREPARING TO READ

Children prepare for learning to read by being read to, listening to stories being told, and enjoying stories with peers and significant adults. Children learn that reading is important when they see that their parents enjoy reading. When they see familiar pictures or symbols with accompanying words, such as in advertising or on traffic signs, they can be encouraged to recognize those words. Activities that encourage children to want to read and give them experience in interpreting the world around them are called **pre-reading activities.**

Should children be taught to read in preschool? Among eight-year-olds, those who learned to read after they started school read just about as well as those who were taught to read in preschool. Hurrying preschool children onto the next developmental level makes them miss some of the important time they need to spend exploring, experimenting, and creating. Experiences during this

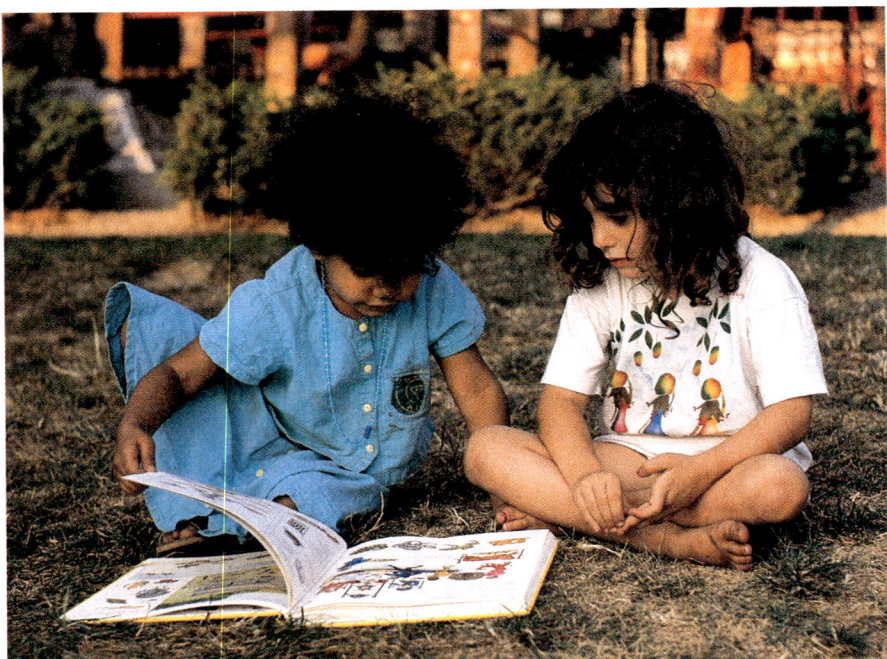

FIGURE 12-5   Although many preschoolers are interested in learning to read, there is no evidence that early reading gives a child an advantage in elementary school.
Source: © S. Rosenberg/International Stock Photography

time are important not only for later reading but for science, math, and social development as well. When preschool teachers push reading, they are limiting the developmentally appropriate activities that should be provided during the preschool years. Thus, in some ways learning to read early interferes with development rather than enhancing it.

Pushing children to read early can actually turn them against reading. When children are pushed to do something before they are ready, they resist learning. A particular task may even become distasteful to them. Some children respond to pressure to learn by learning the skill much later or learning it poorly.

What happens, then, if children show an interest in reading during the preschool years? Teachers of preschoolers simply respond to the children's natural curiosity. When a child requests help with a word or a book, a teacher responds positively to that child's request.

PREPARING TO WRITE

Learning to write begins when children have opportunities to experiment with holding and using writing tools, such as pencils or crayons. This experimenting often occurs in the following sequence:

- Picking up the tool
- Making random marks
- Making dots and lines
- Making circles
- Putting a face in a circle
- Drawing other body parts

Letters usually begin to appear on children's drawings when they are between four and five years old if they see letters regularly. Teachers can stimulate children to try making letters by labeling objects in the room with correct printscript and by putting children's names on papers and possessions, again in correct printscript. Activities that help prepare children to learn to write are called **pre-writing activities.** Making preschool children copy letters printed on a mimeographed sheet is not considered a developmentally appropriate activity for them.

Learning Basic Math Concepts

For preschoolers the purpose of learning simple math concepts is to develop an understanding of numbers. Knowing the number of fingers on a hand involves more than counting how many—it also means understanding what five of something is. Children need a great deal of experience in counting objects to begin to understand the concept of number.

Preschool children are also becoming familiar with basic shapes, such as circles, triangles, and squares. They need experience with parts and whole objects. Activities that help children understand basic math ideas and gain a foundation for developing math skills are called **pre-math activities.**

Learning Basic Science Concepts

Science in the preschool classroom takes the form of discovery. Activities that help children learn about the natural world and how it works are developmentally appropriate. Discovery activities center around water, wind, seasons, plants, rocks, sand, and animals. Appropriate classroom pets such as rabbits and ducks are gentle with children and relatively easy to care for. Adults must exercise care that discovery activities are safe and manageable. Many books are available that offer good suggestions for science and discovery activities.

Developing a Sense of Aesthetics

Aesthetics means the perception and appreciation of beautiful things. Children need opportunities to see beautiful colors and places and to hear and enjoy music. Children need to see colorful flowers, a blanket of fresh snow, running water, singing birds, and other beautiful things from nature. Music for children is selected with an understanding of how it affects them. Soothing music helps them rest; music with a lively beat helps them experience rhythm.

LEARNING CENTERS IN PRESCHOOLS

The preschool environment is organized in learning centers to make it possible for children to choose from a variety of activities. Learning centers are a way of arranging the preschool classroom to encourage children to engage in developmental play and learning, individually or in small groups.

Learning centers are best set up to offer materials that suggest play ideas to children. The furnishings and play materials in the centers are arranged so that children can get to them without adult help and can help clean up and put away the materials.

There are four main types of learning centers. These are the family center, the block and building center, the art center, and the quiet center. Within learning centers, specific areas can be established. **Activity areas** are spaces set up for particular activities, such as playing with water or looking at books.

The Family Center

The family center is usually furnished with child-sized wooden furnishings, most often those of a kitchen. If there is enough space, the family center may be expanded with child-sized sofas, rocking chairs, and beds. Real objects used in the family center encourage children to pretend. These objects can be rotated to encourage new ideas.

Props suggesting a special form of play can be placed in the family center on occasion. These include the following:

- Lunch pails
- Irons and ironing boards
- Warm, soapy water and sponges
- Shaving cream and a bladeless razor
- Bandages, hot water bottles, and other health care items
- Dress-up clothes that indicate adult roles

With supervision, children can help prepare simple snacks in the family center. An adult working with children there can interact with them, asking questions and providing suggestions that extend their play and encourage them to talk and think about family.

The Block and Building Center

Blocks provide a wonderful opportunity for children to create and construct. Creating allows children to use their imaginations. The block and building center contains two kinds of blocks and props that can be used with them.

MATHEMATICALLY SIZED AND SHAPED BLOCKS

Mathematically shaped blocks are made from wood and have standard geometric shapes: squares, rectangles, triangles, and circles. Half-circles and quarter-circles may also be included in larger sets. The blocks fit nicely into children's hands. They are sized so that two of one size and shape laid properly together are the same size and shape as one of a larger kind. As preschoolers use these blocks, they gain experience with adding, subtracting, multiplying, dividing, and the properties of geometric shapes. Although the children will not learn to do the mathematical operations until later, the experiences they have using the blocks stay in their minds and provide a foundation for that later learning.

STRUCTURE BLOCKS

Structure blocks are larger blocks that can be used to build buildings, fences, and roads and may be made of wood or cardboard. Structure blocks give children opportunities to try bigger ideas. Used in combination with the smaller blocks, they allow children to develop some rather complex ideas.

PROPS

Props in the block and building center often include transportation toys such as cars, tractors, and trains. Also provided frequently are sets of small wooden people, hats for role play, and traffic signs. Props can be changed to suggest different occupations.

Special props are sometimes put in the block and building center to suggest specific places. Children enjoy pretending that the center is one of the following:

- Barber or beauty shop
- Clothing store
- Grocery store
- Doctor's office
- School
- Fire station
- Church or synagogue

The Art Center

The art center provides children with the opportunity to experiment with many basic, or raw, materials. To set up an art center, the teacher places various materials where children can get them easily. The teacher shows the children how materials may be used but does not tell them what to make.

For preschool children unpatterned art is developmentally appropriate. **Unpatterned art** is any activity that allows children to use art materials in appropriate ways to design freely. Pre-schoolers should select materials and do their own projects. Such activity helps them learn to use materials effectively and crea-tively and boosts their self-esteem. What a child makes is not as important as the fact that he or she is using imagination and expressing thoughts and feelings in an appropriate way.

Preschool children should not color in printed pictures, cut out designated shapes, or copy teacher-made projects. Doing these kinds of activities keeps preschoolers from developing skill in handling materials. Their limited fine motor skills may make it impossible for them to complete such projects without the teacher's assistance or correction. Their self-esteem can therefore be damaged.

Child-sized furnishings in the art area usually include an easel, a table with chairs, and a shelf containing a variety of materials. Aprons to protect clothing are a must. They should be hung where children can easily reach them. The materials commonly placed in the art center include the following:

- Collage materials (pieces of pretty paper or cloth or other small items to glue onto a paper or structure)
- Blank paper of a variety of colors, sizes, and shapes
- Tempera paint
- Paintbrushes of varying sizes
- Crayons
- Blunt scissors (some for left-handed children)
- Colored chalk
- Fingerpaint
- Glue

All materials do not have to be put out on the shelves every day. Different ways of applying paints should be offered. For example, tempera paint can be put onto paper with a toothbrush rubbed on a screen, with a catsup squeeze bottle, with a clothes-pin holding a piece of sponge, with sponges of different sizes and shapes, or with long-handled brushes designed for children to use when easel painting. All colors of paint do not have to be available every day. Creativity can be encouraged by changing the size and shape of paper. One way to encourage children to think differently in the art center is to cut a small shape, such as a heart or triangle, out of the center of the paper.

Art activities that encourage children's creativity include the following:

- Forming clay (easily homemade)
- Easel painting
- Fingerpainting
- Gluing (collages)
- Cutting paper

Teachers working with children in the art area allow them to choose their own activity. Teachers may need to assist children in putting on their aprons. Teachers supervise children's use of materials only to ensure safety and prevent excess waste or unnecessary mess.

The Quiet Center

The family, block, and art centers are often busy and sometimes noisy since children will often talk while they play or work. An area of the preschool classroom is set aside for a **quiet center.** This center includes a book area, a toy and puzzle area, a discovery area, and a listening area. These areas are for activities that are quieter and usually involve only a few children.

BOOK AREA

The book area has a bookshelf that displays books where children can see and reach them, good lighting, and a soft surface where children can relax with a book. Bean-bag chairs are often used.

TOY AND PUZZLE AREA

The toy and puzzle area offers activities designed to help children strengthen small muscles in the hands and to solve problems. These manipulative activities include puzzles, beads to string, pegboards, nesting blocks, and counting frames. This area is set up with these kinds of toys on a shelf where children can reach them and a table with chairs where children can work.

DISCOVERY AREA

The discovery area gives children an opportunity to discover how the natural world works. This area often has a table where teachers place different objects and tools to use in investigating the properties of the objects. Tools include magnifying glasses, magnets, balance scales, and stethoscopes. Aquariums, enclosed ant farms, plants, and small pet cages may be included in this area. Children need to be guided when helping to take care of living things.

LISTENING AREA

The listening area has a simple tape recorder that older children can operate, tapes (including some that come with books), and earphones. Some centers combine the listening and reading areas.

Other Learning Areas

Sand tables or water tables are sometimes set up in the discovery center or as a separate learning area. Sand can be presented dry or with a bucket of water to make it easier to mold. Equipment can be included to sift, mold, or pour the sand. When a water table or other water activity is offered, the water can be warm or cool, soapy or plain. Equipment included on the water table can be used to pour, measure, or make bubbles.

The carpentry area offers small blocks of soft wood and simple, child-sized tools. This area is always closely supervised by adults and is used mostly with older preschoolers. Wood projects for younger preschoolers and toddlers should be done without tools and limited to gluing.

Large muscle areas are sometimes found indoors in centers that have enough space for them. These areas are particularly useful if outdoor space is limited or weather is harsh. Equipment can include climbers, tumbling mats, balance beams, and small, portable trampolines. Impact-absorbing surfaces—usually mats—are placed under the equipment when it is in use.

Choosing Props for Preschoolers' Learning

The kind and quality of props introduced into children's play is important in shaping that play and can influence values. For example, when a teacher places a lunch pail and hard hat in the family center or block center, children often respond by imagining work situations. Providing children an opportunity to play with work-related props encourages the development of a sense of the value of work.

Inappropriate props can shape play in a way that develops undesirable values. Guns and other war toys may encourage children to imitate killing scenes they have seen on television. This kind of play does not teach children that weapons pose danger to people—that people get hurt and can die when they are shot or stabbed. When this kind of pretending appears in children's play, adults should remind them about the dangers of weapons by saying, for example, "Guns can hurt people and cause them to die."

Another group of props that are inappropriate are toys or play materials designed for older children. These may be physically dangerous to preschoolers. An example is a skateboard. Preschoolers' motor skills are not developed adequately enough to handle skateboards safely.

Some props encourage play that is not developmentally suited to preschoolers. Dolls that have adult body shapes are an example. Dressing adult-shaped figures is different from the game of dress-up in which children wear adult clothing. Wearing such clothing encourages role play that is based on thinking about careers and adult tasks. This is different from the role play that can result from emphasis on body shape. The appropriate time for playing with adult-shaped dolls is during the later elementary years when children's bodies are beginning to change.

Props that encourage the imitation of movie, cartoon, and television characters are usually not the best choice. It is particularly important to avoid selecting characters that are classified as anti-heroes. Role play involving movie, cartoon, and television characters can be violent and represent undesirable values.

Simulation games that encourage children to act out search-and-destroy activities can be particularly harmful. Although most preschoolers will not be able to participate in extended games, short versions of these games may emerge in their play. If they do, the play should be redirected.

THE PRESCHOOL TEACHER'S ROLE

The preschool teacher is responsible for planning the curriculum, leading groups of children, evaluating children's progress, and working with parents.

Planning the Preschool Curriculum

Ms. Martinez was very concerned about planning. She knew that doing a good job of planning would make learning in her classroom much more effective. When evaluation time was approaching, she always felt better about her performance as a teacher if she had done an adequate job of planning.

Teachers do not simply step into a classroom and teach. They must carefully plan. **Curriculum planning** is what the teacher does to design the children's experiences: setting up the environment, establishing schedules and routines, and deciding on and getting ready for activities. Good planning reflects goals, things the teacher wants the children to accomplish. These goals are based on the developmental needs of the children.

Effective curriculum planning requires several steps. These are as follows:

Step 1   Set developmentally based goals.

Step 2   Make a block plan that outlines themes for a block of time, usually from three months to a year. Holidays and special occasions are included in this plan. (A sample three-month block plan is shown in Illustration 12-3.)

Step 3   Make a unit plan outlining the ideas that are to be presented each week.

Step 4   Plan each week, selecting the activities that are to be offered. These activities are chosen to reflect goals and highlight special occasions.

Step 5   Make a daily plan indicating how each day will be approached. Plans for the preschool classroom include the kind of play that will be encouraged in each of the learning centers. Plans for the next day are based on both the weekly plan and an evaluation of the current day. Needs and interests of individual children are taken into consideration, and plans are adjusted as required. (A sample daily plan is presented in Illustration 12-4.)

Step 6   Evaluate the plan by comparing what actually happened to what was planned. Future planning takes into account the knowledge gained from this evaluation process.

LA CASITA CHILDREN'S CENTER

Three-Month Block Plan for the Four-Year-Olds' Room

MONTH	WEEK	THEME	CELEBRATIONS
MARCH		LIVING THINGS	ST. PATRICK'S DAY
	Week 1	Plants	
	Week 2	Animals	
	Week 3	Families	
	Week 4	Homes	
APRIL		SPRING	EASTER
	Week 1	Wind	
	Week 2	Rain	
	Week 3	New Babies	
	Week 4	Growing	
MAY		CULTURES	
	Week 1	Black	MAY DAY
	Week 2	Hispanic	CINCO DE MAYO
	Week 3	Asian	
	Week 4	Caucasian	
	Week 5	Indian	

ILLUSTRATION 12-3   This is an example of a three-month block plan drawn up by a preschool teacher.

SCHEDULING AND ROUTINES

A major responsibility of teachers or directors in child care centers is to set the schedule for the children's day. Schedules and routines give direction to the children's day and provide the teacher with a structure on which to base planning. In preschools the schedule is based on self-care routines and periods of quiet

```
                    LA CASITA CHILDREN'S CENTER

                    Daily Plan for May 5
                 Celebration Day: Cinco de Mayo

  8:45 — 9:00    Large Circle Time

  9:00 — 10:00   Learning Centers

LEARNING
CENTER              ACTIVITY              KEY EXPERIENCES

Art Center          Easel painting        Drawing and painting
                    Salt-flour clay       Making models out of clay
                                          (representing)
Block Center        Gazebo (prop)         Experiencing space, role play
Family Center       Stuff sopaipillas     Recognizing taste
Quiet Center        Mariachi music        Starting and stopping action
                                          on signal

10:00 - 10:30       Snack and review      Describing past events
                      time: Stuffed
                      sopaipillas and
                      pineapple juice
10:30 - 11:00       Outdoor playtime:     Exploring space
                      Breaking the pinata
11:00 — 11:30       Help prepare lunch
11:30 — 12:00       Lunch time
12:00 — 12:30       Clean up, brush teeth
12:30 — 12:45       Story time: Grandma's Listening to stories
                      Adobe Dollhouse
12:45 - 2:30        Nap time
 2:30 - 3:00        Afternoon snack:
                      Jicama and biscochos
 3:00 - 3:15        Brush teeth, clean up
 3:15 - 3:45        Small group activity  Observing seasonal changes
                      activity: Nature
                      walk
 3:45 - 4:30        Outdoor playtime
 4:30 - pick-up     Individual indoor play
```

ILLUSTRATION 12-4 This is a daily plan drawn up by a preschool teacher. (Sopaipillas are deep-fried pieces of dough. Mariachi music, often heard at Mexican-American celebrations, is made by three or four people singing and playing guitars and other instruments. A piñata is a hollow shape made of paper-mache and filled with candy and small toys. Children strike the piñata until it breaks and then rush to pick up the candy and toys. Jicama is a plant root looking somewhat like a potato and having a slightly sweet taste. Biscochos are party cookies.)

and active play. Periods of active play are balanced with periods of quiet play or rest. By alternating these periods, teachers help children manage their energy.

TRANSITION ACTIVITIES

Children need help making the change from active play to quieter play or from quieter times to more active ones. **Transition activities** are planned actions that provide a way to help children make such adjustments. Transition activities very often can be made to fit naturally into the children's day. Transitions are easier if teachers bring the children together and create a feeling of a group activity.

The time between lunch and naptime is a transition. If children are provided with simple tasks, this transition goes more smoothly. They can put dishes away, brush their teeth, get their blankets, and settle into a quiet mood. By teaching children the order of tasks to be done and allowing them to do the tasks themselves or with little help, teachers aid the transition from mealtime to naptime. Some teachers use a story to settle children into a quiet time.

Transition activities can be used to move children from one location to another. For example, teachers can have children form a line by asking them to make a train and then use "chug-chug" noises to "move the train" from the outdoor play area into the classroom.

Transition activities can also prepare children for a listening activity. For example, the teacher might involve children in a finger play that ends with their hands in their laps. Then the teacher can remind the children that their hands need to stay quietly in their laps while they listen to a story.

PLANNING FOR HOLIDAYS AND SPECIAL EVENTS

Holidays shared by nearly all the children in a center are easy to plan for. These generally include the following:

- New Year's Day
- Valentine's Day
- The first day of spring
- Mother's Day
- Father's Day
- Memorial Day
- The Fourth of July
- Labor Day
- Columbus Day
- Thanksgiving

Holidays that may be celebrated by some children but not others include the following:

- Christmas
- Hanukkah
- St. Patrick's Day
- Chinese New Year
- Cinco de Mayo
- Yom Kippur
- Easter

Celebrations create excitement. Children are sometimes more difficult to manage on celebration days. Teachers will need an extra measure of understanding and possibly extra help on special occasions. Young children handle celebrations better when teachers discuss what is going to happen with them ahead of time.

Activities that are normally carried out on holidays may need to be explained to small children. Most activities will need to be adapted to children.

When celebrating holidays that involve gifts, teachers must be very careful to see that all children receive similar gifts. If gifts are donated to the center, the staff has to know what they are and control the way in which they are given.

Every child's birthday is a very special day to him or her. Honoring children's birthdays is a very important activity in preschools. Every child's birthday needs to be observed. It is most important that no child feel slighted because his or her birthday is missed or is not celebrated the same way as the other children's birthdays. Birthdays that occur on weekends or holidays should be observed on the day before the weekend or holiday.

FAMILIES AND CULTURAL BACKGROUNDS

Each child's family is important to him or her. Each family's cultural heritage is important as well. Teachers have a responsibility to value each child within the context of his or her culture.

The preschool curriculum can be planned so that activities reflect the cultural traditions of families and children. Each culture represented in the center is presented positively and with equal time and energy. In some centers a day or a week is set aside in which props, materials, and activities reflect a particular culture.

Religious practice is a part of each child's culture and should be respected. When a center is owned or sponsored by a specific religious group, the teaching of that particular faith or tradition is sometimes a part of the curriculum. When this is the case, it is important that all parents enrolling children are told what is going to be taught.

Some families celebrate holidays in a religious way and others in a nonreligious way. Every child's family practice needs to be taken into consideration when planning for holidays.

Some holidays commonly celebrated may be offensive to some families. One of these is Halloween. There may be other holidays that people in a community might find offensive or might have negative feelings about. Child care teachers need to honor the feelings of the families they serve when planning celebrations.

Teaching Methods and Skills

Teaching methods are the ways teachers work with children to help them learn. Teachers interact with children, ask them questions, and suggest ideas designed to extend learning. This interaction is best done individually or in small groups.

LEADING YOUNG CHILDREN

Good teachers are good leaders. They set the pace in the classroom and manage the children, the schedule, the curriculum, and the environment in a way that helps children learn and develop self-esteem and personal strength.

Leading large groups of children. In many child care centers the children are brought together in large groups, or class groups, once or twice during the day. Large groups give children an opportunity to greet one another and participate in teacher-led activities.

Teachers leading a large group, in what is sometimes called circle time, need to know songs, finger plays, or stories very well before introducing them to the children. Illustration 12-5 lists the steps for teaching children a new song. When repeating a song the children have sung before, tell them you are going to sing the song and sing it through once for them. Some will sing along with you.

Leading small groups of children. Young children function best when they play in small groups or alone. Small groups of children make it possible for teachers to give individual attention. If teachers lead children in a specific activity, they can do it more effectively in a small group. For example, planning and reviewing of playtime as well as special projects such as cooking work best in small groups.

ILLUSTRATION 12-5   A caregiver could use these steps when introducing a new song to a group of children.

Step 1   Choose a short song.

Step 2   Get the children's attention.

Step 3   Tell the children they are going to learn a new song.

Step 4   Ask them to listen while you sing one verse.

Step 5   Sing in a clear voice, pronouncing the words correctly. Look at the children while you sing.

Step 6   Now say the words to the children.

Step 7   Have them say the words with you.

Step 8   Ask them to sing with you.

Step 9   If there are actions, sing the verse again with the actions.

Step 10   Sing the verse again, asking the children to sing along and do the actions.

Step 11   When the children have learned the first verse, and if they are enjoying the song, teach them the words to a second verse.

Step 12   Sing the second verse with them twice.

Step 13   Now sing both verses.

Step 14   Praise them for participation, but do not make them sing or participate. Some children enjoy listening.

SPECIAL SKILLS FOR WORKING WITH YOUNG CHILDREN

Each teacher brings his or her own talents, knowledge, and abilities to the classroom. Teachers can develop additional skills as well. Three skills that are helpful in working with young children are using puppets, storytelling, and singing with the autoharp.

Using puppets. With very young children puppets are best used without a stage or props. Usually teachers use them to talk with the children. Sometimes puppets are used to teach new words or ideas. More about using puppets with preschoolers is presented in the Hands On with Children feature at the end of this chapter.

Storytelling. Children love stories. Being able to tell children a story is a skill well worth developing.

The first step in storytelling is choosing a story that is interesting to tell. A good story has the following features:

- Interesting characters

- A simple, but intriguing plot

- Appeal to the listeners—young children

- Shortness—can be told well in five minutes

- Acceptable values—reflects the kind of values young children need to hear

Telling a story requires knowing the story really well. The storyteller needs to read the story several times until it is familiar. It is then helpful to write out character and plot cards. Once the story is learned thoroughly, these can be discarded.

Preschool children enjoy having stories presented in a variety of ways. The storyteller can use a flannelboard or puppets. Another possibility is for the storyteller to wear a costume related to the story.

Before telling a story, the teacher can use a fun way of calling children together and getting them involved in listening. Some teachers have a storyteller hat or shawl they wear when it is story time.

Some techniques that improve storytelling include the following:

- Use a clear voice.

- Exaggerate facial expressions.

- Introduce the characters as real people or animals, making children feel as though the storyteller might know them personally.

- Use sounds, objects, and even smells to help children get involved in the story.

- Build the story as you go, giving little hints about the end during the telling, without giving away the ending.

Playing the autoharp. The **autoharp** is a stringed instrument that is held on the lap and can be played after only a little practice by people who do not know music. Names of chords are written above words in most children's songs. The names of those chords are also written on a set of keys on the autoharp. To play the autoharp, the teacher presses a key with one hand and strums the strings with the other. Children can help strum using fingers, brushes, or picks if the teacher holds the autoharp. (A pick is a small piece of plastic used for strumming stringed instruments.) Usually the teacher presses the keys.

Evaluating Children's Progress

Evaluating is the way teachers assess children to see how they are doing developmentally. **Assessing** means checking a child's specific characteristics, skills, and abilities using knowledge of children's developmental abilities.

There are many ways to evaluate. Often teachers can tell how children have grown simply by being with them every day and observing their progress. Sometimes teachers record situations and events that happen with young children. These are kept in the child's file. As children change, teachers are able to see changes.

Another way to evaluate children's progress is to use a checklist or rating sheet that lists specific behaviors. Rating the frequency of behaviors is a fairly objective way to evaluate children's progress. An example of a form that could be used to evaluate the developmental progress of four-year-olds is shown in Illustration 12-6. Various sheets similar to this can be purchased. Different developmental descriptions would be used for younger and older children, of course.

Some child care centers may choose to use standardized tests. Results of tests given to preschool children tend not to be as accurate as those from tests given to older children. Parents sometimes place too much importance on test scores and pressure children because of results. Evaluation procedures for young children should be kept simple and uncompetitive.

Records of children's evaluations are used to improve planning, to help ensure each child's optimal development, and to aid

LA CASITA CHILDREN'S CENTER
Developmental Checklist for Four-Year-Olds

Child's Name *Chris Douglas* Age *4 yr. 4 mo.* Date *4/22/91*

Teacher Evaluating Child's Development *Maria Martinez*

DESCRIPTION OF BEHAVIOR	OFTEN	SOMETIMES	NEVER
Physical			
1. Runs smoothly, speeding up and slowing down	✓		
2. Carries things without spilling		✓	
3. Goes up and down stairs using alternating feet	✓		
4. Puts together simple puzzles (6–10 pieces) without help	✓		
Cognitive (Mental)			
5. Draws lines, dots, and circles	✓		
6. Cuts with scissors	✓		
7. Imitates a simple pattern (such as matching a sequence of colors when stringing beads)	✓		
8. Identifies objects as same or different	✓		
Language			
9. Listens to a story	✓		
10. Asks many "how" and "why" questions	✓		
11. Sings simple songs and nursery rhymes	✓		
12. Uses new words, including verbs and pronouns		✓	
Social			
13. Identifies and appreciates own gender	✓		
14. Has conversations with people	✓		
15. Plays with, rather than beside, others	✓		
16. Takes turns	✓		
Self-Help			
17. Feeds self entire meal	✓		
18. Helps put away clothes and toys	✓		
19. Brushes teeth and washes hands	✓		
20. Plays well alone		✓	

ILLUSTRATION 12-6 This rating sheet for evaluating developmental progress is completed by checking the frequency of specific behaviors.

in communicating with parents. All children's records are confidential.

Working with Parents

Many parents consider teachers to be authorities on children. They expect teachers to know and practice good developmental child care. Parents frequently ask teachers for advice.

Advising parents about child-rearing practices can be a tough task. Teachers may be tempted to offer advice that is not asked for. This can cause angry feelings and may even prompt parents to withdraw a child from the center.

There are times when children need teachers to offer parents some assistance. Being available and supportive usually creates an atmosphere that encourages parents to seek advice. Experienced teachers learn how to open a subject with parents and give them the opportunity to ask questions. Indirect guidance is often well received by parents. Some ways this can be offered include the following:

- Comments made when parents are dropping off and picking up children
- Notes, pictures, and articles on bulletin boards
- Articles in a newsletter
- Presentations or announcements at parents' meetings
- Conferences during home visits
- Activities or discussions at parents' workshops

Parents may welcome workshops where they learn more about effective parenting. Workshop topics that may interest parents include discipline, communication, play, language and talking, helping children think, and teaching children values.

Justin worked quietly at the carpentry table for most of playtime, screwing wood screws into balsa wood and gluing pieces together. He left the structure to dry and played for a while in the family center.

When playtime was over, Ms. Martinez led the children in cleaning up. Then the children sat down with her to talk about playtime. Justin brought the wood structure he had been making.

When it was Justin's turn, she said gently, "Justin, tell us about what you did today."

"I made this." Justin held up the glued wood structure so Ms. Martinez and the other children could see it.

"How nice, Justin!" she said warmly. "Tell us about it."

"I glued it and put screws in it for my dad," Justin said proudly.

"He is a lucky dad. What tools did you use?" she said.

"Some wood and a screw and some glue," Justin replied.

"Would you like to have a box to put it in so it will be easier to carry?" Ms. Martinez asked, as she reached behind her for a box.

Justin nodded in agreement. Ms. Martinez helped Justin to set the structure into the box. The day had been a success for Justin, and he felt good about himself. It had been a success for Ms. Martinez, too. The children in her four-year-olds' class had learned and been well cared for.

Summary

The physical and emotional care of preschool children require the teacher to have the ability to balance challenge and safety and to provide adequate adult supervision. The teacher's job is to help preschoolers develop self-care skills, manage their emotions, develop personal strength, and get along with other children.

Children learn through the experience of play. Mental skills developed through play include perception, memory, reasoning, and creativity. Play is based on developmentally appropriate activities. Learning tasks for preschoolers include understanding the concepts of classification, seriation, number, space, and time. Children involved in active learning are more likely to learn. Planning and reviewing with preschool children extend their mental abilities. Play is most beneficial when it provides key experiences.

The curriculum in preschools is designed to develop personal strength and an ability to get along with others. Physical development is geared to improving gross motor skills, fine motor skills, and coordination. These are developed through movement and manipulative activities. Language skills for preschoolers include learning to listen and to speak. They also have experiences that get them ready to learn to read and write. Pre-math activities help children become familiar with the way shapes and numbers work. Science activities are designed to introduce children to the way the natural world works. An introduction to aesthetics encourages children to enjoy beautiful things.

The learning environment of the preschool is set up in learning centers. These include the family center, the block and building center, the art center, and the quiet center. The quiet center usually has several activity areas—the book area, the toy and puzzle area, the discovery area, and the listening area.

Teachers plan for preschoolers' play. They work this into the schedule and routines. They include plans for holidays and special occasions. Children's families and cultures are considered when planning activities and events.

Useful teaching skills include using puppets, storytelling, and playing the autoharp. Working with parents and evaluating children's progress are other teaching skills.

Terms and Concepts

Affirmation

Active learning

Passive learning

Key experiences

Developmental tasks

Perception

Memory

Short-term memory

Long-term memory

Reasoning

Creativity

Imagining

Developmentally appropriate practices

Manipulative activities

Coordination

Pre-reading activities

Pre-writing activities

Pre-math activities

Aesthetics

Activity areas

Structure blocks

Unpatterned art

Quiet center

Curriculum planning

Transition activities

Autoharp

Evaluating

Assessing

Checking Your Understanding

1. How can preschool teachers encourage the development of a sense of self-worth and good social skills?

2. What is the role of play in learning?

3. Name the learning tasks for play.

4. List the curriculum areas for preschool children.

5. What are key experiences? Why are they important?

6. Describe each of the four main learning centers set up in most preschool classrooms.

7. Select one learning center and describe how it might be set up to encourage preschoolers' learning.

8. What are the steps in planning? Why are they important?

9. What methods can be used in teaching preschool children?

10. What methods are used to evaluate preschoolers' progress?

11. Why is working with parents a part of teaching preschoolers?

USING PUPPETS WITH PRESCHOOLERS

Puppets can be easily made from materials found around many homes. An important feature for puppets used with preschoolers is that they have a mouth that moves.

Older preschool children often enjoy a simple puppet play that is performed behind a simple puppet screen. Since children tend to grab at puppets, a second teacher sits in front of the puppet screen with the children.

Teachers using puppets with preschoolers need to set some basic guidelines, such as these:

- Children sit in front of the stage and do not go behind the stage.

- Children may answer puppets when they ask questions, but need to be quiet while puppets talk.

- The teacher sitting in front of the stage will introduce the puppets and the teacher using the puppets to the children.

- Children will have an opportunity to handle puppets with careful supervision and to see how they work, either before or after the story.

- Children are not allowed to damage puppets.

Abdication   Giving up of one's responsibility and authority.

Abstinence   Refraining from sexual intercourse.

Abstract thinking   Thinking that is not tied to the senses, movement, or concrete experiences.

Active learning   Learning by experience and doing.

Activity areas   Spaces in a child care center set up for particular activities, such as playing with water or looking at books.

Adoptive parents   People who adopt a baby or child.

Advocate   A person who speaks for, supports, and intercedes for another person or group of people.

Aesthetics   The perception and appreciation of beautiful things.

Affirmation   Acceptance that is based on a person's worth, rather than on performance.

Afterbirth   The placenta and amniotic sac, which are delivered after a baby is born.

Amniotic fluid   Fluid inside the amniotic sac, which keeps the unborn baby's temperature even, acts as a shock absorber, and helps the baby slip out of the mother's body during delivery.

Amniotic sac   Membrane that surrounds the unborn baby and is filled with amniotic fluid.

Apgar test   A procedure used in many hospitals to check newborns' heart rate, breathing, reflexes, muscle tone, and skin tone.

Appendicitis   An inflammation of a small part of the lower intestine.

Appreciation   Expression of love and positive feelings for another person.

Appropriate touching   Physical contact that feels safe to children and does not harm them.

Assessing   Checking a child's specific characteristics, skills, and abilities, using knowledge of children's development.

Associative play   Play in which children play close by one another but do not cooperate.

Attachment   Secure feeling that babies develop when parents care for them and meet their needs in a helpful, consistent manner; sense of being closely connected to another person.

Autoharp Stringed instrument that is held on the lap.

Autonomy Ability that children develop to assert themselves and care for themselves.

Availability A characteristic of parents that includes spending time with children, being attentive to them, and listening to them.

Babbling Similar to cooing, except sounds usually begin with consonants, for example, "pa" or "ta."

Bilingual teachers Teachers who know two languages well enough to speak and teach in both of them.

Biological causes of handicaps Abnormalities in genes and chromosomes that cause handicaps.

Birth canal Passageway from the uterus to the outside of a woman's body through which the baby must pass during delivery.

Birth parents People who give a baby up for adoption.

Blastocyst The early embryo, formed by the ninth day of conception.

Blended families Families into which at least one parent brings children from a former marriage.

Bonding Feeling of belonging to one another that develops as parents and newborn spend time together.

Brazelton Neonatal Assessment Scale A procedure used by some hospitals to show parents how their newborn infant responds to various actions and to detect problems.

Bread and cereal group Foods that are made from grains and provide iron and B vitamins.

Breech delivery Birth in which the baby's head is not the first part of the body to come through the birth canal.

Car safety seats Restraints designed to reduce or prevent injury to young children if an automobile accident should occur.

Career cluster Group of jobs that are similar or related to one another.

Career goals Statements that spell out what kind of work a person wants to do.

Career ladder Cluster of jobs in a field arranged according to level of responsibility and qualifications.

Caregivers People who care for children away from home, providing for their basic physical and emotional needs.

Cephalocaudal development Pattern of growth in which baby's growth begins at the head and moves toward the feet.

Cervix Opening of the uterus through which the baby must pass during delivery.

Chain of command Organizational structure of business that specifies whom each person supervises and to whom each person reports.

Child care careers Positions in child care such as caregivers, teachers, teacher's aides, cooks, or program directors.

Child development researchers Professionals who study the development and behavior of children.

Child life specialists Child development specialists who work with children and families during children's hospitalization or extended periods of health care.

Child neglect Failure to provide a child with adequate food, shelter, clothing, health care, and/or love.

Child pornography Materials that depict erotic acts involving children.

Childlessness Having no children, either by choice or because of an inability to conceive.

Child-proofing Limiting access to or removing potential hazards in a child's surroundings.

Chronic illness A long, often serious, sickness.

Classification Sorting of objects into categories by their features.

Closeting Locking a child in a confined area; also called confinement.

Code of ethics Written statement that outlines the standards of conduct for a profession.

Commitment A decision that holds families together and involves unconditional love and fidelity.

Communicable diseases Illnesses that are passed from one person to another.

Communication Ability to talk and listen to other people; the exchange of information.

Competence Ability to accomplish tasks and accept responsibility.

Conception Fertilization of the ovum by the sperm.

Confidentiality of files Limiting the disclosure of information in children's files to authorized people.

Confinement Placement of a child in a confined area; also called closeting.

Consistency The performance of activities in the same manner over a period of time.

Continuous and orderly growth Principle that states that growth goes on all the time and progresses in a sequence.

Contraceptives Means of preventing conception; birth control devices.

Contractions Movements of uterine muscles to push the unborn baby toward the birth canal.

Cooing Sounds made up of mostly vowels or vowel-sounding utterances; produced by babies at about three months.

Cooperative centers Child care centers in which parents are expected to assist a certain number of days each month in exchange for lower fees.

Coordination The ability to use several muscles together to accomplish a goal.

Coping skills The ability to deal with crises and stress and to provide support for others or seek support from them when needed.

Creativity The ability to form original ideas from experiences and to express them in a unique way.

Curiosity The desire to know, learn, and explore.

Curriculum planning What teachers do to design children's experiences, set up the environment, establish schedules and routines, and decide on and get ready for activities.

Custodial care programs Child care programs that are aimed at taking care of the physical needs of young children.

Day care centers Child care centers that serve children from birth through age five, have a minimum of ten children, and are open full-time.

Developmental lag Significant slowness in a child's mental, language, motor, or social development in comparison to other children of the same age.

Developmental programs Child care programs that provide both custodial care and activities that encourage children to develop.

Developmental tasks The mental and physical skills that children need to master at specific ages.

Developmentally appropriate activities Activities that are suited to a child's needs and abilities.

Developmentally appropriate practices Provision of opportunities for play and learning that suit children's abilities.

Dilation Opening up of the cervix during labor.

Direct guidance Method of directing children by telling and showing them what is expected.

Directors Managers of a child care center who plan, organize, carry out plans, and evaluate the results.

Discipline The training and correcting of children in a way that encourages them to mature and to learn self-control.

Drop-in centers Centers that provide essentially babysitting services and are usually located in a department store or mall.

Echolalia Imitation by a baby of vocal sounds of others in tones that are conversational.

Effacement Thinning out of the cervix during labor.

Embryo Medical term for a developing baby from implantation until the eighth week of pregnancy.

Emotional child abuse Injury of a child's mental or emotional well-being; also called mental abuse.

Emotional development Development of children's feelings about themselves and their relationships with other people.

Employment history Summary of work experience.

Entrepreneurship Owning and operating a small business.

Environment Everything that surrounds and involves a person.

Environmental causes of handicaps Prenatal and postnatal factors in a person's surroundings that can cause mental or physical problems.

Episiotomy Surgical cut sometimes made during delivery to increase the size of the opening of the birth canal and prevent the mother's tissues from tearing.

Evacuation drill   Practice in getting all the children out of a building safely, in case of a fire or other dangerous situation.

Evaluating   Assessing children to see how they are doing developmentally.

Exploitation   Use of a child's talents, appearance, or ability to make money or gain prestige or position for another person, without regard for the consequences to the child.

Extended family   Relatives other than parents and siblings, such as grandparents and cousins.

Extrinsic valuing   Judging people's worth by what they look like or can do.

Family day homes   Child care centers that serve fewer than ten children and are run in the owner's home.

Fetal monitor   Device used to keep track of uterine contractions and the unborn baby's heartbeat during labor.

Fetus   Medical term for an unborn baby from the eighth week of pregnancy until birth.

Fine motor skills   Motor abilities that involve the muscles of the fingers and hands.

Foster families   Families that provide full-time care for someone else's child for a designated period of time.

Freedom within limits   Way of defining behaviors among which children can choose freely as long as they obey the rules that apply.

Fruit and vegetable group   Foods such as apples, bananas, and oranges and carrots, peas, and greens that provide a variety of vitamins, minerals, natural fiber, and water.

Functions of parents   Duties of parenthood, including establishing and maintaining a secure family, helping children develop a sense of self-worth, teaching children and providing for learning, protecting children, providing for children's physical needs, and guiding and disciplining children.

Gender   The sex of a person, male or female.

Goal   Something a person wants to accomplish.

Grief   Emotional process people go through when they lose someone they love or something they value very much.

Gross motor skills   Motor abilities involving the large muscles.

Guidance   Parents' provision, based on their wisdom and experience, of a direction for their children's lives.

Gynecologists   Doctors who specialize in women's reproductive health.

Handicapped children   Children who have difficulty adjusting or responding to people, objects, and events around them because of physical, mental, or emotional problems.

Hazards   Any situations, objects, or substances that might cause an injury or create an emergency.

Head Start   Federally funded program designed to meet the developmental needs of children from three to five years old from poor families in order to prepare them for school.

Health check   Quick daily procedure carried out by caregivers to determine whether any of the children in a child care center are ill.

Health screenings   Tests that reveal particular problems in young children, such as vision, hearing, or speech problems.

Heredity   The characteristics that a person inherits from his or her parents through the genes and chromosomes.

Home schooling   Teaching of children completely at home, rather than sending them to school.

Hygiene   Conditions or practices that promote good health.

Imagining   Pretending.

Immunity   The ability of the body to resist infection by a specific disease.

Immunization records   Forms used to record vaccinations.

Immunizations   Doses of vaccines.

Impact-absorbing surfaces   Materials, such as sand or shredded tires, that will break a child's fall without injuring the child.

Implantation   The final event of the period of the ovum, in which the blastocyst attaches to the lining of the uterus.

Incest   The sexual abuse of a child by a family member.

Indirect guidance   Method for directing children by controlling their circumstances.

Induced abortion   Intentional separation of a fetus or unborn baby from a woman's body before it is able to live on its own; commonly referred to as abortion.

Infants   Babies from birth until they are almost able to walk (around one year).

Infections   Conditions that are caused by bacteria, viruses, fungi, or parasites and usually affect a limited area of the body.

Insulin reaction   A condition that occurs when there is too much insulin in the blood.

Interacting   Taking turns listening and talking to one another, while giving special attention to each other.

Intrinsic valuing   Valuing people for their uniqueness as individuals.

Job interview   Meeting between an employer and a job applicant for the purpose of exchanging information about the applicant's skills and other qualifications and about the job's benefits and requirements.

Key experiences   Experiences that are basic to children's development and active learning.

Labor   Process by which a baby becomes physically separated from the mother's body.

Lack of supervision   Situation in which children are left without an adult to watch them and protect them from dangers.

Language and speech development   Gaining the ability to communicate with other people.

Lanugo   Soft downy hair that forms on an unborn baby's head.

Latch-key children   Children who come home after school to an empty house and must care for themselves until their parents arrive home from work.

Leadership skills   Qualities and abilities that help make a person effective as a leader.

Legal liability   Responsibility for someone or something that includes having to bear the consequences if the person or thing is harmed.

Lightening   Process in which an unborn baby shifts position about a week before birth, sometimes causing the mother to feel lighter.

Lines of authority   The lines showing the relationships between various positions on an organizational chart.

Listening   A skill that involves both hearing what another person is saying and understanding what he or she is feeling.

Logical consequences   The events that normally follow an action.

Long-term memory   The ability to recall information after a long time.

Manipulative activities   Activities designed to strengthen and coordinate small muscles in the hands.

Mannies   Male nannies.

Maturation   Process of development in which the child's muscles and nervous system get ready to learn.

Meat group   Foods such as chicken, beef, turkey, and pork that provide protein, iron, and B vitamins.

Memory   A person's mental storehouse of experiences and information that can be used at a later time.

Mental development   Development of children's minds, involving moving from simple ways of learning to more complex ones; also called cognitive development.

Milk group   Foods such as milk, yogurt, and cheese that provide calcium, phosphorus, protein, vitamins A and D, and some B vitamins.

Minimum standards   Rules that are developed by a government agency concerned with child care and must be followed by anyone engaged in the business of child care.

Moral development   Development of a sense of right and wrong.

Motor activity   The way muscles and nerves work together to make movement.

Movement activities   Activities designed to get children to move and exercise various parts of their bodies.

Multi-handicapped children   Children who have conditions that affect more than one, or even all, of the developmental areas.

Nannies   Trained professionals who are employed by families to care for children full-time in the home.

Natural birth control   Birth control method in which couples abstain from sexual intercourse during the woman's most fertile period.

Nonorganic failure to thrive syndrome   Failure of young children to grow and develop normally when there is no physical cause.

Obstetricians   Doctors who specialize in delivering babies.

Occupational therapists   Skilled professionals who train children to perform tasks and help them gain skills.

On-the-job training   Learning of new skills while at work.

Open adoption   Type of adoption in which the birth parents and the child given up for adoption can get to know one another, if desired, once the child is grown.

Ovulation   Expulsion of an ovum from a woman's ovary, normally occurring midway between menstrual periods.

Ovum   Female reproductive cell.

Parallel play   Play in which infants play side by side, but do not cooperate with one another or develop games together.

Parental commitment   A choice parents make to act in their child's best interests in spite of the cost to themselves.

Parent's day out centers   Child care centers that provide custodial care and sometimes developmental or educational activities to children on a part-time basis.

Passive learning   Learning that occurs when a child is not actively involved, but just absorbs information.

Pediatricians   Doctors who specialize in caring for babies and children.

Pediatrics   Field of medicine focused on children's health care.

Pedophile   A sexually perverted person who prefers children as sex objects.

Peers   People of similar ages or interests.

Pelvic examination   Procedure in which a doctor checks a woman's reproductive organs.

Perception   Ability to absorb new information through the senses.

Period of incubation   The length of time it takes for a child to come down with an illness after coming into contact with it.

Period of the embryo   The time from implantation until the eighth week of pregnancy.

Period of the fetus   The time from the eighth week of pregnancy until birth.

Period of the ovum   The time from conception until implantation.

Perpetrator   Person who abuses a child.

Philosophy   A way of thinking and believing that often guides decision making.

Physical child abuse   Nonaccidental bodily injury to a child.

Physical development   The development or growth of the body, motor abilities, and coordination.

Physical therapists   Skilled professionals who train children to use muscles that do not work well.

Placenta   A physical connection between a mother and an unborn baby through which oxygen and carbon dioxide and food and waste are exchanged.

Policies of child care centers   Sets of rules that outline how child care centers do business.

Policy handbook   Book outlining a child care center's policies that is distributed by the center to parents.

Positive statements   Sentences that give children a direction in which to go, rather than telling them what not to do.

Postpartum blues   A period of depression, lasting from a few hours to a few weeks, that a woman may enter following the birth of her child.

Pre-math activities   Activities that help children understand basic math ideas and gain a foundation for developing math skills.

Premature infants   Babies who are born before the thirty-sixth week of pregnancy.

Pre-reading activities   Activities that encourage children to want to read and give them experience in interpreting the world around them.

Preschoolers   Children from three to six years old.

Pre-writing activities   Activities that help prepare children to learn to write.

Principles of growth and development   Patterns that children's development follows.

Procedures   Established techniques for carrying out necessary tasks in the most effective and efficient way possible.

Productive language   Speaking, or the ability to form words purposefully.

Professional liability insurance   Insurance that provides legal aid when a child care center or caregiver is sued.

Props   Objects that encourage children in their play.

Proximodistal development   Pattern in which growth begins in the trunk area and proceeds to the limbs.

Punishment Correction of children in ways that are harmful to them and do not contribute to their growth; action by an adult who is taking out feelings of anger or frustration on a child.

Quality time Time that parents and children spend together that provides a sense of closeness, communication, and learning.

Quantity time Amount of time parents spend with their children.

Quickening First movement of an unborn baby that can be felt by the mother; usually occurs in the fourth month of pregnancy.

Quiet center Area of a preschool classroom set aside for quiet activities, such as a book area or listening area.

Rate of development The speed at which children develop, which differs for each child.

Readiness State of being ready to learn.

Reasoning Mental process used to figure out how the world operates and to organize information in a way that makes it useful.

Receptive language The ability to understand or receive what someone says.

Redirection Giving a child another option for his or her effort or behavior when it is not successful or desirable.

Reflexes Automatic responses to stimuli.

Reinforcement Method for strengthening a desired behavior in a child.

Respiratory distress Difficulty in breathing.

Resumé Document that is prepared by a person to show a potential employer that he or she is qualified for a job.

Roles of parents Ideas of what mothers or fathers should do.

Routines Established methods and times for performing activities, giving children a sense of sameness and security.

Sanitation The act of keeping surfaces free from bacteria and viruses that might make people sick.

Self-care routines Ways children learn to care for their own health.

Self-concept A person's view of himself or herself.

Self-help skills Abilities that children must acquire in order to care for themselves.

Sensorimotor thinking Early thinking that is tied to contact with the senses or the body's movements.

Sensory disorders Deficiency in hearing or sight.

Separation anxiety Insecurity and fear experienced by some children when away from parents.

Seriation Arrangement of things into an orderly sequence.

Sexual child abuse Any action in which an adult uses a child for sexual purposes.

Short-term memory Ability to remember specific information for a short period of time.

Siblings Brothers and sisters.

SIDS monitor Device that flashes a light and sounds an alarm if a baby stops breathing.

Significant people People who are important to a child emotionally and have an influence in his or her life.

Simple to complex development Principle stating that a child progresses from simple abilities to more complex ones.

Single-parent families Families in which one parent has sole responsibility for the family.

Social development Development of children's capacity to care for, get along with, and love other people.

Social services Public agencies that serve children and families.

Solitary play Play in which a child engages alone, without paying attention to other children.

Special needs programs Programs that help developmentally delayed or handicapped children to function more effectively.

Speech therapists Skilled professionals who help children to correct problems with learning to speak well.

Sperm Male reproductive cell.

Spiritual development Attaining of an awareness of life's meanings and the personal strength to live consistently within one's beliefs.

Spiritual wellness State of having convictions that guide and provide purpose for one's life.

Spontaneous abortion Medical term for a miscarriage; occurs when an unborn baby is expelled from a woman's body before the twentieth week of pregnancy.

Stages of development Steps in development, defined by the characteristics of different age groups.

Stereotyping Categorizing or labeling people rather than viewing them as individuals.

Stranger anxiety Negative reaction of babies and toddlers to strangers.

Structure blocks Blocks that are made of cardboard or wood and can be used to build buildings, fences, and roads.

Structured choices Choices that are limited to a set of acceptable alternatives in order to give children the opportunity to act with autonomy while following an adult's leadership.

Structured educational programs Programs that teach children specific skills, such as early reading or dancing.

Sudden infant death syndrome (SIDS) Condition that causes some infants to die because breathing stops.

Supervising adult A full-grown person who is familiar with children's abilities, recognizes hazards, watches children carefully, and can act appropriately in case of immediate danger.

Teachers Caregivers who also teach and guide children.

Temper tantrum Outburst of emotion, sometimes spontaneous and sometimes intentional, in which a child may cry expressively, kick, throw things, bite, or bang his or her head against something.

Temperament Tendency of a person to act, feel, and think in consistent ways throughout a lifetime.

Termination of parental rights The permanent, legal removal of a child from his or her parents.

Tethering Tying children to furniture or other objects to keep them from getting into things or making messes.

Theory of development Statement or set of statements intended to explain how a particular type of development progresses.

Thermometers Devices for measuring temperature.

Time out Guidance method by which a child who has behaved unacceptably must spend a short amount of time sitting apart from other children.

Time together Time families spend together.

Toddlers Young children, ranging from those just beginning to walk to those who can walk and talk fairly well (about age three).

Tracking Ability of newborn babies to follow an object with their eyes if it is moved slowly at the right distance.

Transition activities Planned actions that provide a way to help children make the adjustment from one activity to another.

Transition times Periods of time between activities.

Transitions Changes in situations, such as moving from home to a child care center, or vice versa.

Trial-and-error learning Process in which children experiment to find solutions to problems.

Trimesters Three time periods about three months long that make up the full nine-month period of a pregnancy.

Tubal ligation A surgical procedure that makes a woman unable to conceive.

Twos Toddlers between 24 and 36 months old.

Umbilical cord Cord that attaches the unborn baby to the placenta and contains two arteries and a vein to transport blood.

Unconditional love Kind of love children get from parents; does not change because of circumstances or children's actions.

Unpatterned art Any activity that allows children to use art materials in appropriate ways to design freely.

Uterus Part of a woman's body where a baby develops until birth.

Utterance Something a baby says; a sound or group of sounds that may or may not resemble words.

Vaccines Low-level doses of active or inactive viruses given to children to help them establish immunity to diseases.

Vasectomy A surgical procedure that makes a man unable to impregnate a woman.

Vernix caseosa A waxy substance that covers and protects the skin of an unborn baby.

Vulnerability The characteristic of being easily hurt.

Work-based centers Day care centers that are set up by a business for its employees.

Zygote The first cell formed after the ovum and sperm have fused.

INDEX